Fundamentals of Anaesthesia and Acute Medicine

Cardiovascular Physiology

Fundamentals of Anaesthesia and Acute Medicine

Cardiovascular Physiology

Edited by
Hans-Joachim Priebe
Professor of Anaesthesia, University Hospital, Freiburg, Germany

and

Karl Skarvan
Professor of Anaesthesia, University of Basel, Switzerland

Series editors
Ronald M Jones
Professor of Anaesthetics, St Mary's Hospital Medical School, London

Alan R Aitkenhead
Professor of Anaesthesia, University of Nottingham

and

Pierre Foëx
Professor of Anaesthetics, University of Oxford

© BMJ Publishing Group 1995

First published in 1995
by the BMJ Publishing Group, BMA House, Tavistock Square,
London WC1H 9JR

British Library Cataloguing in Publication Data
A catalogue record for this book is available
from the British Library

ISBN 0-7279-0781-6

Typeset in Great Britain by
Apek Typesetters Ltd, Nailsea, Avon
Printed and bound in Great Britain by Latimer Trend & Co., Plymouth

Contents

Contributors

John Atlee III, MD
Professor of Anesthesiology
Medical College of Wisconsin, Milwaukee, USA

James E Baumgardner, PhD, MD
Assistant Professor of Anesthesia and Bioengineering
Hospital of the University of Pennsylvania, Philadelphia, USA

Wolfgang Buhre, MD
Department of Anaesthesia, Georg-August-Universität Göttingen,
Germany

Christopher P Harkin, MD
Research Fellow, Department of Anesthesiology, Medical College of
Wisconsin, Milwaukee, USA

Andreas Hoeft, MD
Department of Anaesthesia, Georg-August-Universität Göttingen,
Germany

Nguyen D Kien, PhD
Associate Professor of Anesthesiology
University of California, USA

David E Longnecker, MD
Robert Dunning Dripps Professor and Chairman, Department of
Anesthesia
Hospital of the University of Pennsylvania, Philadelphia, USA

David K Menon, MD, MRCP, FRCA
Lecturer in Anaesthesia, University of Cambridge; Consultant,
Neurosciences Intensive Case Unit, Department of Anaesthesia,
Addenbrooke's Hospital, Cambridge, UK

Hans-Joachim Priebe, MD
Professor of Anesthesiology
University Hospital, Freiburg, Germany

CONTRIBUTORS

John A Reitan, MD
Professor of Anesthesiology
University of California, USA

Karl Skarvan, MD
Professor of Anaesthesia
Department of Anaesthesia, University of Basel, Switzerland

Keith Sykes, MB BChir, FRCA
Emeritus Professor, Nuffield Department of Anaesthetics
University of Oxford, UK

Heinrich Taegtmeyer, MD, DPhil
Professor of Medicine
Division of Cardiology, University of Texas Houston Medical Center,
USA

David C Warltier, PhD, MD
Professor of Anesthesiology, Cardiology and Pharmacology
Medical College of Wisconsin, USA

Foreword

The pace of change within the biological sciences continues to increase and nowhere is this more apparent than in the specialties of anaesthesia, acute medicine, and intensive care. Although many practitioners continue to rely on comprehensive but bulky texts for reference, the accelerating rate of biomedical advances makes this source of information increasingly likely to be dated, even if the latest edition is used. The series *Fundamentals of anaesthesia and acute medicine* aims to bring to the reader up to date and authoritative reviews of the principal clinical topics which make up the specialties. Each volume will cover the fundamentals of the topic in a comprehensive manner but will also emphasise recent developments or controversial issues.

International differences in the practice of anaesthesia and intensive care are now much less than in the past, and the editors of each volume have commissioned chapters from acknowledged authorities throughout the world to assemble contributions of the highest possible calibre. Three volumes will appear annually and, as the pace and extent of clinically significant advances varies among the individual topics, new editions will be commissioned to ensure that practitioners will be in a position to keep abreast of the important developments within the specialties.

Not only does the pace of advance in biomedical science serve to justify the appearance of an international series of this nature but the current awareness of the need for more formal continuing education also underlines the timeliness of its appearance. The editors would welcome feedback from readers about the series, which is aimed at both established practitioners and trainees preparing for degrees and diplomas in anaesthesia and intensive care.

RONALD M JONES
ALAN R AITKENHEAD
PIERRE FOËX
May 1995

Preface

Is it necessary to understand the cardiac action potential, ventriculoarterial coupling, or coronary steal to become a good anaesthetist or intensive care physician? Probably not; but an understanding of cardiovascular physiology may help you to deliver better care. Too many patients still develop perioperative cardiac complications that require prolonged hospital stays and expensive intensive care, which may result in chronic disability or death, and increase the cost of health care. Such costs can possibly be reduced by optimising perioperative patient care.

Perioperative care should be based on a profound understanding of normal cardiovascular function and the derangements that are caused by anaesthesia, surgery, and trauma. This monograph will, we hope, serve as a framework to help anaesthetists and intensive care physicians towards better comprehension of the normal cardiovascular physiology before they address the complex problems of patients with heart disease and impaired cardiac reserve. It is intended to provide an overview of some basic aspects of cardiovascular physiology relevant to those anaesthetists and intensive care physicians in training who are caring for patients with cardiovascular disease.

In the past few years, advances in the understanding of cardiovascular physiology have been rapid and dramatic. The enormous body of information in this area has required selectivity in the choice of topics and, undoubtedly, a certain degree of simplification in the interests of didactics and space. Each chapter could easily be the subject of a separate textbook. The need to present only the essentials must not distract from the fact that many basic concepts in cardiovascular physiology are under continuing intensive investigation, and that, at times, many controversies exist.

A broad range of topics is discussed – from microcirculation and cardiac metabolism to regional circulation and cardiac performance. This text therefore provides physiological fundamentals, and discussion about the cardiovascular effects of various anaesthetic drugs or diseases of the cardiovascular system is not a primary goal of this monograph.

The topics selected reflect their clinical importance. Anaesthetics and many other drugs may themselves modify and interfere with cardiac metabolism, cardiac electrophysiology, cardiac performance, cardiovascular control mechanisms, and different regional circulations. As examples of each of these topics, discussions concerning anaesthetic effects on the ischaemic myocardium, their arrhythmogenic or antiarrhythmogenic potential, their myocardial depressant properties, their interference with the autonomic nervous system, or their effect on the coronary circulation may be mentioned. So, chapters dealing with the physiological fundamentals of cardiac metabolism, electrophysiology, and performance of overall cardiovascular control mechanisms and different regional circulations have been included.

There has been an explosion of microvascular research over the past two decades. We have become increasingly aware that anaesthetics and critical illness may interfere with the microcirculation. Consequently, a separate chapter on the microcirculation has been included. We are also beginning to learn that not only anaesthetic drugs, but the anaesthetic state as such may elicit cardiovascular effects, and this is dealt with in the final chapter.

We wish to thank all contributors sincerely. Without them this book would not have been possible.

We hope that this text will provide a summary of the fundamental aspects of cardiovascular physiology that are useful and necessary for the anaesthetist and the intensive care physician.

HANS-JOACHIM PRIEBE
KARL SKARAVAN

1: Cardiac cellular physiology and metabolism

HEINRICH TAEGTMEYER

New horizons

Cardiac cellular physiology and metabolism have long been considered areas of physiology that are of interest to only a small group of basic scientists. Although clinicians have laid the foundations for much of the work in this area,[1 2] their research has been descriptive; the clinical usefulness has therefore been limited to the detection of coronary artery disease by the release of lactate or alanine from the ischaemic myocardium.[3-5] When it was shown (using isotopic methods) that lactate release occurred in the presence of net lactate extraction by the normal human heart,[6] it seemed that the usefulness of the invasive assessment of cardiac metabolism to detect coronary artery or other forms of heart disease had come to an end.

A number of technical advances in the diagnosis and treatment of heart disease have resulted in renewed interest in cardiac metabolism by both clinical investigators and basic scientists alike. The most dramatic recent examples include reports on enhanced myocardial function in transgenic mice overexpressing the β_2-adrenergic receptor,[7] highly efficient gene transfer into adult ventricular myocytes,[8] and the grafting of fetal myocytes into adult host myocardium.[9]

It seems, however, that the ultimate success of gene therapy for the failing heart continues to be constrained by an inadequate understanding of the underlying pathophysiological events. New insights into cellular physiology and pathophysiology have come from the use of positron labelled metabolic tracers or tracer analogues for the non-invasive assessment of regional myocardial blood flow and metabolism as a tool to differentiate between reversible and irreversible myocardial ischaemia.[10-12] Other examples also include the use of tomographic nuclear magnetic resonance (NMR) spectroscopy for the early detection of contractile dysfunction in the pressure overloaded left ventricle.[13] Furthermore, cellular mechanisms of adaptations to ischaemia, reperfusion, and reperfusion injury have come into focus when it became possible to reverse the deleterious effects of compromised or absent blood flow. Even cardiovascular scientists often find this emerging area of cellular and metabolic pathophysiology confusing.[14]

1

The message is nevertheless clear: modern management of patients with overt or latent cardiac dysfunction includes physiological approaches which were unthinkable only a decade ago. Hence, it is appropriate to review some of the salient concepts of cellular function and energy transfer in heart muscle and relate them to specific clinical situations, which will be addressed in the second half of this chapter. The interested reader may also wish to refer to the literature for more detailed information.[15]

Principles of energy transfer in heart muscle

Heart muscle consists of a complex, but efficient, system of energy transfer, at the centre of which is a network of enzyme catalysed reactions. Although bewildering at first glance, the purpose of this network is easy to understand, and a number of simple principles on function and metabolism of the heart are worth remembering. These are listed in the box and discussed below.

Salient features of heart muscle

- Consumer and provider of energy
- High rate of energy turnover
- Metabolic omnivore
- Depends on oxygen for energy production
- Only limited endogenous fuel reserves
- Wide range of adaptations

The heart, like all organs of the mammalian body, consists of a number of different components, all of which are in a constant state of flux. These include:

- interactive proteins
- purine bases
- energy providing intermediates
- membranes
- ions
- signal molecules.

In addition, heart muscle has retained its ability to adapt to environmental changes by altering the synthesis and/or degradation rates of specific proteins or, acutely, by changing flux through metabolic pathways to maintain its state of equilibrium. Only the most severe environmental changes, such as those induced by an interruption of oxygen supply, result in a collapse of

2

energy production and, consequently, in a collapse of the blood circulation. This example illustrates that cardiac metabolism cannot be separated from function of the heart, on the one hand, and from function of the body as a whole, on the other.

Heart muscle is both a consumer and a provider of energy. The heart consumes energy locked in the chemical bonds of fuels through their controlled combustion, and converts chemical energy into physical energy. The predominant form of physical energy of the heart consists of pump work. In this respect, the heart can be considered as a transducer—that is, a device that receives energy from one system and transmits it to another system. As a result of its ability to convert chemical energy into mechanical energy, the heart also provides energy in the form of substrates and oxygen both for itself and to the rest of the body. In this context, two important concepts emerge:

1 The heart is a "hot spot" of metabolic activity, because ATP (adenosine triphosphate), the chemical energy available for conversion to mechanical energy at the contractile site, has to be continuously resynthesised from its breakdown products ADP and P_i (inorganic phosphate). The greater the work output, the higher the rate of ATP turnover.

2 When the heart's ability to convert chemical into mechanical energy is reduced (for whatever reason), the consequences result in functional and metabolic abnormalities in the rest of the body, commonly referred to as "heart failure."

Hence, there is virtually no organ in the human body which is not affected by an impairment of energy transfer in the heart.

The role of ATP as the main provider of chemical energy for support of various cell functions was first postulated by Lipmann[16] when he drew attention to the biological importance of the ATP–ADP couple. The rate of ATP turnover in the heart is far greater than in other organs of the mammalian body and is often underestimated. A simple calculation, based on measurements of myocardial oxygen consumption, indicates that in the course of 24 hours the human heart produces (and uses) 35 kg of ATP, that is, more than $100\times$ its own weight in ATP and more than $100\,000\times$ the amount of ATP stored in the heart and readily available for hydrolysis. Although the human heart accounts for only 0.5% of the total body weight, it claims 10% of the body's oxygen consumption. It is also important to remember that the *rate of energy turnover*, and not the tissue content of ATP, is the determinant of myocardial energy metabolism.[16-18] The studies by Clarke *et al*[18] on the temporal relationship between energy metabolism and myocardial function have demonstrated (by NMR spectroscopy using phosphorus-31) that the phosphorylation potential—the ratio of high energy phosphates—is the only parameter to change faster than contractile function in the setting of ischaemia and reperfusion.

3

As the heart meets the bulk of its energy needs by oxidative phosphorylation of ADP, it is not surprising that heart muscle cells are richly endowed with mitochondria, the cell organelles that contain the enzymes of oxidative metabolism. A close correlation exists among mitochondrial volume fraction, heart rate, and total body oxygen consumption, with mitochondrial volume fractions ranging from 25% in humans to 38% in mice.[19] Cardiac mitochondria are not only abundant in number; they also contain a far larger number of cristae (that is, the morphological sites of the respiratory chain enzymes) than mitochondria of other organs such as liver, brain, or skeletal muscle.[20]

Finally, energy metabolism of the heart must also be considered in the context of energy transfer in biological systems in general. Knowledge of the vast array of metabolic pathways in the cell is often regarded as a horror by students of biochemistry. The complexities of pathways become comprehensible the moment the following three general principles are considered:

1 The first law of thermodynamics
2 The second law of thermodynamics
3 The principle of moiety conservation.

Understanding these principles also makes it easier to understand the clinical relevance of deranged myocardial metabolism in myocardial ischaemia, infarction, or reperfusion.

Thermodynamic aspects of energy transfer in biological systems

Energy transfer in biological systems obeys the first and second laws of thermodynamics. These two laws state that, within a closed system, energy can only be converted from one form into another, and a process only occurs spontaneously if it is associated with an increase in disorder (or entropy) of the system. Energy is captured in the form of $-CH_2-$ bonds through the process of photosynthesis, which also generates oxygen from water and carbon dioxide. The captured energy is, in turn, released through the reactions of intermediary metabolism which produces reducing equivalents to combine with molecular oxygen to form water (see below). Most dehydrogenase reactions are also linked to decarboxylation reactions (for example, pyruvate dehydrogenase, isocitrate dehydrogenase, and 2-oxoglutarate dehydrogenase) resulting in the liberation of carbon dioxide. Carbon dioxide and water are, in turn, substrates for photosynthesis. The description of this simple energy cycle emphasises the fact that, in a biological environment, molecules are recycled.

Metabolic pathways and moiety conserved cycles

It is a characteristic property of all living cells, including heart muscle, to allow complex chemical reactions to proceed quickly at relatively low temperatures and low concentrations of substrates. The efficient transfer of energy occurs though enzyme catalysed metabolic pathways, at the centre of which are moiety conserved cycles; these permit multiple use of given resources and are in all likelihood the result of evolutionary selection.[21 22]

A metabolic pathway is defined as a series of enzyme catalysed reactions that start with a flux generating step, usually a reaction catalysed by either a non-equilibrium reaction or transport of the metabolite across a membrane, and ends with the removal of a product (for details see the literature[23 24]). A characteristic feature of most metabolic pathways is that, once flux is initiated, there is a rapid and concerted response of the entire pathway.

Biochemists have learned to distinguish between *control* and *regulation* of metabolism as they determine energy transfer in the cell.[22] In heart muscle, *control* of a metabolic pathway means that a change in the level of a control factor (for example, work load, hormones or drugs, substrate concentration, coronary flow, or oxygen availability) will change the rate of substrate flux. In contrast, *regulation* of a metabolic pathway means that flux of a substrate in a metabolic pathway is dictated by the activity of enzymes, regulators of enzymes, cofactors, and signal transduction pathways.

Many, but not all, of the regulators of energy transfer pathways are part of *moiety conserved cycles*, that is, dynamic cycles in which the essential parts remain unchanged. The first moiety conserved cycle consists of the circulation itself, where erythrocytes and plasma serve as vehicles for the transport of oxygen and substrates and the removal of carbon dioxide and metabolic end products. Inside the myocardial cell, hydrolysis of ATP through cross bridge cycling:

- decreases the proton gradient
- increases the oxidation of NADH
- increases flux through the citric acid cycle
- increases acetyl-CoA utilisation
- increases substrate consumption.

Thus, it is convenient to view energy transfer in heart muscle as a "three-ring-circus," which consists of systemic circulation, cellular metabolism, and cross bridge cycling (fig 1.1). The cycles interact in such a way that an increase in contractile force and cross bridge cycling leads to an increase in systemic circulation and coronary blood flow, and an increase in cellular metabolism and energy turnover (fig 1.2). Conversely, it has been pointed out that, in animals with long circulation times, less substrate and less oxygen are delivered to the cell and, as both limit the rate of the metabolic reaction, the rate is slow. In animals with short circulation times, all the necessary components of the reactions are delivered to the site in a continuous rapid stream and reactions occur almost explosively.[25]

Another moiety conserved cycle, which is often overlooked in a discussion of cardiac metabolism, is the cycle that governs intracellular calcium

5

homoeostasis. According to Barry and Bridge[26] calcium homoeostasis in cardiac myocytes is of functional importance for at least three reasons:

1 The resting cystosolic calcium concentration ($[Ca^{2+}]$) of less than 0·2 μmol/l necessary to allow the contractile elements to relax during diastole must be maintained against a 5000-fold gradient across the sarcolemma ($[Ca^{2+}] > 1$ mmol/l).

2 Excitation–contraction coupling involves a complex interaction of membrane electric elements mediated by specific ion channels. This results in Ca^{2+} influx, which triggers the release of large amounts of Ca^{2+} from the sarcoplasmic reticulum via Ca^{2+} specific release channels[27] and subsequent extrusion of Ca^{2+}. To maintain steady state homoeostasis in this cycle, the amount of Ca^{2+} entering the cell with each contraction must be extruded before the next contraction. Likewise, the large amount of Ca^{2+} released from the sarcoplasmic reticulum must be pumped back into the storage compartment. As a net result, only small amounts of Ca^{2+} enter and leave the cell with each cardiac cycle.

3 The force of contraction in the cardiac myocyte is modulated by variations in the magnitude of the Ca^{2+} transient. Hormones or drugs that modify calcium homoeostasis may significantly alter the force of contraction. In addition, cytosolic Ca^{2+} may be taken up into the mitochondria. Although the mitochondrial Ca^{2+} stores are only indirectly related to the contraction–relaxation cycle, calcium ions are regulators of a number of intramitochondrial enzymes which are activated by Ca^{2+}.[28]

Thus calcium ions may constitute a link between the use and production of ATP. Although this hypothesis has not yet been proved,[29] Denton and McCormack[30] have proposed that the main role of the Ca^{2+} transporting system within the inner mitochondrial membrane is a means by which changes in the cytosolic concentration of Ca^{2+} could be relayed into

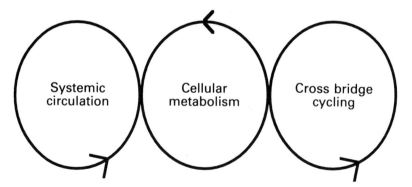

Fig 1.1 Energy transfer in heart muscle: efficient energy transfer occurs in moiety conserved cycles.

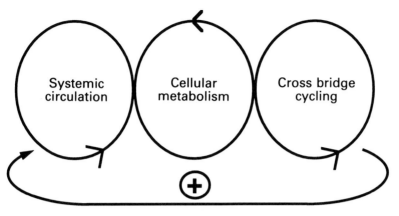

Fig 1.2 Interaction of cycles involved in energy transfer: feedback control of cycles is illustrated by the example of increased contractile activity.

mitochondria, hence influencing the activity of the intramitochondrial Ca^{2+} sensitive dehydrogenases. As Ca^{2+} is the only second messenger for hormones that is transferred across the inner mitochondrial membrane, an important feature of this hypothesis is a suggested mechanism whereby mitochondrial oxidative metabolism and, hence, ATP supply could be stimulated to meet increased demands for ATP that are associated with the stimulation of processes promoted by increases in cytosolic Ca^{2+}.[28] The same authors suggest that, when the Ca^{2+} dependent mechanism for activating oxidative metabolism is available (that is, via the mitochondrial matrix Ca^{2+} sensitive enzymes), then it is the preferred mechanism for promoting the overall process of oxidative phosphorylation.[28]

The sliding filament model of contraction represents another example of a moiety conserved cycle. The molecular mechanisms involved in the sliding filament model of cross bridge formation between actin and myosin have recently been elucidated by the group of Rayment and Holden from the University of Wisconsin at Madison.[31] The essence of the sliding filament model is that the myosin head binds to the actin filament in one orientation, rotates to a second orientation, and then detaches. The cycle is driven in one direction by coupling these transitions to the steps of ATP hydrolysis. Elucidation of the structure of myosin and a model for the actomyosin complex during contraction, including the description of an ATP binding pocket, has advanced the understanding of the molecular design of muscles.

One important consequence of energy transfer through moiety conserved cycles is that the loss of a moiety in any one of the cycles may lead to a loss of energy transfer within the cell.

Examples of loss of a moiety include:

1 The loss of contractile proteins as a result of degradation in excess of

synthesis—for example, in certain forms of dilated cardiomyopathy or chronic myocardial ischaemia.

2 The loss of oxaloacetate from the citric acid cycle through either side reactions, such as transamination, or the inhibition of one or more of the cycle enzymes.

Loss of a moiety is recovered through its resynthesis from precursors via a series of reactions termed "anaplerosis". Hans Kornberg has defined anaplerosis as the replenishment of a depleted cycle by an intermediate precursor.[32] An example of this is shown by the contractile dysfunction of the isolated working rat heart perfused with acetoacetate, which is completely reversed by the addition of glucose as a second substrate.[33] The contractile dysfunction is caused by an inhibition of the enzyme 2-oxoglutarate dehydrogenase as a result of sequestration of free coenzyme A,[34 35] resulting in a shortage of oxaloacetate for the citrate synthase reaction.[36] The normalisation of contractile function with the addition of glucose is the result of the carboxylation of pyruvate through the NADP dependent malic enzyme reaction.[37]

As ischaemia also depletes the citric acid cycle of its intermediates, especially succinate,[38] it is tempting to speculate that the increased glucose and/or lactate requirement in postischaemic myocardium[39–41] may be a reflection of the increased need for replenishment of the depleted citric acid cycle.

A second important consequence of energy transfer through moiety conserved cycles is the effective *recycling of moieties*. These moieties not only involve larger carbon molecules such as glucose and fatty acids, but also the smaller organic acids of the citric acid cycle, particularly recycling of carbon dioxide and water. Without recycling of water, ATP production in the citric acid cycle would be 60% less (6 versus 15 mol ATP per mol pyruvate oxidised). As Ephraim Racker[42] wrote:

> "Mitochondria cleave water without the drama of sunlight and chlorophyll. They perform this task, unnoticed by textbooks, in the quiet and unobtrusive manner characteristic of Hans Krebs and his cycle."

It stands to reason that, under certain circumstances, the *excess of a moiety* may also lead to contractile dysfunction of the heart. This is the case, for example, in ischaemia, reperfusion, and myocardial stunning, where the cells and their organelles may be flooded with Ca^{2+},[43–45] oxygen derived free radicals,[46–49] and protons,[50 51] resulting in cell swelling, osmotic stress, acidosis, and membrane damage.[52]

Catabolism of substrates

In the heart, most enzyme catalysed reactions are catabolic, that is, substrates with high potential energy are broken down to products with low potential energy. Synthetic, or anabolic, reactions such as those serving protein, glycogen, or triglyceride synthesis are less important quantitatively. Even these synthetic reactions on the whole ultimately serve to improve the efficiency of energy production in heart muscle. Thus, heart muscle is endowed with an efficient system of energy transfer which liberates energy locked in chemical bonds through the generation of reducing equivalents and their reaction with molecular oxygen in the respiratory chain. It should be reiterated here that the main purpose of intermediary metabolism in normal heart muscle is the production of reducing equivalents for ATP synthesis by oxidative phosphorylation of ADP.

As proposed by Lehninger,[50] it is convenient to group the breakdown of substrates into three stages:

1 The first stage consists of the breakdown of substrates to acetyl-CoA.
2 The second stage is the oxidation of acetyl-CoA in the citric acid cycle.
3 The third stage is the reaction between reducing equivalents and molecular oxygen in the respiratory chain, where electron transfer is coupled to rephosphorylation of ADP to ATP.

As ATP production is tightly coupled to ATP use, so substrate oxidation is tightly coupled to cardiac work.[33 51 53–56] In the presence of adequate substrate supply, the maximal rate of oxidation of substrate is determined by the capacity of the 2-oxoglutarate dehydrogenase reaction in the citric acid cycle.[57] The exact mechanism by which respiration is coupled to energy expenditure in vivo is, however, not known.[58] In contrast, the efficiency of oxidative phosphorylation for energy production is well established:

$$1 \text{ mol glucose} \xrightarrow[\text{(aerobic)}]{\text{Oxidation}} 36 \text{ mol ATP}$$

$$1 \text{ mol glucose} \xrightarrow[\substack{\text{to lactate} \\ \text{(anaerobic)}}]{\text{Metabolism}} 2 \text{ mol ATP}$$

On a mole for mole basis, the energy yield from the oxidation of long chain fatty acids is even greater than that from glucose or lactate.

Nutrition of the heart and myocardial protein turnover

The recent interest in healthy nutrition for the heart has almost exclusively focused on cholesterol because of its role in the development of coronary artery disease. There is little appreciation of the fact that, in terms of general descriptors of energy metabolism, heart muscle does not function simply as a conformer in response to substrate availability,[59] but that substrate use is controlled by the physiological demands on the system. There is also little

9

appreciation of the fact that the heart stores endogenous substrates such as glycogen and triglycerides, in response to changes in the dietary state.[60][61] In contrast to skeletal muscle, starvation increases the tissue content of both glycogen and triglycerides in heart muscle, an observation consistent with a biologist's definition of true "hibernation."

The heart continuously synthesises and degrades its own constituent proteins,[62] a little appreciated process that is significantly slowed down by myocardial ischaemia.[63][64] Although protein turnover is perhaps the most difficult metabolic process to study in the heart in vivo, and although it appears that each protein has its own characteristic half life,[65] recent estimates indicate that 4·8% of myocardial protein is synthesised per day,[66] that is, the mammalian heart regenerates itself completely over a period of three weeks. As the net muscle mass results from a balance of synthesis and degradation, hypertrophy may be the result of either increased rates of protein synthesis or decreased rates of protein degradation. Although acute volume overload of the myocardium leads to an increase in synthesis, chronic volume overload seems to lead to suppression of protein degradation.[66] The pathways linking mechanical signals to changes in cardiac myocyte degradation rates are not known,[67] and the unravelling of mechanisms involved in myocardial protein degradation continue to pose a challenge to cellular and molecular biologists.

Substrate competition

As a result of the omnivorous nature of the heart, glucose, lactate, fatty acids, ketone bodies, and, under certain circumstances, amino acids are all converted to acetyl-CoA and compete for the fuel of respiration (fig 1.3). The relative predominance of one fuel over another depends on the arterial substrate concentration, which, in the case of fatty acids, ketone bodies, and lactate, can vary over a wide range (table 1.1), on hormonal influences, on work load, and on oxygen supply. Likewise, the use of specific substrates by the heart varies with the physiological state of its environment. When Bing[1] cannulated the coronary sinus and measured aorta–coronary sinus differences in substrate concentrations across the heart, he observed a proportional relationship between substrate concentration in the blood and substrate uptake by the heart for all substrates investigated, that is, glucose, lactate, fatty acids, ketone bodies, and amino acids. Subsequent work by Keul et al[2] has established that the contribution of fuels to the heart's respiratory fuel depends on the physiological state of the whole body, which can vary enormously. The data from Keul's work are of interest, because they show a relatively constant glucose uptake (16–31%), whereas the uptake of fatty acids plus ketone bodies, and the uptake of lactate, vary considerably (from 25% to 63%, and from 5% to 61%, respectively). This observation is of relevance with respect to fatty acids and ketone bodies. Although fatty acid oxidation can be almost completely suppressed when lactate and fatty acids are abundant, there is a consistent rate of carbohydrate use. The need for glucose or lactate is most probably given by the need for pyruvate carboxylation and the anaplerosis of the citric acid cycle. In keeping with this hypothesis the author's group has recently shown that lactate (40 mmol/l) suppresses glucose uptake by the isolated working rat heart by 90%, whereas 3-hydroxybutyrate at the same concentration suppresses glucose uptake by only 64%.[68] Collectively these findings suggest that the fuels for cardiac energy metabolism can be grouped into *essential fuels* which provide both acetyl-CoA and oxaloacetate:

- glucose
- lactate
- pyruvate
- certain amino acids

and into *non-essential fuels*, which provide only acetyl-CoA (fig 1.3):

- fatty acids of all chain lengths
- ketone bodies
- leucine.

Fatty acids are the preferred fuel for respiration in the fasted state,[69] but

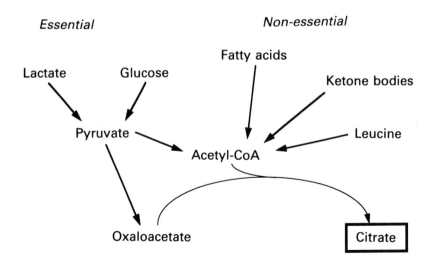

Fig 1.3 Essential and non-essential fuels for cardiac energy production. Note that glucose, lactate, and pyruvate provide both substrates for the citrate synthase reaction, acetyl-CoA, and oxaloacetate. Carboxylation of pyruvate leading to the formation of oxaloacetate is an anaplerotic pathway. The importance of anaplerosis of normal contractile function of the heart has recently been elucidated.[37]

Table 1.1 Metabolite concentrations in human plasma under various conditions.

	Glucose (μmol/l)	Lactate (μmol/l)	Free fatty acids (μmol/l)	Ketone bodies (μmol/l)
Rest (postabsorptive)	5·0	0·5	0·1	0·1
Running (90 min)	5·0	5·0	1·7	1·8
Fasting	4·5	1·0	1·6	4·5
Diabetic ketoacidosis	30·0	1·0	1·7	10·0

Reproduced with permission from Taegtmeyer H. *Basic Res Cardiol* 1984; **79**: 322–36.

even when fatty acid or ketone body concentrations are high, a certain amount of glucose continues to be oxidised.[33][70] Conversely, high lactate concentrations as observed with strenuous exercise can provide almost all[71] or the bulk of the fuel for respiration.[70]

Even amino acids, when present in very high concentrations, can become a fuel for respiration in heart muscle.[1] In this respect, the heart is not different from the body as a whole. When an omnivorous animal consumes a normal meal containing protein, carboydrate, and fat, the degradation of any excess amino acids (that is, amino acids not needed for growth and replacement) takes precedence over the degradation of carbohydrates and fats.[72] This phenomenon is the result of a strict control of amino acid metabolism by their K_m values (the Michaelis constant or the concentration of substrate required for half maximal velocity of an enzyme catalysed reaction) and reveals an *important principle of metabolic control*. As dietary protein or amino acids cannot be stored in large quantities, the amino acids from intestinal digestion are distributed between blood plasma and tissues. By contrast, the products of the digestion of carbohydrate and fat leaving the intestine after absorption can be stored rapidly as either glycogen or triglycerides. As this storage process starts immediately, fluctuations in plasma glucose and fatty acid levels are moderate and transient compared with fluctuations in amino acid levels. The increased amino acid concentrations in blood and tissues automatically cause an increased rate of amino acid degradation because the K_m values of the enzymes initiating amino acid degradation are in general high and exceed the concentration of amino acids in the tissues.

In summary, many factors contribute to the selection of energy providing fuels for the heart. According to Krebs,[72] they may be classified under three main categories:

1 Concentration of the direct fuel in the tissue.
2 The presence, in the tissue, of the enzymes required for the degradation.
3 The kinetic properties of the key enzymes, especially of those that initiate the release of energy.

Each of these three main factors is, in turn, complex and depends on a variety of components. The entry of fuels into the cell, as well as synthesis

12

and degradation of stored fuel reserves, is controlled by hormones such as insulin and adrenaline as well as other environmental factors, with a cAMP (cyclic $3':5'$-adenosine monophosphate) and a cascade of intracellular signals acting as second messengers. Among the kinetic properties of the key enzymes, the important ones are the K_m values (see above), and the inhibition and activation of enzymes by tissue constituents which exercise either feedback inhibition or allosteric control through allosteric effectors or covalent modification.

Clinical relevance of myocardial metabolism

Altered energy metabolism is the cause of many clinical forms of heart disease (summarised in the box). In his recent review on myocardial metabolism, Lionel Opie[73 74] referred to a "decline and resurgence of myocardial metabolism" and pointed to several problems of interest to the clinician. We have identified three areas of clinical relevance:

1 The first area is the tracing of metabolic pathways for the diagnosis of ischaemia and other forms of heart disease.
2 The second area is best identified under the heading "metabolic mechanisms of heart disease," where contractile failure represents the end result of profound metabolic derangements.
3 The third area of relevance to the clinician is best described as metabolic support for the failing heart and includes replenishment of cofactors or intermediary metabolites in certain forms of dilated cardiomyopathy with resultant improvement in contractile performance.

Most importantly, it includes the concept of metabolic support for the failing heart after prolonged periods of ischaemia such as hypothermic ischaemic arrest. This chapter does not intend to duplicate the very detailed pathophysiological and clinical discussions by Opie, cited earlier.[73 74]

Tracing metabolic pathways in the intact heart

A detailed knowledge of the pathways of individual substrates for energy production is normally not required for the clinician diagnosing or treating patients with heart disease. Metabolism comes under scrutiny, however, when coronary arteries are not (or are no longer) obstructed and the heart fails to contract, as is the case, for example, in cardiomyopathies or in reperfused myocardium after complete coronary occlusion. More importantly, substrate metabolism has come into focus through the development of new, non-destructive imaging techniques such as NMR spectroscopy and positron emission tomography (PET) which permit the assessment of regional metabolic processes in the beating heart in vitro and in vivo.[12 75–84]

Altered energy metabolism in clinical forms of heart disease

I *Myocardial ischaemia*
    Latent ischaemia
    Hibernation
    Myocardial infarction
    Reperfusion/reperfusion injury
    Stunning/postischaemic dysfunction
    Preconditioning/stress response

II *Cardiomyopathies*
    Dilated cardiomyopathies
    Systolic dysfunction
    Hormonal or nutritional deficiencies

III *Hypertrophy*
    Adaptation
    Maladaptation
    Diastolic/systolic dysfunction

Although NMR spectroscopy holds the promise of detecting derangements in energy rich phosphate metabolism before the development of contractile dysfunction,[13] PET imaging holds the promise of detecting reversibly ischaemic, viable myocardium.[85–87]

NMR spectroscopy

The basis of NMR spectroscopy is relatively simple: although all nuclei of atoms have an overall positive charge, some also have a "spin" which gives them a magnetic moment.[88] A powerful magnetic field orients the nuclear spins and, hence, establishes their different energy states. Transitions between adjacent energy states are induced by the application of an oscillating magnetic (or radiofrequency) field. The device that provides the radiofrequency field is also used to detect the result and signal or resonance (hence, the name radiofrequency coil or probe). Biologically important nuclei with a spin are ^1H, ^2H, ^{13}C, ^{15}N, ^{17}O, ^{31}P, ^{23}Na, ^{39}K, ^{87}Rb, and ^{19}F. Selective enrichment of low abundance nuclei (for example, ^{13}C) leads to an increase in their sensitivity.

Natural abundance NMR spectroscopy is most commonly used in the form of ^{31}P NMR spectroscopy, which yields distinct, quantitative resonance peaks for monophosphate esters, inorganic phosphates, phosphocreatinine, and ATP. Analysis of energy rich phosphates in the beating heart in vivo by ^{31}P NMR spectroscopy[80] supports the view that, over a relatively wide range, the tissue content of ATP does not correlate with the rate of energy use as measured by the rate of ATP turnover, that is, oxygen consumption or contractile performance of the heart. The recent introduction of a tomographic (spatial stacked plot) analysis of ^{31}P NMR spectra has added a new dimension to the analysis of energy rich phosphates in vivo. When this technique was applied to a group of patients with left ventricular hypertrophy caused by aortic stenosis and/or insufficiency, heart failure was characterised by a decline in the phosphocreatinine:ATP ratio.[13] The recent adaptation of isotopomer analysis of ^{13}C natural abundance or labelled compounds permits the analysis of flux through specific pathways, especially the citric acid cycle and glycogen turnover, through the acquisition of serial spectra.[84 89-91] A main advantage of NMR spectroscopy is the specificity of the technique which allows tracing of the flux of specific metabolites into and out of metabolic pools. The isotopomeric enrichment of glutamate as an index for flux through the citric acid cycle may serve as an example.

Positron emission tomography

Tracing of metabolic pathways with short lived positron emitting tracers has thus far been more successful in its clinical application than NMR spectroscopy, mainly because technology exists which makes it possible to assess regional differences of metabolic activity of the heart by visual inspection and quantitative analysis of radioactivity in "regions of interest."[12 92] Two types of approaches can be distinguished:

1 *Uptake and retention* of a tracer analogue such as fluorodeoxyglucose (FDG).
2 *Uptake and clearance* of tracers such as ^{11}C-labelled fatty acids, where the rapid phase of clearance from the tissue represents either β oxidation and oxidation in the citric acid cycle (in the case of long chain fatty acids), or oxidation in the citric acid cycle alone (in the case of acetate).

Whereas the uptake and retention of FDG is linear with time and follows zero order kinetics, the clearance of labelled fatty acids is biexponential,[93-95] suggesting both rapid and slow turnover pools for long and short chain fatty acids. Relative size and slope of each of the exponential components of the ^{11}C time–activity curve relate to oxidation and release from storage of the labelled compound. Both FDG and ^{11}C-labelled fatty acids have been used clinically to assess substrate metabolism in normal and ischaemic myocardium.

At the time of writing, the argument about whether enhanced glucose uptake (assessed with FDG) or residual oxidative capacity (assessed by the early, rapid clearance phase of [^{11}C]acetate) constitutes the gold standard for reversible tissue injury in ischaemic, reperfused, or "hibernating" myocardium has not been settled. The clinical utility of perfusion–metabolism mismatching is, however, clear: preserved metabolic activity (in this case, manifested by the retention of FDG), in the absence of significant coronary flow (in this case, manifested by the absent uptake of the flow marker ^{13}NH$_3$), which strongly suggests that myocardium has the potential of resuming

15

normal contractile function (and, hence, oxidative metabolism) upon restoration of blood flow and oxygen supply. It appears, however, that the usefulness of imaging regional metabolic activity in heart muscle is limited, because the same functional information can be obtained with less expensive, more direct methods such as assessment of contractile reserve.

Metabolic adaptation and deadaptation: the cellular consequences of ischaemia and reperfusion

Heart muscle regulates its energy supply by regulating coronary flow in accordance with the energy needs of the cell. For example, under resting conditions, coronary flow is about 1 ml/min per g wet weight in humans, and it increases in parallel with myocardial oxygen consumption, that is, when oxygen consumption doubles, coronary flow doubles, and so on. Conversely, a reduction of coronary flow results in a reduction of myocardial oxygen delivery and a consequent reduction in contractile force. In clinical practice, this relationship manifests itself as stress induced asynergy or "hibernating myocardium."

The earliest forms of ischaemia, defined as lack of oxygen supply as a result of inadequate blood flow, occur in patients unable to increase coronary flow in response to increased energy demands. As resting coronary flow is normal in this setting, this form of ischaemia is sometimes referred to as "normal flow" ischaemia. By contrast, when coronary flow is reduced at rest, the term "low flow ischaemia" has been used. The extreme form of ischaemia is, of course, reached by the complete occlusion of a coronary artery with subsequent necrosis of the tissue supplied. Thus there is a continuum of ischaemia, with mild, "normal flow" ischaemia at one end and the extreme situation of a myocardial infarction at the other end of the spectrum.

Ischaemia affects myocardial energy metabolism by slowing down aerobic metabolism of substrates, reducing the tissue content of phosphocreatinine and adenine nucleotides, and first increasing and then slowing down anaerobic metabolism of substrates. Just as there is a continuum of the relative restriction of oxygen delivery, one might expect a continuum of metabolic responses to ischaemia. With "normal flow" ischaemia, heart muscle is still capable of oxidising fatty acids and glucose under resting conditions. Opie and co-workers[96] have shown that, as coronary blood flow decreases, the relative contribution of glucose to the residual oxidative metabolism increases and oxidation of glucose accounts for a greater percentage of aerobic ATP production. Increased uptake of a glucose analogue by ischaemic myocardium has also been found when the energy demand for the heart was increased by pacing or exercise.[6 97] There is increased lactate release from the stressed myocardium[6 98] and increased glucose uptake, especially when fatty acid levels are low.[99] Possible reasons for increased glucose uptake with stress and ischaemia are as follows:

1 Glucose makes better use of the limited amount of oxygen available to the myocyte. If blood supply is mildly reduced, the heart switches from fatty acids to glucose as the preferred fuel for respiration.
2 Glycolysis yields a small amount of ATP through substrate level phosphorylation in the cytosol, independent of the availability of oxygen (2 mol ATP/mol glucose, whereas 36 mol ATP are produced per mol glucose oxidised).
3 Glucose transport is enhanced in oxygen deprived tissue. Thus more glucose enters the cell, and glucose is preferred over fatty acids as substrate for energy production.

The regulation of intermediary metabolism of glucose, fatty acids, and amino acids during ischaemia is complex and requires further discussion with respect to accumulation of intermediary metabolites and reversibility of ischaemic tissue damage. When oxygen becomes rate limiting for energy production, flux through the electron transport system of the respiratory chain slows down and the ratio of the reduced form of nicotinamide adenine dinucleotide (NAD) to the oxidised form ($[NADH]:[NAD^+]$) increases. This reduced state reflects a lack of ATP production by oxidative phosphorylation, which is accompanied by a loss of contractile function.

The exact biochemical mechanisms responsible for the rapid loss of contractile function are not yet known with certainty; some workers implicate the loss of ATP[100] and others implicate the accumulation of potentially toxic intermediary products such as H^+ [101][102] or lactate.[103] Kübler and Katz[104] thought it unlikely that decreased ATP supplies for energy consuming reactions in the myocardial cell cause the observed decrease in myocardial contractility because of the low K_m for ATP at the substrate binding sites of energy consuming reactions in the heart. In other words, at prevailing concentrations of ATP in the ischaemic, non-contracting tissue, enzymes such as myosin ATPase should still operate at near maximal velocity. These authors therefore speculated that small changes in ATP may already exert modulatory effects on ion fluxes, and the large amount of inorganic phosphate may form insoluble calcium–phosphate precipitates which trap calcium in the sarcoplasmic reticulum, and mitochondria.[104] Another possible explanation for the discrepancy between ATP content and ATP conversion into useful energy for the heart is the trapping, or "compartmentation," of ATP in a compartment that is inaccessible to the enzymes of the contractile apparatus or ion pumps (for example, mitochondria). Examining the acute effects of ischaemia on phosphocreatinine and ATP, Gudbjarnason et al[105] found that breakdown of phosphocreatinine was more rapid than the breakdown of ATP. The kinetic heterogeneity of ATP and phosphocreatinine depletion seems to indicate an inhibition of transfer ATP from mitochondria to the cytosol, and it has been speculated that the reduction in regeneration of cytosolic ATP causes the early cessation of

17

contractile activity in ischaemic myocardium. It is reasonable to state that the actual biochemical mechanism for contractile failure in the ischaemic and infarcted myocardium continues to remain elusive. Recent experimental work has emphasised the phenomenon of ischaemic preconditioning[106] and the role of stress proteins in myocardial protection.[107] Work from the author's and other laboratories has renewed attention to the fact that, of all substrates used for energy production by the myocardium, glucose is, with the exception of glutamate, the only substrate yielding ATP by anaerobic substrate level phosphorylation.[15]

Metabolic support of the acutely ischaemic myocardium

The use of glucose, insulin, and potassium (GIK) as inotropic metabolic support for the acutely ischaemic, reperfused myocardium is controversial and has largely been abandoned on the basis of theoretical[108] and experimental[103] argument. Likewise, the use of GIK in the setting of acute myocardial infarction, first proposed by Sodi-Pallares and his co-workers in Mexico (1962), and further developed by Rackley and his co-workers in the USA,[109-111] has not been generally accepted because of inconclusive evidence in earlier clinical trials.[112] In spite of substantial experimental evidence in support of beneficial effects of substrate manipulation, especially promoting glucose metabolism in myocardial ischaemia,[113-116] the concept of metabolic support for the failing ischaemic (or postischaemic) myocardium has been relegated to the antics of medical therapy.

The starting point for the interest of the author's laboratory in GIK was the observation that "glycogen loading" of rat hearts 90 min before hypothermic ischaemic arrest significantly improves ischaemia tolerance as evidenced by a return of normal left ventricular function after 12 h of ischaemia (instead of 3 h in controls).[117] In contrast, glycogen depletion before ischaemia failed to improve left ventricular function of rabbit heart after hypothermic ischaemic arrest.[118] The author's studies demonstrated a correlation between glycogen content on the one hand and the tissue content of energy rich phosphates and recovery of function with reperfusion on the other, although they were not able to identify the mechanism for the protective effect of GIK.

In a subsequent series of experiments, the author's group therefore examined the effect of glycogen loading on recovery of function and associated biochemical parameters after a brief (15 min) period of normothermic ischaemia and reperfusion in rat hearts.[119 120] It was found that glycogen loaded hearts recovered faster than their controls, used more glucose, maintained normal energy rich phosphate levels, and lost a significantly smaller amount of marker proteins (myoglobin, lactate dehydrogenase, citrate synthase) with reperfusion. Although these studies are largely descriptive, they point to a physiological role for glycogen which complements its role as endogenous substrate but is still elusive to a mechanistic analysis.

As there were no prospective, controlled, clinical studies examining the efficacy of GIK in patients with refractory left ventricular failure after cardiopulmonary bypass and hypothermic ischaemic arrest for aortocoronary bypass surgery, the author's group undertook a limited randomised clinical trial on 22 patients who required postoperative intra-aortic balloon counter-pulsation for a cardiac index of 2·5 l/min per m² or less. Half of the patients received GIK (for dose, see below) for up to 48 h.[121] The results were so striking (a 50% increase in cardiac index, a 30% decrease in the requirement for inotropic drugs, and a 75% decrease in 30 day mortality rate) that surgeons at the University of Texas Medical School at Houston and the Texas Heart Institute have started to include GIK in the management of postoperative refractory left ventricular failure. In addition, protocols of preoperative glycogen loading are being developed for the ex vivo preservation of donor heart for heart transplantations and for high risk patients with compromised left ventricular function (left ventricular ejection fraction of less than 30% before surgery of any conceivable aetiology). To a large extent, these protocols are now employed on an empirical basis with good success, but so far, for the most part, without the benefit of rigorous scientific scrutiny.

Conclusions

The heart is both a consumer and a provider of energy. Energy transfer in heart muscle is highly efficient and occurs through a series of moiety conserved cycles. New methods developed during the past decade have resulted in a better understanding of the physiology of myocardial cell function, and gene therapy for the contraction of cellular defects is looming on the horizon. The ultimate success of new treatment modalities is, however, still constrained by the inadequate understanding of the underlying pathophysiological events. Often more acute interventions are necessary. These recent developments point to a need to re-examine the concept and utility of metabolic support for the failing myocardium in defined clinical settings, such as reperfusion after an acute ischaemic event or controlled hypothermic ischaemic arrest.

The author's laboratory is supported by a grant from the US Public Health Service, National Institutes of Health (R01-HL 43113) and by a grant-in-aid from the American Heart Association, National Center.

1 Bing RJ. The metabolism of the heart. *Harvey Lect* 1955; **50**: 27–70.
2 Keul J, Doll E, Steim H, Homburger H, Kern H, Reindell H. Über den Stoffwechsel des menschlichen Herzens I. *Pflügers Arch Ges Physiol* 1965; **282**: 1–27.
3 Gorlin R, Brachfeld N, Messer JV, Turner JD. Physiologic and biochemical aspects of disordered coronary circulation. *Ann Intern Med* 1959; **51**: 698–706.
4 Krasnow N, Neill WA, Messer JV, Gorlin R. Myocardial lactate and pyruvate metabolism. *J Clin Invest* 1962; **41**: 2075–85.
5 Mudge GH, Mills RM, Taegtmeyer H, Gorlin R, Lesch M. Alterations of myocardial amino acid metabolism in chronic ischemic heart disease. *J Clin Invest* 1976; **58**: 1185–92.

6 Gertz EW, Wisneski JA, Neese RA, Bristow JD, Searle GL, Hanlon JT. Myocardial lactate metabolism: Evidence of lactate release during net chemical extraction in man. *Circulation* 1981; **63**: 1273–9.

7 Milano CA, Allen LF, Rockman HA, *et al.* Enhanced myocardial function in transgenic mice overexpressing the β_2-adrenergic receptor. *Science* 1994; **264**: 582–6.

8 Kirshenbaum LS, MacLellan WR, Mazur W, French BA, Schneider MD. Highly efficient gene transfer into adult ventricular myocytes by recombinant adenovirus. *J Clin Invest* 1993; **92**: 381–7.

9 Soonpaa MH, Koh GY, Klug MG, Field LJ. Formation of nascent intercalated disks between grafted fetal cardiomyocytes and host myocardium. *Science* 1994; **264**: 98–101.

10 Schelbert HR, Schwaiger M. Positron emission tomography studies of the heart. In: Phelps M, Mazziota J, Schelbert H, eds, *Positron emission tomography and autoradiography: principles and applications for the brain and the heart.* New York: Raven Press, 1986: 581–661.

11 Bergmann SR. Clinical applications of assessments of myocardial substrate utilization with positron emission tomography. *Mol Cell Biochem* 1989; **88**: 201–8.

12 Schwaiger M, Hicks R. The clinical role of metabolic imaging of the heart by positron emission tomography. *J Nucl Med* 1991; **32**: 565–78.

13 Conway MA, Allis J, Duwerkerk R, Niioua T, Rajagopalan B, Radda GK. Low phosphocreatine/ATP ratio detected *in vivo* in the failing hypertrophied human myocardium using ^{31}P magnetic resonance spectroscopy. *Lancet* 1991; **338**: 973–6.

14 Kloner RA, Przyklenk K. Understanding the jargon: a glossary of terms used (and misused) in the study of ischaemia and reperfusion. *Cardiovasc Res* 1993; **27**: 162–6.

15 Taegtmeyer H. Energy metabolism of the heart: From basic concepts to clinical applications. *Curr Prob Cardiol* 1994; **19**: 57–116.

16 Lipmann F. Metabolic generation and utilization of phosphate bond energy. *Adv Enzymol* 1941; **1**: 99–165.

17 Taegtmeyer H. Cardiac preconditioning does not require myocardial stunning. *Ann Thorac Surg* 1993; **55**: 400.

18 Clarke K, O'Conner AJ, Willis RJ. Temporal relation between energy metabolism and myocardial function during ischemia and reperfusion. *Am J Physiol* 1987; **253**: H412–21.

19 Barth E, Stämmler G, Speiser B, Schaper J. Ultrastructural quantitation of mitochondria and myofilaments in cardiac muscle from 10 different animal species including man. *J Mol Cell Cardiol* 1992; **24**: 669–81.

20 McNutt NS, Fawcett DW. Myocardial ultrastructure. In: Lauger G, Brady A, eds, *The mammalian myocardium.* New York: John Wiley & Sons, 1974: 1–49.

21 Baldwin JE, Krebs HA. The evolution of metabolic cycles. *Nature* 1981; **291**: 381–2.

22 Brown GC. Control of respiration and ATP synthesis in mammalian mitochondria and cells. *Biochem J* 1992; **284**: 1–13.

23 Newsholme EA, Start C. *Regulation in metabolism.* London: J. Wiley & Sons, 1973: 349 PP.

24 Newsholme EA, Leech AR. *Biochemistry for the medical sciences.* Chichester: J Wiley, 1983: 952 PP.

25 Coulson RA, Hernandez T, Herbert JD. Metabolic rate, enzyme kinetics *in vivo. Comp Biochem Physiol* 1977; **56A**: 251–62.

26 Barry WH, Bridge JHB. Intracellular calcium homeostasis in cardiac myocytes. *Circulation* 1993; **87**: 1806–15.

27 Fabiato A. Calcium induced release of calcium from the cardiac sarcoplasmic reticulum. *Am J Physiol* 1983; **245**: C1–14.

28 McCormack JG, Halestrap AP, Denton RM. Role of calcium ions in reperfusion of mammalian intramitochondrial metabolism. *Physiol Rev* 1990; **70**: 391–425.

29 Lehninger AL, Reynafarie B, Vercesi A. Transport and accumulation of calcium in mitochondria. *Ann NY Acad Sci* 1978; **307**: 160–76.

30 Denton RM, McCormack JG. On the role of the calcium transport cycle in the heart and other mammalian mitochondria. *FEBS Lett* 1980; **119**: 1–8.

31 Rayment I, Holden HM, Whittacker M, *et al.* Structure of actin–myosin complex and its implications for muscle contraction. *Science* 1993; **261**: 58–65.

32 Kornberg HL. Anaplerotic sequences and their role in metabolism. *Essays Biochem* 1966; **2**: 1–31.

33 Taegtmeyer H, Hems R, Krebs HA. Utilization of energy providing substrates in the isolated working rat heart. *Biochem J* 1980; **186**: 701–11.

34 Taegtmeyer H. On the inability of ketone bodies to serve as the only energy providing substrate for rat heart at physiological work load. *Basic Res Cardiol* 1983; **78**: 435–50.

35 Russell RR, Taegtmeyer H. Coenzyme A sequestration in rat hearts oxidizing ketone bodies. *J Clin Invest* 1992; **89**: 968–73.

36 Russell RR, Taegtmeyer H. Changes in citric acid cycle flux and anaplerosis antedate the functional decline in isolated rate hearts utilizing acetoacetate. *J Clin Invest* 1991; **87**: 384–90.

37 Russell RR, Taegtmeyer H. Pyruvate carboxylation prevents the decline in contractile function of rat hearts oxidizing acetoacetate. *Am J Physiol* 1991; **30**: H756–62.

38 Taegtmeyer H. Metabolic responses to cardiac hypoxia: Increased production of succinate by rabbit papillary muscles. *Circ Res* 1978; **43**: 808–15.

39 Schwaiger M, Schelbert H, Ellison D, *et al*. Sustained regional abnormalities in cardiac metabolism after transient ischemia in the chronic dog model. *J Am Coll Cardiol* 1985; **6**: 337–47.

40 Schwaiger M, Neese RA, Araujo L, *et al*. Sustained nonoxidative glucose utilization and depletion of glycogen in reperfused canine myocardium. *J Am Coll Cardiol* 1989; **13**: 745–54.

41 Czernin J, Porenta G, Brunken R, *et al*. Regional blood flow, oxidative metabolism, and glucose utilization in patients with recent myocardial infarction. *Circulation* 1993; **88**: 884–95.

42 Racker E. Energy cycles in health and disease. *Curr Top Cell Regul* 1981; **18**: 361–75.

43 Steenbergen C, Murphy E, Levy L, London RE. Elevation in cytosolic free calcium concentration early in myocardial ischemia in perfused rat heart. *Circ Res* 1987; **60**: 700–7.

44 Tani M, Neely JR. Role of intracellular Na^+ in Ca^{2+} overload and depressed recovery of ventricular function of reperfused ischemic rat hearts. Possible involvement of H^+-Na^+ and Na^+-Ca^{2+}. *Circ Res* 1989; **65**: 1045–56.

45 Marban E, Kitakaze M, Koretsune Y, Yue DT, Chacko VP, Pike MM. Quantification of $[Ca^{2+}]_i$ in perfused hearts. Critical evaluation of the 5F-BAPTA and nuclear magnetic response method as applied to the study of ischemia and reperfusion. *Circ Res* 1990; **66**: 1255–67.

46 Rao PS, Cohen MV, Mueller HS. Production of free radicals and lipid peroxides in early experimental myocardial ischemia. *J Mol Cell Cardiol* 1983; **15**: 713–16.

47 Kloner RA, Przyklenk K, Whittacker P. Deleterious effects of oxygen radicals in ischemia/reperfusion. Resolved and unresolved issues. *Circulation* 1989; **80**: 1115–27.

48 Ferrari R, Alfieri O, Curello S, *et al*. Occurrence of oxidative stress during reperfusion in human heart. *Circulation* 1990; **81**: 201–11.

49 Bolli R. Mechanism of myocardial "stunning". *Circulation* 1990; **82**: 723–38.

50 Lehninger AL. *Biochemistry*, 1st edn. New York: Worth Publishers, 1970: 1013 PP.

51 Winterstein H. Ueber die Sauerstoffatmung des isolierten Säugetierherzens. *Zeitschrift für Allgemeine Physiologie* 1904; **4**: 333–59.

52 Jennings RB, Reimer KA, Steenbergen C. Myocardial ischemia revisited. The osmolar load, membrane damage, and reperfusion. *J Mol Cell Cardiol* 1986; **18**: 769–80.

53 Rohde E. Über den Einfluss der mechanischen Bedingungen auf die Tätigkeit und den Sauerstoffverbrauch des Warmblüterherzens. *Naunyn-Schmiedeberg's Arch Pharmakol Exp Pathol* 1912; **68**: 401–10.

54 Evans CL. The effect of glucose on the gaseous metabolism of the isolated mammalian heart. *J Physiol (Lond)* 1914; **47**: 407–18.

55 Neely JR, Liebermeister H, Battersby EJ, Morgan HE. Effect of pressure development on oxygen consumption by isolated rat heart. *Am J Physiol* 1967; **212**: 804–14.

56 Nguyên VTB, Mossberg KA, Tewson T, *et al*. Temporal analysis of myocardial glucose metabolism by ^{18}F-2-deoxy-2-fluoro-D-glucose. *Am J Physiol* 1990; **259**: H1022–31.

57 Cooney GJ, Taegtmeyer H, Newsholme EA. Tricarboxylic acid cycle flux and enzyme activities in the isolated working rat heart. *Biochem J* 1981; **200**: 701–3.

58 Balaban RS. Regulation of oxidative phosphorylation in the mammalian cell. *Am J Physiol* 1990; **258**: C377–89.

59 Jones BP, Shan X, Park Y. Coordinated multisite regulation of cellular energy metabolism. *Annu Rev Nutr* 1992; **12**: 327–43.

60 Evans G. The glycogen content of the rat heart. *J Physiol (Lond)* 1934; **82**: 468–80.

61 Denton RM, Randle PJ. Concentrations of glycerides and phospholipids in rat heart and gastrocnemius muscles. *Biochem J* 1967; **104**: 416–22.

62 Gevers W. Protein metabolism of the heart. *J Mol Cell Cardiol* 1984; **16**: 3–32.

63 Lesch M, Taegtmeyer H, Peterson MB, Vernick R. Studies on the mechanism of the inhibition of myocardial protein synthesis during oxygen deprivation. *Am J Physiol* 1976; **230**: 120–6.

64 Taegtmeyer H, Lesch M. Altered protein and amino acid metabolism in myocardial hypoxia and ischemia. In: Wildenthal K, ed, *Degradative processes in heart and skeletal muscle*. Amsterdam: Elsevier/North Holland, 1980: 347–60.

65 Morgan HE, Rannels DE, McKee EE. Protein metabolism of the heart. In: Berne R, ed, *Handbook of physiology: The cardiovascular system: The heart*. Washington, DC: American Physiology Society, 1979: 845–71.

66 Magid NM, Borer JS, Young MS, Wallerson DC, Demonteiro, C. Suppression of protein degradation in progressive cardiac hypertrophy of chronic aortic regurgitation. *Circulation* 1993; **87**: 1249–57.

67 Samarel AM. Hemodynamic overloaded the regulation of myofibrillar protein degradation. *Circulation* 1993; **87**: 1418–20.

68 Taegtmeyer H, Doenst T, Mommessin JI, Guthrie PH, Williams CM. Further evidence for the importance of anaplerosis in the isolated working rat heart: A tracer kinetic study with [^{18}F] fluoro-2-deoxyglucose (FDG) (abstract). *Circulation* 1993; **88**: I-284.

69 Rothlin ME, Bing RJ. Extraction and release of individual free fatty acids by the heart and fat deposits. *J Clin Invest* 1961; **40**: 1380–5.

70 Keul J, Doll E, Keppler D. *Energy metabolism of human muscle*. Basel: S Karger, 1972: 313 PP.

71 Drake AJ, Haines JR, Noble MM. Preferential uptake of lactate by the normal myocardium in dogs. *Cardiovasc Res* 1980; **14**: 65–72.

72 Krebs HA, Williamson DH, Bates MW, Page MA, Hawkins RA. The role of ketone bodies in caloric homeostasis. In: Weber G, ed, *Advances in enzyme regulations*, Vol. 9. New York: Pergamon Press, 1971: 387–409.

73 Opie LH. Cardiac metabolism—emergence, decline, and resurgence. Part I. *Cardiovasc Res* 1992; **26**: 721–33.

74 Opie LH. Cardiac metabolism—emergence, decline, and resurgence. Part II. *Cardiovasc Res* 1992; **26**: 817–30.

75 Gadian DG, Hoult DI, Radda GK, Seeley PJ, Chance B, Barlow C. Phosphorous nuclear magnetic resonance studies in normoxic and ischemic cardiac tissue. *Proc Natl Acad Sci USA* 1976; **73**: 291–332.

76 Weiss ES, Hoffman EJ, Phelps ME, *et al.* External detection and visualization of myocardial ischemia with ^{11}C substrates in vitro and in vivo. *Circ Res* 1976; **39**: 24–32.

77 Jacobus WE, Taylor G, Hollis DP, Nunnally RL. Phosphorous nuclear magnetic resonance of perfused working rat hearts. *Nature* 1977; **265**: 756–8.

78 Ingwall JS. Phosphorous nuclear magnetic resonance spectroscopy of cardiac and skeletal muscles. *Am J Physiol* 1982; **242**: H729–44.

79 Bottomley PA. Noninvasive study of high energy phosphate metabolism in human heart by depth-resolved ^{31}P NMR spectroscopy. *Science* 1985; **229**: 769–72.

80 Balaban RS, Kontor HL, Katz LA, Briggs RW. Relation between work and phosphate metabolite in the in vivo paced mammalian heart. *Science* 1986; **232**: 1121–3.

81 Schelbert HR. Assessment of myocardial metabolism by PET: A sophisticated dream or clinical reality? *Eur J Nucl Med* 1986; **12**: 570–5.

82 McMillin-Wood JB. Biochemical approaches in metabolism: application to positron emission tomography. *Circulation* 1985; **72**: IV145–50.

83 Taegtmeyer H, Mossberg KA, Nguyen VTB. Positron labelled tracers: A window for the assessment of energy metabolism in heart and skeletal muscle. *Acta Radiol* 1991; **376**(suppl): 40–4.

84 Lewandowski ED. Nuclear magnetic resonance evaluation of metabolic and respiratory support of work load in intact rabbit hearts. *Circ Res* 1992; **70**: 576–82.

85 Tillisch J, Brunken R, Marshall R, *et al*. Prediction of reversibility of cardiac wall motion abnormalities predicted by positron tomography, ^{18}fluoro-deoxyglucose, and ^{13}NH$_3$. *N Engl J Med* 1986; **314**: 884–8.

86 Gould KL, Yoshida K, Haynie M, Hess MJ, Mullani NA, Smalling RW. Myocardial metabolism of fluoro-deoxyglucose compared to cell membrane integrity for the potassium analogue R6-82 for assessing viability and infarct size in man by PET. *J Nucl Med* 1991; **32**: 1–9.

87 Yoshida K, Gould KL. Quantitative relation of myocardial infarct size and myocardial viability by positron emission tomography of left ventricular ejection fraction and 3-year mortality with and without revascularization. *J Am Coll Cardiol* 1993; **22**: 984–97.

88 Radda GU. Control, bioenergetics, and adaptation in health and disease: noninvasive biochemistry from nuclear magnetic resonance. *FASEB J* 1992; **6**: 3032–8.

89 Malloy CR, Sherry AD, Jeffrey FMH. Carbon flux through citric acid cycle pathways in perfused heart by ^{13}C NMR spectroscopy. *FEBS Lett* 1987; **212**: 58–62.

90 Weiss RG, Gloth ST, Kalil-Filho R, Chacko VP, Stern MD, Gerstenblith G. Indexing tricarboxylic acid cycle flux in intact hearts by carbon-13 nuclear magnetic resonance. *Circ Res* 1992; **70**: 392–408.

91 Laughlin MR, Fleming Taylor J, Cresnik AS, Balaban RS. Regulation of glycogen metabolism in canine myocardium: Effects of insulin and epinephrine in vivo. Am J Physiol 1992; **262**: E875–83.

92 Bergman RN. Toward physiological understanding of glucose tolerance. *Diabetes* 1989; **38**: 1512–27.

93 Schelbert H, Henze E, Sochor H. Effects of substrate availability on myocardial ^{11}C palmitate kinetics by positron emission tomography in normal subjects and patients with ventricular dysfunction. *Am Heart J* 1986; **111**: 1055–65.

94 Brown MA, Marshall DR, Sobel BE, Bergmann SR. Delineation of myocardial oxygen utilization with carbon-11 labelled acetate. *Circulation* 1987; **76**: 687–96.

95 Buxton DB, Schwaiger M, Nguyen NA, Phelps ME, Schelbert HR. Radiolabelled acetate as a tracer of myocardial tricarboxylic acid cycle flux. *Circ Res* 1988; **63**: 628–34.

96 Opie LH, Owen P, Thomas M, Samson R. Coronary sinus lactate measurements in assessment of myocardial ischemia: Comparison with changes in lactate/pyruvate and β-hydroxybutyrate/acetoacetate ratios and with release of hydrogen, phosphate, and potassium from the heart. *Am J Cardiol* 1973; **32**: 295–305.

97 Schelbert, HR. The heart. In *Computed emission tomography*, Eds, Ell P, Holman B, Oxford: Oxford University Press, 1982: 91–133.

98 Gertz EW, Wisneski JA, Neese R. Myocardial lactate extraction: Multidetermined metabolic function. *Circulation* 1980; **61**: 256–61.

99 Wisneski JA, Gertz EW, Neese RA, Gruenke LD, Morris DL, Craig JC. Metabolic fate of extracted glucose in normal human myocardium. *J Clin Invest* 1985; **76**: 1819–27.

100 Hearse DJ. Myocardial enzyme leakage. *J Mol Med* 1977; **2**: 185–200.

101 Katz AM, Hecht HH. The early "pump" failure of the ischemic heart. *Am J Med* 1969; **47**: 497–502.

102 Williamson JR, Shaffer SW, Ford C, Safer B. Contribution of tissue acidosis to ischemic injury in the perfused rat heart. *Circulation* 1976; **53**: 3–14.

103 Neely JR, Grotyohann LW. Role of glycolytic products in damage to myocardium: Dissociation of adenosine triphosphate levels and recovery of function of reperfused canine myocardium. *Circ Res* 1984; **55**: 816–24.

104 Kübler W, Katz AM. Mechanism of early "pump" failure of the ischemic heart: Possible role of adenosine triphosphate depletion and inorganic phosphate accumulation. *Am J Cardiol* 1977; **40**: 467–71.

105 Gudbjarnason S, Mathes P, Ravens KG. Functional compartmentation of ATP and creatine phosphate in heart muscle. *J Mol Cell Cardiol* 1970; **1**: 325–39.

106 Murry CE, Jennings RB, Reimer KA. Preconditioning with ischemia: a delay of lethal cell injury in ischemic myocardium. *Circulation* 1986; **74**: 1124–36.

107 Marber MS. Stress proteins and myocardial protection. *Clin Sci* 1994; **86**: 375–81.

108 Neely JR, Morgan HE. Relationship between carbohydrate and lipid metabolism and the energy balance of heart muscle. *Annu Rev Physiol* 1974; **36**: 413–39.
109 Rogers WJ, Stanley AW, Breing JB, *et al*. Reduction of hospital mortality rate of acute myocardial infarction with glucose-insulin-potassium infusion. *Am Heart J* 1976; **92**: 441–54.
110 Rackley CE, Russell RO, Rogers WJ, Papapierto SE. Clinical experience with glucose–insulin–potassium therapy in acute myocardial infarction. *Am Heart J* 1981; **102**: 1038–49.
111 Whitlow PL, Rogers WJ, Smith LR, *et al*. Enhancement of left ventricular function by glucose–insulin–potassium infusion in acute myocardial infarction. *Am J Cardiol* 1982; **49**: 811–20.
112 Medical Research Council Working Party. Potassium, glucose, and insulin treatment for acute myocardial infarction. *Lancet* 1968; **ii**: 1355–60.
113 Opie LH. The glucose hypothesis: Relation to acute myocardial ischemia. *J Mol Cell Cardiol* 1970; **1**: 107–15.
114 Hearse DJ, Chain EB. The role of glucose in the survival and "recovery" of the anoxic isolated perfused rat heart. *Biochem J* 1972; **128**: 1125–33.
115 Opie LH, Bruyneel K, Owen P. Effects of glucose, insulin, potassium infusion and tissue metabolic changes within first hour of myocardial infarction in the baboon. *Circulation* 1975; **52**: 49–57.
116 Apstein CS, Gravino FN, Haudenschild CC. Determinants of a protective effect of glucose and insulin on the ischemic myocardium. Effects on contractile function, diastolic compliance, metabolism, and ultrastructure during ischemia and reperfusion. *Circ Res* 1983; **52**: 515–26.
117 McElroy DD, Walker WE, Taegtmeyer H. Glycogen loading improves left ventricular function of the rabbit heart after hypothermic ischemic arrest. *J Appl Cardiol* 1989; **4**: 455–65.
118 Lagerstrom CF, Walker WE, Taegtmeyer H. Failure of glycogen depletion to improve left ventricular function of the rabbit heart after hypothermic ischemic arrest. *Circ Res* 1988; **63**: 81–6.
119 Schneider CA, Nguyên VTB, Taegtmeyer H. Feeding and fasting determine postischemic glucose utilization in isolated working rat hearts. *Am J Physiol* 1991; **260**: H542–8.
120 Schneider CA, Taegtmeyer H. Fasting in vivo delays myocardial cell damage after brief periods of ischemia in the isolated working rat heart. *Circ Res* 1991; **68**: 1045–50.
121 Gradinak S, Coleman GM, Taegtmeyer H, Sweeney MS, Frazier OH. Improved cardiac function with glucose–insulin–potassium after coronary bypass surgery. *Ann Thorac Surg* 1989; **48**: 484–9.

2: Ventricular performance

KARL SKARVAN

Anaesthetists are keenly aware of the importance of ventricular performance and that preservation of optimal heart function represents one of the foremost goals of anaesthetic management during the perioperative period. Only rarely does the heart work under such challenging and often untoward conditions as occur during this time. Acute changes in ventricular loading, gas exchange, intrathoracic pressure, autonomic nervous tone, as well as the effects of anaesthetic and other drugs and various mediators, all put a substantial stress on the heart. This may give rise to cardiac morbidity even in patients with normal hearts, whilst patients with limited contractile and coronary reserve are, of course, at a much higher risk. Hence, a proper understanding of ventricular function is a prerequisite to correct evaluation and optimisation of cardiac function in the perioperative period. With regard to the predominant role of the left ventricle in the pumping function of the heart, this chapter focuses on the normal performance of the left ventricle and the assessment of the determinants of its function.

Ventricle as a muscle

The fundamental properties of the myocardium have been thoroughly studied in isolated animal and human heart muscle preparations. The *resting length* of the unstressed muscle strip represents the starting point for the following considerations (fig 2.1). This resting length can be increased by attaching a small weight to one end of the muscle. This weight will stretch the muscle to a longer resting length in proportion to the weight itself, as well as the elastic properties of the muscle. This distending force or weight (expressed in grams) is called the *preload* of the muscle. The preload, which is related to the resting length of the sarcomeres, has an important influence on the following contraction of the muscle.[1] When the muscle is prevented from shortening (isometric contraction), the active tension or force developed during contraction is directly proportional to preload or resting length. If the muscle is allowed to shorten (isotonic contraction), both the extent and velocity of shortening will increase in proportion to resting length. This dependence of contraction on resting length (preload) is a fundamental property of the myocardium and is known as the force–length relationship.[1,2] The property of the myocardium to develop progressively more energy with increasing sarcomere length has been also termed "length dependent activa-

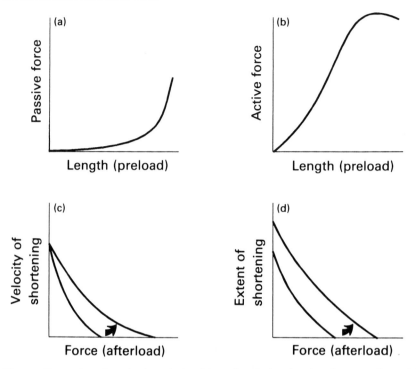

Fig 2.1 Force–length–velocity relationships of an isolated strip of myocardium. (a) Passive force builds up with increasing resting length; (b) active developed force increases with increasing resting length; (c) shortening velocity decreases with increasing load; (d) extent of shortening decreases with increasing load. Arrows indicate alterations caused by an increase in myocardial contractility.

tion" and appears to be related to an increase in the number of actin–myosin cross bridges, increased sensitivity to intracellular calcium, and increased calcium release from sarcoplasmic reticulum.[3]

A second weight can be attached to the moving end of the isotonically contracting muscle strip. This additional weight is engaged only during contraction when it is lifted by the shortening muscle, and hence ensures a constant tension in the muscle during its shortening. This second weight represents the *afterload* of the muscle. Similar to preload, afterload also has an important influence on contraction. Both the extent of muscle shortening and shortening velocity are inversely related to afterload. Thus, an increase in afterload decreases, whereas a decrease in afterload increases, the extent and velocity of shortening.[1] The dependence of contractile performance on the shortening load is the second fundamental property of the myocardium.[4–6] The reduced shortening resulting from increased afterload can be reversed up to a given limit by an appropriate augmentation of preload.[7]

When preload and afterload are maintained at constant levels, the developed tension (in isometric contraction) or extent and velocity of shortening (in isotonic contraction) can be increased by increasing the *inotropic state* of the muscle, for example, by adding calcium to the bath.[1] Thus the contractile behaviour of the isolated heart muscle can be exhaustively analysed within the framework of a force–length relationship. It is determined by the interplay of preload, afterload, and contractility. We shall see that this concept is also most useful for evaluation of the intact ventricle.[14]

Isolated ventricle

How can the principles governing contraction of an isolated strip of myocardium be applied to the intact ventricle? The ventricle can also contract either isometrically (for example, against an infinite resistance of an aortic clamp) or isotonically (when it is allowed to eject against a variable resistance). The resting fibre length can be increased by increasing either the blood volume in the ventricle or the volume of saline in a balloon positioned in the ventricle in the isovolumic preparation. The passive distension of the ventricle induced by the increased filling volume leads to a progressive increase in the passive force in the ventricular wall and in pressure in the ventricular cavity, depending on the elastic properties of the ventricular wall. The relation between resting pressure (P) and volume (V) is known as a diastolic P/V relationship and describes the chamber elasticity. During contraction, force is generated in the ventricular wall and transferred to the blood contained in the cavity, causing the ventricular pressure to rise (fig 2.2). If the ventricle were severed into two equal parts along an imaginary plane, the intracavitary pressure would immediately tear both halves apart. Consequently, an opposing force of equal dimension must be operational in the dividing plane of the ventricle to hold both parts together. On the basis of this assumption, mathematical models were developed that allow net wall forces to be calculated.[45] Depending on the orientation of the imaginary plane, circumferential, meridional, and radial forces can be calculated. Thus, in an intact ventricle, the resting volume corresponds to the resting fibre length, and the developed pressure or the calculated force corresponds to the force measured in the isolated muscle.

During isovolumetric contraction (analogue of isometric contraction), the developed ventricular pressure and wall force are directly proportional to the filling volume of the ventricle.[148] At a given filling volume, the maximal developed pressure will increase with positive inotropic stimulation. The ventricle, which is allowed to eject, also contracts under isovolumetric conditions until the aortic valve opens. During this isovolumetric contraction, the pressure increases while the ventricular volume remains unchanged, although the fibre length may change because the ventricle changes its geometry and assumes a more spherical shape. After the opening of the aortic

27

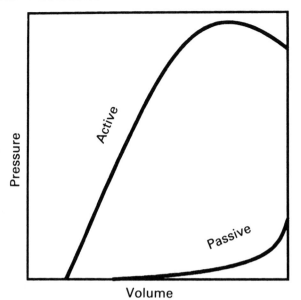

Fig 2.2 Passive (diastolic) and active (systolic) pressure–volume relationships of the ventricle. Curves illustrate filling and contractile behaviour of the ventricle for a given inotropic state.

valve, myocardial fibres begin to shorten and volume (stroke volume) is expelled from the ventricle into the aorta. The fibres stop shortening because there is only one end systolic force that can be sustained by the myocardial fibres at a given contractile state. This force is defined by the systolic P/V relationship of the isovolumetrically contracting ventricle and is independent of preload. When this level of force is reached in the course of contraction, the shortening stops and the myocardium begins to relax. Thus, the ventricle operates within the boundaries determined by the passive (diastolic) and active (systolic) P/V relationship.[9][10] For teaching purposes, maximal isovolumetric and end systolic force–length relationships can be considered as equivalent. Similar to an isolated muscle and an isovolumetric preparation, the contractile behaviour of the ejecting ventricle is controlled by fibre length (preload), instantaneous wall force (afterload), and contractile state.[15] The wall force during ejection is a function of ventricular size and geometry, and of developed pressure. As ventricular size decreases in the course of ejection, the instantaneous wall force and hence the afterload decreases. A normally contracting ventricle "unloads itself."[4]

Ventricle in situ

The function of the left ventricle is usually described in terms of pressure and volume. Both variables are used for the construction of the pressure–

volume diagram, an analogue of the force–length diagram. In the pressure–volume (P/V) diagram, the pressure plotted on the y axis corresponds to the force, and the volume plotted on the x axis corresponds to the myocardial fibre length.[9] During one cardiac cycle of the ejecting heart, a P/V loop is inscribed (fig 2.3). The cycle begins at end diastole, characterised by end diastolic volume and corresponding end diastolic pressure (fig 2.3, point 1). During isovolumetric contraction, pressure increases while volume remains constant until the aortic valve opens (fig 2.3, point 2) and ejection starts. Ejection stops when the active end systolic P/V relationship is reached (fig 2.3, point 3). Ventricular relaxation causes the aortic valve to close and the pressure to fall without changes in volume (isovolumetric relaxation). When the ventricular pressure falls below the atrial pressure, the mitral valve opens (fig 2.3, point 4) and ventricular filling starts.[9–11] In the context of the P/V diagram, the effects of the three major determinants of the ventricular function—preload, afterload, and contractile state—can be illustrated.

Preload

An increase in end diastolic volume (preload) shifts the starting point of the loop to the right along the passive P/V relationship whereas the end systolic point remains unchanged. This results in an increase in ejected volume

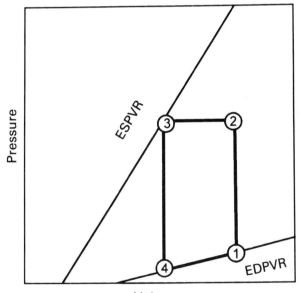

Fig 2.3 Left ventricular pressure–volume relationship. Points 1 to 4 demarcate the pressure–volume loop that is explained in the text. ESPVR (end systolic pressure–volume relationship) and EDPVR (end diastolic pressure–volume relationship) are curvilinear, but on this diagram, for simplification, they are approximated by straight lines.

(stroke volume). The ejection fraction (stroke volume divided by end diastolic volume) increases.

Afterload

An increase in ejected stroke volume can also be achieved by a decrease in afterload. A decrease in the wall force facilitating ejection can be caused by a decrease in ventricular volume, pressure, or both.[12] In any case, this will be reflected by a downward shift of the end systolic point of the loop along the active end systolic *P/V* relationship associated with the increase in stroke volume and ejection fraction. This phenomenon is the basis for treating the failing ventricle by *afterload reduction*. In contrast, an increase in afterload will cause an upward shift of the end systolic point. As a consequence, stroke volume and ejection fraction decrease. A normal left ventricle responds to an acute increase in afterload by an immediate increase in end diastolic volume. This decrease, in turn, restores the stroke volume. The so called homoeometric regulation or Anrep effect will subsequently restore the end diastolic volume, in spite of the persisting higher afterload, by adjusting the intrinsic myocardial contractility.[13] A failing ventricle is deprived of these compensatory mechanisms and, consequently, becomes exquisitely sensitive to any increase in the shortening load.

Contractile state

The third major determinant of ventricular function is the contractile state. A change in the contractile state will breech the confines of the diastolic and end systolic *P/V* relationships. With an increase in contractility, the end systolic points of the *P/V* loop will be shifted upwards and to the left of the original active end systolic *P/V* relationship; consequently, stroke volume and ejection fraction will increase. The new end systolic *P/V* relationship, which now determines the extent of ejection, is shifted to the left and its slope is steeper. Thus, the positive inotropic stimulation causes the ventricle to empty more efficiently to a smaller end systolic volume.[9–11] With limited ventricular filling, for example, low venous return resulting from hypovolaemia or shortened diastolic filling time caused by tachycardia, the end diastolic point of the *P/V* loop will also shift to the left. At this point, the positive inotropic intervention will become evident by an increase in pressure rather than by an increase in stroke volume. The common positive inotropic agents may also exert vasodilating, afterload reducing, and positive lusitropic effects. This last effect, by virtue of improving ventricular relaxation, shifts the diastolic *P/V* relationship downwards, which facilitates ventricular filling and further enhances ejection, provided the blood volume and venous return are adequate.

Thus, *P/V* diagrams help the anaesthetist to have a better understanding of changes in ventricular function under rapidly changing loading conditions. *P/V* diagrams do not, however, account for the fourth major determinant of ventricular function, the heart rate, and they also do not depict the rate related phenomena such as shortening velocity or rate of pressure change.

The heart as a pump

Functioning as a pump, the ventricle generates pressure and displaces volume. The mechanical properties of the ventricular pump are elasticity, resistance, and inertance:[4 12]

- Elasticity reflects the rate independent relationship between pressure and volume in the ventricle and determines the volume displaced from the ventricle during systole (stroke volume).
- Ventricular resistance is rate dependent (changing with flow velocity), and it is related to the viscous properties of the ventricular pump that is operational during ejection.
- Inertance describes the force required to accelerate the mass of the ventricle and the blood contained within it at end diastole.

These three properties of the ventricular pump determine the amount of pressure generated. In an isovolumetrically contracting ventricle, the maximal pressure is determined solely by the elasticity. In contrast, the ejecting ventricle develops less pressure because part of its contractile energy is used to overcome the resistive and inertial forces.[4]

The pump function of the ventricle can be described by means of a pump function graph plotting pressure against flow (fig 2.4). The graph shows an inverse curvilinear (parabolic) relationship between mean left ventricular pressure and flow. Increased ventricular filling shifts the curve upwards and

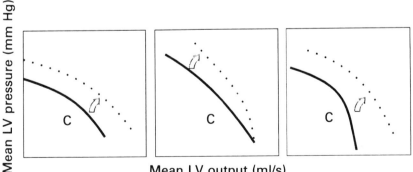

Fig 2.4 Pump function curve of the left ventricle. Ventricular pump output decreases with increasing developed pressure and eventually ceases when the pressure necessary to generate flow exceeds the capacity of the ventricular pump. Arrows indicate the effects of increased ventricular filling (left), contractility (middle), and heart rate (right).[14]

to the right; an increase in heart rate has the same effect. An increase in contractility causes the curve to rotate to the right around the flow axis intercept.[14] Power output of the ventricular pump can be calculated as the product of mean ventricular pressure and flow. Knowing the myocardial oxygen consumption, which represents the power input, the efficiency of the ventricular pump can be calculated. On the basis of this pump model applied to a cat heart, an efficiency of 20% was estimated.[15] It was also shown that the left ventricle tends to work at maximal power output while minimising its volume.

Clinical evaluation of global ventricular pump function

During anaesthesia the blood pressure resulting from the interaction between the left ventricle and the systemic vasculature often represents the only, although remote, index of ventricular performance. Nevertheless, when normal values of blood pressure are accompanied by clinical signs of an adequate peripheral circulation (pulse quality, capillary refill time, skin temperature, etc), it can be assumed that ventricular performance is satisfactory. Visual analysis of the intra-arterial pressure waveform, with regard to rate of pressure rise, amplitude, and width of the pressure wave, as well as to respiratory pressure variation, provides additional useful information. The use of a thermodilution pulmonary artery catheter allows measurement of cardiac output, stroke volume (SV), and left and right ventricular stroke work. When evaluating the adequacy of these flows and work data, the corresponding filling pressures of both ventricles (wedge and right atrial pressure) and blood gases (mixed venous oxygen saturation or tension and pH) must be taken into consideration. The most commonly used quantitative measure of ventricular performance is the ejection fraction (EF):[16]

$$EF = \frac{\text{Stroke volume}}{\text{End diastolic volume}} = \frac{SV}{EDV}.$$

Usually measured by radionuclide ventriculography during preoperative evaluation, it can also be assessed in the perioperative period by echocardiography. The calculation of ejection fraction from echocardiographic data is, however, time consuming and therefore not suitable for on line monitoring. The changes in left ventricular cross sectional area at the midpapillary, muscle level can, however, be monitored continuously. The left ventricular fractional area change (FAC) obtained by transoesophageal echocardiography correlates reasonably well with a simultaneously measured radionuclide ejection fraction:[17-19]

32

$$FAC = \frac{\text{End diastolic area} - \text{End systolic area}}{\text{End diastolic area}}$$

Normal value > 0.5 or 50%.

Determinants of ventricular function

What appears to be simple and easily understandable in an isolated papillary muscle preparation becomes a complex and sometimes controversial issue in the clinic. On the one hand, the indiscriminate use of the physiologically well defined terms of preload, afterload, and contractility by clinicians occasionally gives rise to criticism and confusion; on the other, many useful concepts of perioperative management are based on the interplay of these major determinants of ventricular function. Therefore, a detailed review of the determinants of ventricular function and of the methods used for their assessment is indicated.

Preload

Strictly speaking, preload is the force that stretches the resting myocardium and determines the resting length of its contractile fibres. In an intact ventricle, ventricular end diastolic volume is proportional to the preload.[1 4 6 9] The measurement of end diastolic volume in patients is difficult. Most data in the literature are based on contrast ventriculography. Ventriculography requires radiography apparatus, heart catheterisation, and an injection of contrast medium; it cannot be used for multiple measurements. Moreover, the calculated volumes depend on the ventricular geometry, model and formula used, and accurate identification of the endocardial borders. Inclusion of the volume of papillary muscle and trabeculae into the ventricular volume may lead to an overestimation of the volume. Furthermore, only a limited number of beats can be evaluated. Nevertheless, results obtained from ventriculography represent the standard to which the other results from less invasive methods have been compared. Recently ultra fast computed tomography and magnetic resonance imaging have also been used for measurement of ventricular volumes.[20] Neither of these methods, although accurate, can be used in the perioperative setting.

Equilibrium and first pass radionuclide cineangiography have, however, been used in intensive care units. Although accurate with regard to determination of ejection fraction, radionuclide cineangiography can only approximate the absolute ventricular volume using either the geometric (length–area) or a count based method. A real breakthrough in perioperative assessment of ventricular end diastolic size was the introduction of transoesophageal echocardiography. Several studies have shown a good correlation between left ventricular volumes assessed by transoesophageal echocardiography and those obtained by contrast or radionuclide ventriculography or transthoracic echocardiography.[17] [19] [21] The use of a biplane transoesophageal probe improves the accuracy of volume measurements.[22] In spite of the good correlations found, transoesophageal echocardiography appears to underestimate left ventricular volume systematically. This results, in part, from exclusion of papillary muscles and trabeculae from the cavitary volume and foreshortening of the ventricular cavity on its long axis.

For perioperative on line estimation of left ventricular filling volume, however, the calculation of end diastolic volume is not necessary. The area of the cross sectional view of the left ventricle in the transgastric short axis view has been shown to reflect left ventricular filling reasonably well. The recently introduced and commercially available automated border detection method traces the changes of the left ventricular area throughout the cardiac cycle and displays in real time the end diastolic and end systolic area values together with the fractional area change (fig 2.5).[23] [24] Findings of small

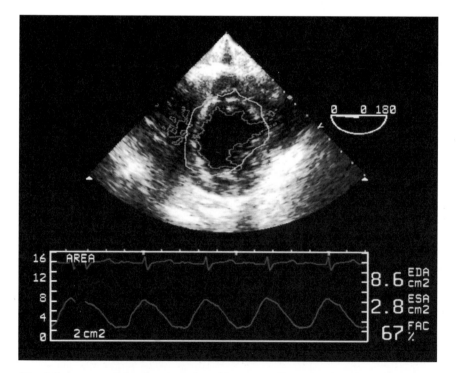

Fig 2.5 Automated border detection. Top: two dimensional, echocardiographic, short axis view of the left ventricle with left ventricular cavity area encircled by endocardial borders and the line drawn around the region of interest. Bottom: electrocardiogram and left ventricular area waveform—EDA (end diastolic area), ESA (end systolic area), and FAC (fractional area change).

ventricular size at end diastole, partial or complete obliteration of left ventricular cavity at end systole, and the "kissing papillary muscles" sign, all of which can be assessed usually by the naked eye, are most useful in the clinical diagnosis of an inadequate filling volume. The dimensional data obtained by transoesophageal echocardiography (cavity radius and wall thickness), together with the measured filling pressure (wedge pressure or mean left atrial pressure), allow calculation of the end diastolic wall stress which may correlate even better with the end diastolic fibre length than the end diastolic volume.[25]

Without the possibility of monitoring left ventricular size, the filling pressure, usually measured as the mean capillary pulmonary wedge pressure, remains the only means of estimating left ventricular filling volume during the perioperative period. The limitations of the wedge pressure as a measure of preload must, however, be kept in mind. The relationship between pressure and volume in diastole is curvilinear and changes when the ventricle moves along the P/V relationship.[9 10] Moreover, acute changes in ventricular stiffness may also substantially alter the relationship between filling pressure and volume (see section on "Diastolic performance").

Afterload

It is difficult to apply laboratory results that describe ventricular afterload in an isolated heart muscle to the evaluation of ventricular function in patients. In heart muscle in vitro, the afterload remains constant during shortening and can be defined by a single value of force. In the intact ventricle in situ, afterload also represents the force opposing the shortening and ejection of blood during ventricular contraction. Its assessment is, however, much more complex and depends on factors both internal and external to the myocardium:

1 The internal factor (muscle load) refers to the instantaneous force or tension within the ventricular wall that is related to the size and shape of the chamber and the pressure within it.[4 6 12]
2 The external factor (arterial load) refers to the physical properties of the arterial system which the ventricle encounters during ejection.[26]

Another, although similar, concept of systolic loading describes the total ventricular systolic load comprising intrinsic and extrinsic components:

1 The intrinsic component corresponds to intraventricular pressure gradients
2 The extrinsic component is related to aortic root pressure waveform resulting from the interaction between ventricular ejection and aortic input impedance.[27]

This total ventricular load and the changing ventricular geometry determine the total muscle load expressed in terms of systolic wall stresses. These

35

stresses, in turn, determine the contractile behaviour of the ventricle within the framework of a force–velocity–length relationship. The novel aspect of this concept of the left ventricular systolic load is the incorporation of transient intraventricular pressure gradients related to blood inertia and impulsive flows in the early ejection and to the convective flow acceleration in the left ventricular outflow tract at peak ejection. Instantaneous high fidelity measurements of pressure and flow indeed demonstrated significant inhomo-geneity of intraventricular pressure during ejection with local gradients up to 8 mg Hg at rest and 16 mg Hg at exercise.[27] These pressure gradients increase with diminishing chamber volume and with positive inotropic stimulation. These findings are the basis for understanding the phenomenon of dynamic intraventricular obstruction associated with hypovolaemia and high adrenergic tone, which occasionally develops in the perioperative period.

Also new and clinically important is the recognition that the intrinsic and extrinsic loads are complementary and competitive. Thus a reduction in the extrinsic load by a vasodilator can be offset by a compensatory increase in the intrinsic component of the total load.[27]

How can left ventricular afterload be assessed in the clinic? All of the following have been proposed as a measure of left ventricular afterload:

- arterial and ventricular pressures
- peripheral vascular resistance
- aortic input impedance
- systolic wall stress
- effective arterial elastance.

The meaning and the clinical utility of each of these parameters are discussed below.

Arterial and ventricular pressures—The peripheral arterial pressure is an unreliable index of left ventricular afterload. The arterial pressure waveform results from a complex interaction between cardiac and peripheral factors. Arterial pressure can remain unchanged in spite of relevant changes in the systolic load. Of all the ventricular pressures that can be measured (instan-taneous, peak, end systolic, and mean), the mean left ventricular pressure reflects the afterload best.[28] The left ventricular pressure measurement is, however, limited to the heart catheterisation laboratory.

Peripheral vascular resistance—The peripheral resistance is calculated as the ratio of mean arterial pressure divided by flow (cardiac output) and is inversely related to the fourth power of the radius of the vascular bed. In a steady flow system, the peripheral resistance indeed represents the total load imposed on the pump. In the presence of intermittent ejection of blood into a distensible reservoir and of pulsatile flow, however, the total external load also includes elastic properties of the arterial system and wave reflections.[26 28]

Aortic input impedance—The use of aortic input impedance instead of peripheral resistance as a measure of the total load was proposed.[28][29] In general, impedance is a measure of opposition to flow presented by a system. In contrast to resistance which refers to non-oscillatory steady motion, impedance is confined to the oscillatory motion of blood. In the arterial system, oscillatory waveforms are superimposed on a mean non-pulsatile (steady) component, and the total opposition to flow is a sum of both components. The aortic input impedance relates the oscillatory or sinusoidal pressure in the aorta to the oscillatory flow, and is influenced by distensibility (compliance) of blood vessels and inertia of the blood. In the presence of high impedance to flow, there are wide fluctuations of pressure in the aorta:

$$\text{Magnitude of impedance} = \frac{\text{Amplitude of pressure sine wave}}{\text{Amplitude of flow sine wave}}$$

$$= \text{Modulus of impedance.}$$

The modulus of zero frequency harmonic (mean pressure/mean flow) corresponds to the peripheral resistance. The characteristic impedance, which quantifies the oscillatory component of the load, is the ratio of pulsatile pressure and flow in the absence of reflected waves; it is calculated as the arithmetic mean of the impedance moduli above 2–4 Hz.

Steps in calculating input impedance

1 Reduce the original pressure and flow waveforms to a finite number (10–18) of constituent sinus waves with increasing frequencies by means of the Fourier analysis.
2 Characterise each resulting sinus wave (*harmonic*) by its frequency, which is a multiple of the frequency of the original waveform.
3 Calculate for each frequency the impedance moduli.
4 Plot the impedance moduli of the sine waves against their respective frequencies to obtain an *impedance spectrum* (fig 2.6).

Hence the complete description of aortic input impedance includes peripheral resistance and a series of values for impedance moduli at increasing frequencies.[28][30] Aortic impedance moduli are not stable but oscillate around the characteristic impedance value as a result of the reflected waves. A decrease in resistance or an increase in aortic compliance will decrease the amplitude of reflected waves and moduli oscillation whereas an increase in resistance or a decrease in aortic compliance will have the opposite effect. The reflected waves exert a prominent influence on impedance moduli, particularly at low frequencies, and represent an additional compo-

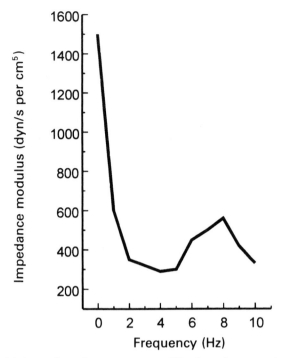

Fig 2.6 Arterial input impedance spectrum. The impedance moduli are plotted against their respective frequencies. The impedance modulus at zero frequency represents the peripheral vascular resistance. The impedance minimum for this example is 4 Hz.

nent of ventricular afterload.[31] The overall contribution of the frequency dependent (oscillatory) impedance to flow in the normal systemic circulation is, however, only approximately 10% of the total external load.

In a study in normal subjects, the impedance modulus fell from the high level at zero frequency (peripheral resistance) to a minimum at 4 Hz and slightly increased again. The characteristic impedance was 90 ± 34 dyn/s per cm^5, which corresponded to 8% of the total peripheral resistance.[30] The aortic input impedance was shown to be a major determinant of left ventricular load and function. An increase in characteristic impedance with constant resistance clearly reduced the extent and velocity of shortening and decreased cardiac output.[29] [32] However attractive from the physiological point of view, its cumbersome calculation renders the aortic input impedance unsuitable for assessment of ventricular afterload under clinical conditions.

Systolic wall stresses—The measurement of ventricular size and wall thickness by echocardiography allows assessment of the ventricular afterload by calculating the forces acting across the ventricular wall as systolic wall stresses.[25] [33] Stress is defined as the force acting on a surface divided by the

38

cross sectional area over which the force acts. The total stress can usually be reduced to component stresses acting perpendicular or parallel to the surface. The units of stress are dyn/cm^2 or g/cm^2. The theoretical calculation of ventricular wall stress relies on complex mathematical models. In practice, assumptions for simplification are inevitable. The left ventricular geometry is usually approximated by a sphere or a prolate ellipsoid; the ellipsoid has a stress distribution between that of a sphere and that of a cylinder. In the human ventricle, the stress distribution at the equator more closely resembles that of a cylinder. Consequently, the models based on an ellipsoid or a sphere tend to underestimate the circumferential and overestimate the longitudinal (meridional) stress. According to Laplace's law, the tension or force in the wall of a hollow, thin walled structure is proportional to the transmural pressure and the principal radii of curvature. In a thin walled structure the bending and radial stresses can be neglected. The meridional and circumferential stresses in the wall of a prolate, thin walled ellipsoid can be calculated when systolic pressure, corresponding radii of the curvature, and wall thickness are known.[33]

The basic assumption of the thin walled models is that the wall is thin relative to the diameter. In an attempt to obtain a better approximation to the real stresses and to study the stress distribution across the wall, thick walled ventricular models were developed. The earlier models, which assumed isotropic (homogeneous) properties of the myocardium, showed that the stresses are apparently higher in the inner layers of the ventricular wall than in the outer layers. Newer models incorporating anisotropic properties of the myocardium, cylindrical geometry, and fibre direction revealed uniform distribution of stress across the ventricular wall.[34] The mechanism keeping the transmural distribution of the stress uniform is related to the interplay of the field of deformation and regional fibre orientation. When change in ventricular volume induces transmural gradients in fibre strain (relative elongation), an appropriate amount of torsion redistributes the fibre strain from the inner to the outer layers and equalises wall stresses. This uniformity of the mechanical load in the myocardium is not restricted to the left ventricular wall alone but is also found in the papillary muscles and the free right ventricular wall.[34]

In animal experiments, systolic wall stress was compared with the aortic input impedance with regard to the estimation of left ventricular afterload. It was found that alterations in ventricular stress more accurately predicted alterations in ventricular shortening than the aortic input impedance. On the other hand, systolic wall stress, which represents the internal load imposed on the contracting myocardium, also appears to reflect alterations in the external load.[32]

In echocardiographic studies, the meridional end systolic wall stress (WS) is usually calculated in dyn/cm^2 according to the angiographically validated formula

$$WS = \frac{P \times D \times 1 \cdot 33}{4WT(1 + [WT/D])}$$

where P is end systolic pressure, D is the end systolic left ventricular diameter, and WT the end systolic wall thickness.[21] Although it is rather difficult to calculate the systolic wall stress in the perioperative setting, knowledge of at least directional changes of left ventricular afterload may help to evaluate the effects of therapeutic interventions and to optimise left ventricular function. For this purpose the directional changes of the simple ratio $P \times D/WT$ obtained by echocardiography should give sufficient reflection of changes in left ventricular afterload. In the absence of major alterations in arterial pressure, even the end systolic size (dimension or cross sectional area) of the left ventricle alone will help to estimate on line the directional changes in afterload.

Effective arterial elastance—Another measure of left ventricular afterload has been introduced within the framework of the time varying elastance (see section on "Ventriculoarterial coupling"). It is the effective arterial elastance (E_a) that relates end systolic arterial pressure to stroke volume. The concept of arterial elastance is a reflection of pressure that will be generated when the stroke volume is ejected into the arterial system. The greater the stroke volume ejected and the greater the opposition of the arterial system to the ejection, the greater the pressure increase in the arterial system. By plotting generated pressures at end systole against varying stroke volumes, the arterial pressure–volume relationship is constructed. The term for the slope of this linear relationship is "effective arterial elastance" and it is used in the end systolic P/V diagram as a measure of afterload to analyse the coupling of the left ventricle with the arterial system.[35]

Contractility

As previously mentioned, contractility is one of the fundamental properties of the heart muscle manifesting itself through the velocity and extent of shortening. To ascribe an observed change in shortening to a change in contractility, preload, afterload, and heart rate must be held constant. This requirement disqualifies the ejection phase parameters such as stroke volume, ejection fraction, or the first derivative of the left ventricular pressure, dP/dt_{max}, as reliable measures of myocardial contractility.[36]

Currently the most common way of assessing myocardial contractility is the determination of time varying elastance by means of an end systolic P/V relationship.[35 37 38] The slope of the end systolic P/V relationship is the end systolic elastance (E_{es}) or maximal elastance (E_{max}) (fig 2.7). In isolated ejecting ventricles, E_{max} and E_{es} are nearly identical over a wide range of varying preloads. When afterload is altered, they may differ considerably. This is frequently observed in vivo and is probably caused by resistive and

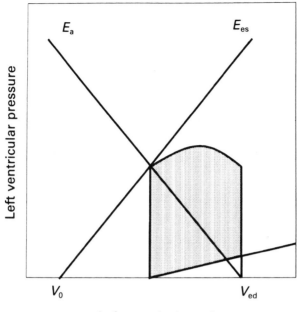

E_a E_{es}

Left ventricular pressure

V_0 V_{ed}

Left ventricular volume

Fig 2.7 End systolic pressure–volume relationship and ventriculoarterial coupling. V_{ed} (left ventricular end diastolic volume), V_0 (volume intercept of the end systolic pressure–volume relationship), E_{es} (end systolic elastance), E_a (effective arterial elastance), grey area (area of the left ventricular pressure–volume loop). The intersection of the E_{es} and E_a lines defines the effective stroke volume.

inertial influences on the end systolic pressures and by the changes in time required to reach end systole as a function of load.[39] In this case, E_{max} is steeper and does not fall on the end systolic (corner) points of the P/V relationship. As E_{es} can be determined more easily, it represents the preferred index of myocardial contractility. To construct an end systolic P/V relationship in an isolated heart, the preload can be varied by changing the volume of saline in the balloon placed in the ventricle. During open chest conditions, preload is usually changed by tightening a ligature around the inferior vena cava. In closed chest conditions, such as in human studies, venous return and preload can be changed by inflating a balloon at the tip of a catheter introduced into the inferior vena cava. Another possibility is to vary preload and/or afterload pharmacologically, for instance with glyceryl trinitrate (nitroglycerin) and phenylephrine.

It has been commonly assumed that the end systolic P/V relationship is linear and, therefore, can be described by two parameters: slope (E_{es}) and volume axis intercept (V_0).[40] Recent studies, however, demonstrated significant non-linearity of the relationship under different conditions, for instance during myocardial ischaemia or a high contractile state.[39 41] Moreover, the end systolic P/V relationship is not completely load insensitive. Changes in afterload can induce parallel shifts of the relationship and alter the slope. The changes in P/V relationships caused by the potential load dependence have, however, been shown to be of minor importance compared with the substantial changes brought about by variation in the inotropic state.[39]

The development of the *conductance catheter* allows determination of E_{es} in animal experiments as well as in patients.[42] In the normal left ventricle, E_{es} values of 3·5–4·5 mm Hg/ml were found, decreasing to 2·5 mm Hg/ml in patients with mildly depressed left ventricular function and to 1·5 mm Hg/ml in patients with severely depressed left ventricular function.[43] The determination of E_{es} by means of the conductance catheter was used for evaluation of myocardial contractility in patients before and after open heart surgery. The E_{es} varied between 0·9 and 5·6 mm Hg/ml with a mean of $2·5 \pm 1·5$ SD (standard deviation), and showed individually variable changes after cardiopulmonary bypass.[44] E_{es} is very sensitive to positive inotropic stimulation, for example, to dobutamine which clearly increases the slope without changes in V_0.[45] It has been recently shown that the use of a conductance catheter to measure ventricular volume can be replaced by the on line measurement of a cross sectional left ventricular area using transoesophageal echocardiography and automated border detection (fig 2.8).

In an open chest study on a dog using instantaneous left ventricular area

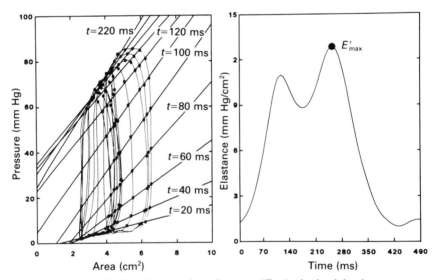

Fig 2.8 Left ventricular time varying elastance (E_{max}) obtained by instantaneous pressure–area relationship. Left: left ventricular pressure–area relationship demonstrating the increasing slope of the relationship (E) from the onset to the end of ejection. Right: the change in elastance (E) plotted against time with the maximal value of the elastance (E_{max}) occurring 250 ms after the onset of ejection. (Reproduced with permission from Gorcsan *et al*.[47])

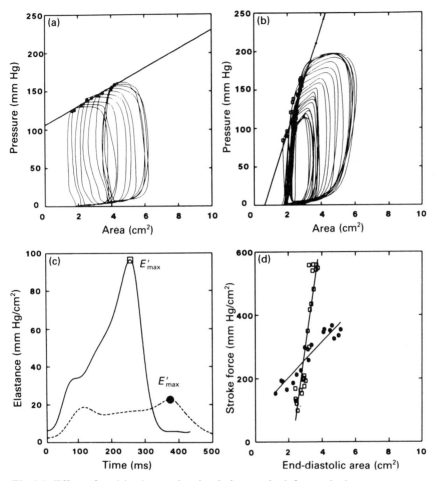

Fig 2.9 Effect of positive inotropic stimulation on the left ventricular pressure–area relationship (E_{max}). (a) Pressure–area loops and slope of the end systolic pressure–area relationship at control. (b) Increase in slope of the end systolic pressure–area relationship (E_{max}) after dobutamine administration. (c) Increase in E_{max} and shortening of the time to E_{max} after dobutamine administration (——) compared with control (– – –). (d) Increase in the slope of the stroke–force end diastolic area relationship after dobutamine administration ($\square$) compared with control ($\bullet$). (Reproduced with permission from Gorcsan et al.[46])

instead of volume, dobutamine (2–5 μg/kg per min) increased E_{es} and E_{max} by 120% of control values (fig 2.9).[46] In a study in patients undergoing open heart surgery, significant decreases in both E_{es} and E_{max} following cardiopulmonary bypass were observed. Such evidence of impaired left ventricular performance was not reflected in any other haemodynamic parameters such as cardiac output, stroke work, or ejection fraction.[47]

In patients with heart disease, the end systolic pressure may be an inaccurate index of ventricular afterload. In aortic stenosis or hypertensive cardiomyopathy, the end systolic pressure is high, although the afterload may be normal as a result of the development of ventricular hypertrophy which is able to normalise the stress. Therefore, in these patients the systolic (peak or end systolic) wall stress is a more reliable reflection of ventricular afterload and should replace end systolic pressure when plotting the P/V diagram. The end systolic wall stress/area relationship was used for estimating left ventricular contractility in patients undergoing aortocoronary bypass surgery.[48] The relationship between end systolic pressure or wall stress and area or diameter can be constructed non-invasively using cuff pressure and echocardiography. The use of systolic cuff blood pressure instead of end systolic pressure does not significantly alter the relationship. When the pressure in the radial artery is recorded perioperatively, the left ventricular end systolic pressure can be approximated with reasonable accuracy from the dicrotic notch pressure by simply adding 8 mm Hg.[49]

In the daily practice of anaesthesia as well as cardiology, it is, of course, not possible to analyse the end systolic stress/volume relationship, and it has been suggested that the simple ratio of end systolic stress to end systolic volume, obtained with the help of echocardiography, may be useful in evaluating left ventricular performance at the bedside. Although such a simple ratio of afterload to end systolic volume must not be used as a substitute for the slope of the pressure or stress/volume relationship, it can, however, provide simple but important information: a ventricle that can shorten to a small end systolic volume at a high end systolic pressure or wall stress is in a better contractile state than a ventricle that remains large at end systole in spite of a similar or even lower pressure.[50 51] The maintenance of a low end systolic size (in the presence of an adequate filling volume) should be the goal of perioperative haemodynamic management in patients with heart disease.

Recently another index of myocardial contractile performance has been validated in patients. It is based on the linear relationship between left ventricular stroke work and left ventricular end diastolic volume. This relationship has been termed the "preload recruitable stroke work relationship."[52] The left ventricular stroke work is calculated as the area of the P/V loops obtained at varying end diastolic volumes. The slope of the stroke work/volume relationship (denoted as M_w) is a measure of myocardial contractility. The relationship is highly linear and, in addition, the slopes and volume–axis intercepts of the preload recruitable stroke work are less variable than those of the end systolic P/V relationships.[53] In a study in patients, both preload recruitable stroke work and end systolic P/V relationships showed high and comparable degrees of linearity and both responded to dobutamine (5 μg/kg per min) by a 125% increase in the slopes of E_{max} and M_w.

44

Following afterload reduction with captopril, the preload recruitable stroke work remained unchanged whereas the end systolic P/V relationship tended to shift to the right.[54] Echocardiography with automated border detection allows assessment of preload recruitable stroke force. End diastolic volume and stroke work are replaced by end diastolic area and stroke force (stroke force is the integral of the pressure–area loop). In experiments performed in dogs, the slope of the preload recruitable stroke force increased 143% after dobutamine (see fig 2.9). In patients, a marked decrease in the slope of the preload recruitable stroke work relationship after cardiopulmonary bypass, not reflected by standard haemodynamic indices, was found.[46 47]

There are additional approved methods that make use of the general principle of relating the parameters of left ventricular function to left ventricular afterload for assessment of ventricular contractility. One of these methods, relying on echocardiographic data, can be useful in the perioperative period. It relates the shortening velocity of circumferential fibres (V_{cf}) to end systolic wall stress.

$$V_{cf} = \frac{\text{Endocardial diastolic circumference} - \text{Endocardial systolic circumference}}{\text{End diastolic circumference} \times \text{Ejection time}}$$

$V_{cf} \times \sqrt{RR}$ is independent of heart rate

where RR is the cardiac cycle.

The relationship between end systolic stress and V_{cf}, reflecting the force–velocity relationship, is linear and inverse, and is shifted upwards by a positive inotropic intervention.[55] A similar relationship exists between end systolic wall stress and ejection fraction.

Heart rate

An isolated strip of heart muscle responds to increasing frequency of electrical stimulation by increasing developed tension or force. This is known as force–interval, strength–interval, or force–frequency relationship. The dependency of the contractile force on the stimulation frequency, known also as Bowditch's positive staircase phenomenon, can be easily demonstrated in isolated muscle strip or heart preparations. This phenomenon is more pronounced in the anaesthetised animal. In intact, conscious animals or in human beings, the staircase phenomenon is weak or absent.[56] In papillary muscles obtained from failing explanted human hearts, a decrease in contractile force with increasing frequency was even found representing a

45

negative staircase effect.[57] The earlier studies in conscious animals and humans were, however, based on unreliable, load dependent indices of myocardial contractility.

In a more recent study in conscious dogs, the end systolic P/V relationship was used as a load insensitive index of myocardial contractility to evaluate the influence of heart rate. The E_{max} increased by more than 200% of control values at the peak pacing rate. In the range 120–180, the pacing rate exhibited a significant correlation with the heart rate. In addition, the volume intercept of the end systolic P/V relationship, V_0, shifted to the right from its control position.[58] This effect may be partly responsible for the changes of stroke volume with changing heart rate. The increased slope of E_{max} and the rightward shift of the V_0 intercept result in an increase in stroke volume at high end systolic pressures, and in a decrease in stroke volume at low end systolic pressures.[58] The enhancement of contractile force by increasing heart frequency has been attributed to an increased availability of calcium to the contractile proteins.[56]

Except for patients with severe bradycardia, it is not a common practice to use cardiac pacing to improve systolic ventricular performance. The development of myocardial stunning or even heart failure during prolonged experimental pacing points to the adverse effect of increased heart rate, which may lead to an exhaustion of myocardial energy reserves.[59] In contrast, paired pacing related to the phenomenon of postextrasystolic potentiation was successfully applied, in patients with severe heart failure, to enhance ventricular pump function.

Ventriculoarterial coupling

The coupling of the left ventricle with the vascular system has been intensively studied in terms of the end systolic P/V relationship described above.[60] In this model both the left ventricle and the arterial system are treated as elastic chambers. The distribution of blood between these two chambers is determined by their relative elastances. The elastance E is a measure of respective chamber stiffness and is represented by the slope of the P/V relationship (see fig 2.7). The pressure varies inversely and linearly with the stroke volume according to the following equation:

$$P_{es} = E_{es} (V_{ed} - SV - V_0),$$

where E_{es} is the ventricular elastance that characterises the contractile properties of the ventricle, P_{es} = end systolic ventricular pressure, V_{ed} = end diastolic volume, SV = stroke volume, and V_0 = volume–axis intercept of the P/V relationship.

The arterial system is characterised in this model by the relationship between end systolic pressure and stroke volume. The slope of this relationship, its effective arterial elastance (E_a), serves as an index of the total external load opposing ejection. E_a comprises the resistance, compliance, and characteristic impedance of the arterial vascular bed. During the ejection phase, elastance varies with time; throughout ejection E_{es} progressively increases from the onset to the end of ejection whereas E_a progressively decreases (time varying elastance). The effective stroke volume resulting from the ventriculoarterial coupling is located at the intersection of the ventricular end systolic P/V and arterial end systolic P/V relationships.[45 60] Graphic analysis of the ventriculoarterial coupling provides expeditious information on left ventricular function and its determinants during acute changes in loading conditions.[35 42] The left ventricle delivers maximal external (stroke) work when the E_a/E_{es} ratio approximates 1. The mechanical efficiency of the ventricle, relating work to the amount of energy consumed, is maximal when E_a is approximately half of E_{es}.[61] In normal subjects, E_{es} and E_a values of 3·5–7·0 and 1·6–4·0 mm Hg/ml, respectively, were found.[43 62] The E_a/E_{es} ratio was 0·4–0·6 and increased significantly with increasing afterload (with methoxamine) as the result of increased E_a. A reduction in load with nitroprusside caused both E_a and the E_a/E_{es} to decrease. Positive inotropic stimulation with dobutamine also decreased E_a/E_{es}, predominantly by an increase in E_{es}.[62]

The end systolic P/V relationship was also used to estimate contractile efficiency. The left ventricular pressure/volume area (PVA) encompassed by the end systolic and diastolic P/V relationship and the systolic part of the P/V loop can be divided into the external (stroke) work and the potential energy (fig 2.10). PVA, which represents the total mechanical energy of ventricular contraction, was shown to correlate directly with myocardial oxygen consumption ($M\dot{V}o_2$).[63–65] The reciprocal of the slope of the linear $M\dot{V}o_2$/PVA relationship is considered to be an index of contractile efficiency. Using this approach, a contractile efficiency of 40% was found in patients with normal left ventricular function.[66] A decrease of efficiency from 46% to 35% was demonstrated in healthy volunteers during positive inotropic stimulation with dobutamine.[67] The ratio of external work (stroke work) to PVA (which represents the total mechanical energy) is considered to reflect the mechanical or work efficiency of the left ventricle. The ratio of 0·6 in patients with normal ventricular function decreased significantly with an increase in afterload and increased when afterload was reduced.[62]

Ventricular function curves and the Frank–Starling law of the heart

Clinical evaluation of overall pump function of the heart is usually based on the ventricular function curve, which relates a measure of ventricular performance (cardiac output, stroke volume, or stroke work) as a dependent variable to a measure of ventricular preload, such as ventricular filling pressure, end diastolic volume, end diastolic cross sectional area, or end diastolic stress.[9][10][68] The ventricular function curve describes the fundamental dependence of ventricular performance on ventricular preload and represents an expression of the Frank–Starling law of the heart (fig 2.11):[69] "the energy of contraction is a function of the length of the muscle fibre."

The dependence of ventricular performance on afterload and contractile state becomes evident as displacement of the ventricular function curve with changing contractility and/or afterload. For example, with decreasing afterload and/or increasing contractility the curve is shifted upwards and to the left. An opposite shift is observed with increasing afterload and/or deteriorating contractility.[68] Hence the function of the ventricle cannot be described by one function curve; instead, a family of ventricular function curves, reflecting the changing load and inotropic states, characterises the ventricular function better.[68][69] Incremental pacing also shifts the cardiac output curve upwards; the magnitude of the shift is, however, less than during exercise at a comparable heart rate as a result of an additional positive inotropic effect of increased sympathetic tone during exercise.[70] At higher preloads the ventricular function curve reaches a plateau where further augmentation in

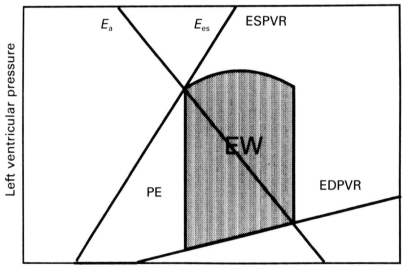

Fig 2.10 Left ventricular pressure–volume relationship and pressure–volume area (PVA): ESPVR (end systolic pressure–volume relationship), EDPVR (end diastolic pressure–volume relationship), E_{es} (end systolic elastance), E_a (effective arterial elastance), EW (left ventricular external work (stroke work)), PE (left ventricular potential energy). The PVA is the sum of EW and PE areas.

Left atrial pressure

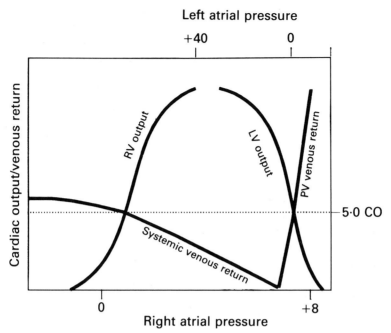

Fig 2.11 Guyton's diagram showing right and left ventricular function curves. At steady state, the output of both ventricles is identical and corresponds to cardiac output (CO). The outputs of the right and left ventricles are determined by the intersections of ventricular output curves with the corresponding systemic and pulmonary venous (PV) return curves.[68]

ventricular filling does not enhance ventricular performance. The so called "descending limb of the Starling curve," which gave rise to considerable controversy in the past, is now considered to be an artefact caused by non-physiological experimental conditions.[69]

Internal control mechanism

Cardiac pump function or its output (cardiac output) is regulated by internal and external factors. The Frank–Starling mechanism represents the internal control mechanism of the pump. It plays an eminent role in the maintenance of the balance between left and right ventricular outputs, and the distribution of blood between the systemic and pulmonary circulation.[10 68 71] The Frank–Starling mechanism has also been shown to be used during early stages of upright exercise, possibly because of a delay in sympathetic activation, but it does not play a role during later stages of vigorous exercise.[72] In normal supine subjects, both in dogs and in humans, and in the presence of normal filling (end diastolic) pressures (10–12 mm Hg), the ventricle operates close to the maximum of its function

49

curve. Attempts to increase filling volume lead to an increase in filling pressure and only modest improvement in ventricular performance.[73 74] In the presence of lower than normal filling pressures, however, the ventricle clearly operates on the ascending limb of the function curve and fluid administration can markedly enhance pump function. In the presence of myocardial depression, for example, as a result of anaesthesia and obtunded baroreflex function, the role played by the Frank–Starling mechanism becomes more important.[13]

External control mechanism

In contrast to the internal control provided by the Frank–Starling mechanism, the external control mechanism of the heart pump resides within the systemic circulation and its interaction with the ventricular function.[68] During the steady state, the heart cannot pump more blood than it receives from the periphery. The flow of blood returning from the periphery is known as *venous return* and is equivalent to cardiac output except for very short periods of time, as during transient compression of the vena cava. Systemic venous return is described by the *venous return curve*, relating flow to right atrial pressure. In the negative filling pressure range, the venous return is maximal, but levels out because of the limiting effect of venous collapse at the thoracic inlet. In the positive pressure range, there is a linear decrease in venous return with increasing atrial pressure until a point is reached when the flow ceases. The corresponding pressure is the *mean systemic pressure*. Venous return to the heart is directly proportional to this mean systemic pressure which, in turn, depends on:

- blood volume
- vascular, notably venous, tone
- external compression of the vessels.

There is a linear relationship between the *pressure gradient* (mean systemic pressure − right atrial pressure) and the venous return. The complex interplay of all major factors involved in cardiac output regulation can be studied on Guyton's graph where both ventricular function curves and venous return curves are combined. The points at which the curves cross represent the equilibrium and determine the actual value of cardiac output (see fig 2.11).

Afterload mismatch

As long as there is a preload reserve, the ventricular performance (produced stroke volume) does not decrease with increasing pressure loading (afterload). The ventricle maintains the stroke volume by mobilising its *preload reserve* and making use of the Frank–Starling mechanism. When the preload reserve is exhausted, for instance by overtransfusion or inadequate venous return, stroke volume becomes dependent on systolic pressure and linearly declines with any further increase in afterload. This can produce an apparent descending limb of the ventricular function curve.[74] This condition has been termed "afterload mismatch" and can be described as the inability of the ventricle at a given level of myocardial contractility to maintain a normal stroke volume against the prevailing systolic load.[75] A change in myocardial contractility will alter the afterload sensitivity of the ventricle and the afterload mismatch will occur at different levels of systolic pressure and stroke volume. The concept of afterload mismatch is useful in the haemodynamic management of the perioperative phase even in patients with normal ventricular function. These patients may have a normal preload reserve but peripheral circulatory factors may generate a venous return that is inadequate to maintain the end diastolic volume needed for normal ventricular performance.[74]

Ventricular diastolic performance

The ventricle can pump only the amount of blood that it has received during diastole. Furthermore, the ventricle which fails to fill properly is deprived of its intrinsic ability to increase the strength of contraction by increasing the length of its contractile fibres (preload). Therefore, the diastolic function of the ventricle is as important as the systolic one.[76 77] A normal diastolic function can be defined as the amount of filling of the ventricle that is necessary to produce cardiac output commensurate with the body needs at normal pulmonary venous pressure.[78] Traditionally, diastole is defined as the part of the cardiac cycle between closure of the aortic valve and closure of the mitral valve. It comprises:

- isovolumic relaxation period
- rapid filling
- slow filling (diastasis)
- atrial systole.

An alternative concept assigns ventricular relaxation, which is an active, energy consuming process of myocardial inactivation, to the systole which, in turn, extends into the rapid filling phase.[79] The major determinants of diastolic performance are:

- myocardial relaxation and elastic recoil
- passive filling characteristics of the ventricle
- atrial function
- heart rate.

Isovolumic relaxation period
During relaxation, ventricular pressure is determined by two overlapping

processes: the decay of the actively developed pressure and the build up of passive filling pressure. Together, these two components result in the effective pressure of the relaxation period. The rapid fall in pressure can be approximated by a monoexponential curve and quantified by its time constant "τ".[77] Maximal negative dP/dt and the duration of the isovolumic relaxation period have been also used for the evaluation of ventricular relaxation. The rate of relaxation is modulated by sympathetic tone and circulating catecholamines. It increases with positive inotropic stimulation and increasing heart rate. Interventions causing an increase in rate and extent of relaxation are called positive lusitropic effects.

A delay of ventricular relaxation can be caused by pressure or volume overload, which primarily prolongs the contraction. The *delayed relaxation* can affect the early rapid filling but does not cause diastolic failure. In contrast, the real impairment in the rate and extent of relaxation will compromise diastolic function. Such impairment becomes evident as an upward shift of the entire diastolic P/V relationship reflecting increased resistance to ventricular filling.[80] Diastolic dysfunction and failure may result from disturbances of the mechanisms that control myocardial relaxation. They include activation–inactivation processes which involve calcium homoeostasis, the function of sarcoplasmic reticulum and contractile proteins, loading conditions, and uniformity of relaxation.[81 82] The most common cause of impaired relaxation in the perioperative period is myocardial ischaemia.

Rapid filling

The driving force of *early* rapid filling is the atrioventricular pressure gradient. This gradient is enhanced by the ventricular elastic recoil or suction. During contraction, potential energy is stored at end systole in the form of a longitudinal gradient of circumferential rotation (twist) and released during early diastole as elastic recoil.[83] During the first one third of the diastole, 60–80% of the stroke volume enters the ventricle.[78]

Slow filling

The following phase of slow filling, diastasis, is characterised by only modest increases in pressure and volume associated with venous or pulmonary venous return. At the end of diastole, atrial contraction raises the atrial pressure and hence the filling pressure gradient, and finishes the filling. Atrial contraction represents a diastolic function reserve which becomes increasingly important in the course of progressive deterioration of diastolic function (atrial booster pump).

Ventricular diastolic function further depends on passive characteristics of the ventricle. These are determined by:

- elastic properties of the myocardium

52

- geometry and thickness of the ventricular wall
- viscoelastic (flow velocity dependent) effects
- external constraints (pericardium, lungs).

These properties, taken together, can be expressed by chamber stiffness which relates the instantaneous change in filling pressure to instantaneous change in filling volume (dP/dV) and reflects the pressure change induced by a unit change in volume (fig 2.12). Chamber compliance (dV/dP) is the reciprocal of chamber stiffness.[84] The diastolic P/V relationship is exponential in shape and its slope increases as the end diastolic pressure increases. The slope of the relationship at any part of the curve correlates linearly with the end diastolic pressure, allowing the calculation of the modulus of chamber stiffness as the slope of the $(dP/dV)/P$ relationship.[84] Changes in chamber stiffness may occur as a consequence of changes in operating end diastolic pressure (preload). With progressive increases in diastolic volume and a rightward shift of the actual P/V loop along the diastolic P/V relationship, the chamber becomes stiffer. In contrast, with a real alteration of chamber stiffness, the whole diastolic P/V relationship and its slope (modulus of chamber stiffness) are altered.

Ventricular hypertrophy and myocardial infarction with ensuing remodelling processes represent the most common causes of increased chamber

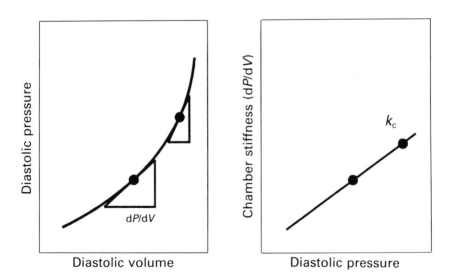

Fig 2.12 Diastolic (passive) pressure–volume relationship. Left: the slope of the pressure–volume relationship (dP/dV) represents the chamber stiffness and increases with increasing diastolic volume. Right: the relationship between chamber stiffness (dP/dV) and diastolic pressure is linear and its slope represents the chamber stiffness constant k_c.[85]

stiffness and diastolic dysfunction. In contrast to chamber stiffness, which is a measure of the ability of the ventricle to oppose distension, myocardial stiffness is a measure of the resistance to stretch of the myocardium itself, when subjected to stress.[77 85] The ventricular diastolic wall stress (σ), similar to systolic stress, is defined as force per unit cross sectional area of the wall and is related to cavity pressure, radius, and wall thickness. Strain (ε) is the change in length with respect to a reference length and is expressed as a percentage. The stress/strain relationship (σ/ε) of the myocardium is non-linear and resembles the diastolic P/V curve in shape. The slope of any part of this exponential curve is termed "elastic stiffness of the myocardium" ($d\sigma/d\varepsilon$). When elastic stiffness is plotted against stress, the relationship becomes linear and its slope can be quantified by a single stiffness constant. An increase in the stiffness constant represents an increase in myocardial stiffness which is usually caused by myocardial fibrosis.[25 77]

Heart rate

Heart rate is also a major determinant of diastolic performance. With excessive heart rate the diastolic reserve based on increased rate of relaxation and atrial booster becomes exhausted and cardiac output falls, even in patients with normal ventricular function. In patients with impaired diastolic performance at rest cardiac output may fall even at modestly increased heart rate.

By providing the anaesthetist with clinically relevant data on ventricular size, wall thickness, and transvalvular filling velocity patterns, transoesophageal two dimensional and Doppler echocardiography have the potential to shed more light on to perioperative changes in diastolic function.

Right ventricular performance

The right ventricle receives systemic and coronary venous return and pumps it into the left ventricle across the pulmonary vascular bed. The right and left ventricles can be described as two pumps in series coupled by the lungs and operating as one functional unit. Both parts of this unit have a common blood supply, a common muscular septum separating both cavities, and common intertwining myocardial bundles. Moreover, both ventricles are confined within a common pericardium and exposed to the same changes in intrathoracic pressure and lung volume. There are, however, important differences between both ventricles. Anatomically, the right ventricle has a crescent shape and consists of the inflow tract (sinus) and outflow tract (conus); the conus is an embryological relic of the bulbus cordis.[86] The outflow tract contracts with a delay of up to 25–50 ms; this asynchrony causes the outflow tract to expand during the contraction of the inflow tract and to maintain right ventricular ejection at a time when the inflow tract is already relaxed. Under intense sympathetic stimulation, significant pressure gradients between inflow and outflow tracts can occur.[87–89]

The wall thickness and myocardial mass of the right ventricle are considerably less than those of the left ventricle, reflecting the lower external work of the former. Although the right ventricle pumps the same amount of blood (cardiac output) as the left ventricle, it does so into a low pressure pulmonary vascular bed with low resistance to flow. The pulmonary input impedance, representing the external load of the right ventricle, differs from the aortic impedance in that the oscillatory component (characteristic impedance) is relatively greater and makes up to 25–30% of the total pulmonary resistance.[90] As a result of the low intraventricular and consequently low intramural pressure, the coronary blood flow in the right ventricle is continuous throughout the cardiac cycle. In spite of these differences the mechanical behaviour of the right ventricle closely resembles that of the left ventricle. An increase in right ventricular filling, reflected by increases in end diastolic volume and/or pressure, and associated with an increase in resting fibre length, leads to an augmentation of right ventricular stroke volume and stroke work according to the Frank–Starling law. Similar to the left ventricle, there is an inverse relationship between the pressure opposing ejection and the produced stroke volume of the right ventricle.

An augmentation of filling volume (preload) and positive inotropic interventions will improve right ventricular performance.[87 89] The right ventricle is, however, more sensitive to afterload then the left one. With increasing resistance to ejection (for example, pulmonary hypertension), the right ventricle readily uses up its preload reserve and dilates. As a result of the high diastolic compliance of the thin walled right ventricular wall, the increase in end diastolic volume can be more pronounced than the increase in filling pressure. Thus, the right ventricle is able to maintain normal pulmonary blood flow and left ventricular filling without an undue increase in central venous pressure. The right ventricular ejection fraction will, however, exhibit a linear decrease with increasing afterload.[87 89] A prerequisite to the maintenance of flow is an adequate preload reserve. Yet there is a limitation to right ventricular performance. A normal, non-hypertrophied, right ventricle will not sustain an acute increase in peak systolic pressure of more than about 70 mm Hg without failing.[89]

Similar to the left ventricle and the systemic circulation, the coupling of the right ventricle and the pulmonary vasculature was studied by means of the time varying elastance model which revealed an optimal matching between the right ventricle and its load under physiological conditions.[90] The right ventricle appears to have better tolerance of the acute decreases in pulmonary compliance (for example, occlusion of a pulmonary artery branch) than increases in resistance (for example, peripheral embolisation or lung inflation).[91 92]

On consideration of the close anatomical relationship between both ventricles, it is not surprising that changes in geometry, pressure, and volume of one ventricle directly affect the function of the other. This is known as ventricular interdependence, and occurs in both diastole and systole.[93][94] An increase in filling volume of one ventricle causes an upward shift of the diastolic P/V relationship, a decrease in diastolic chamber compliance, and an impaired filling of the other ventricle. For instance, an increase in right ventricular diastolic volume and pressure leads to an inversion of the diastolic trans-septal pressure gradient, flattening of the septum curvature, and a leftward shift of the septum during diastole; these effects increase the stiffness of the left ventricle and limit its filling. This diastolic interdependence is more pronounced with an intact pericardium.[95][96]

An example of systolic interdependence is the contribution of the left ventricle to right ventricular ejection. This is accomplished by pulling the right ventricular free wall against the septum during the contraction of intertwining muscle bundles shared by both ventricles.[95][97] This mechanism of "left ventricular assistance" to the right ventricle together with the force acting from behind, which is imparted by left ventricular contraction, explains why there is only a modest depression of haemodynamic function after total exclusion of the right ventricular free wall.[98] The right ventricle can indeed be considered a potentially dispensable organ as long as pulmonary vascular resistance is low.

The right ventricle plays an important role in critical care medicine where often acute changes in loading conditions, gas exchange, and coronary blood flow can eventually cause right ventricular failure. To treat a failing right ventricle properly, reliable data about its function must be obtained, including:

- central venous or right atrial pressure as an index of right ventricular preload
- pulmonary artery or right ventricular systolic pressure as a measure of both the resistance to right ventricular ejection and the generated force
- cardiac output enabling the assessment of right ventricular stroke work, pulmonary vascular resistance, and global cardiac performance.

The use of fast thermistor pulmonary catheters and the thermodilution method for assessment of right ventricular ejection fraction and volumes can provide additional useful information. The most reliable information on the structure and function of the right ventricle at the bedside is obtained by transthoracic and transoesophageal echocardiography. With these methods, end diastolic and end systolic size of the right ventricle, fractional area change, regional wall motion, septum shift, and presence of tricuspid regurgitation can all be evaluated in most patients. First pass or equilibrium radionuclide cineangiography provides an accurate estimation of right ventricular ejection fraction but this is not suitable for monitoring or frequent repeated measurements in the perioperative period.

1 Braunwald E, Ross J Jr, Sonnenblick EH. *Mechanisms of contraction of the normal and failing heart*. Boston: Little, Brown & Company, 1968: 31–76.
2 Brady AJ. Mechanical properties of cardiac fibers. In: Berne RM, ed, *Handbook of physiology, Section 2, Cardiovascular system, The heart*, Vol 1. Bethesda: American Physiological Society, 1979: 461–74.
3 Lew WYW. Mechanisms of volume-induced increase in left ventricular contractility. *Am J Physiol* 1993; **265**: H1778–86.
4 Weber KT, Janicki JS, Hunter WC, Shroff S, Pearlman ES, Fishman AP. The contractile behavior of the heart and its functional coupling to the circulation. *Prog Cardiovasc Dis* 1982; **XXIV**: 375–400.
5 Weber KT, Janicki JS. The dynamics of ventricular contraction: force, length, and shortening. *Fed Proc* 1980; **39**: 188–95.
6 Weber KT, Hawthorne EW. Descriptors and determinants of cardiac shape: an overview. *Fed Proc* 1981; **40**: 2005–10.
7 Strobeck JE, Krueger J, Sonnenblick EH. Load and time considerations in the force–length relation of cardiac muscle. *Fed Proc* 1980; **39**: 175–82.
8 Weber KT, Janicki JS. The metabolic demand and oxygen supply of the heart: physiologic and clinical considerations. *Am J Cardiol* 1979; **44**: 722–9.
9 Parmley WW, Talbot L. Heart as a pump. In: Berne RM, Ed. *Handbook of physiology, Section 2, The heart*, Volume 1. Bethesda: American Physiological Society, 1979: 429–60.
10 Braunwald E, Ross J Jr. Control of cardiac performance. In: Berne RM, ed, *Handbook of physiology, Section 2, Cardiovascular system, The heart*, Vol 1. Bethesda: American Physiological Society, 1979: 533–80.
11 Katz AM. Influence of altered inotropy and lusitropy on ventricular pressure-volume loops. *J Am Coll Cardiol* 1988; **11**: 438–45.
12 Weber KT, Janicki JS. The heart as a muscle-pump system, and the concept of heart failure. *Am Heart J* 1979; **98**: 371–84.
13 Vatner SFE, Braunwald E. Cardiovascular control mechanisms in the conscious state. *N Engl J Med* 1975; **293**: 970–6.
14 Westerhof N, Elzinga G. Cardiac pump function. In: Strackee J, Westerhof N, eds, *The physics of heart and circulation*. Bristol: Institute of Physics, 1993: 207–21.
15 Toorop GP, Van Den Horn GJ, Elzinga G, Westerhof N. Matching between feline left ventricle and arterial load: optimal power or efficiency? *Am J Physiol* 1988; **254**; H279–85.
16 Robotham JL, Takata M, Berman M, Harasawa Y. Ejection fraction revisited. *Anesthesiology* 1991; **74**: 172–83.
17 Clements FM, Harpole DH, Quill T, Jones RH, McCann RL. Estimation of left ventricular volume and ejection fraction by two-dimensional transoesophageal echocardiography: comparison of short axis imaging and simultaneous radionuclide angiography. *Br J Anaesth* 1990; **64**: 331–6.
18 Urbanowitz JH, Cahalan MK, Chatterjee KL, Schiller NB. Comparison of transoesophageal echocardiographic and scintigraphic estimates of left ventricular end-diastolic volume index and ejection fraction in patients following coronary artery bypass grafting. *Anesthesiology* 1990; **72**: 607–12.
19 Smith MD, MacPhail B, Harrison MR, Lenhoff SJ, DeMaria AN. Value and limitations of transesophageal echocardiography in determination of left ventricular volumes and ejection fraction. *J Am Coll Cardiol* 1992; **19**: 1213–22.
20 Pohost GM, O'Rourke RA. *Principles and practice of cardiovascular imaging*. Boston: Little, Brown & Co, 1991: 383–503.
21 Leung JM, Schiller NB, Mangano D. Assessment of left ventricular function using two-dimensional transesophageal echocardiography. In: de Bruijn NP, Clements FM, eds, *Intraoperative use of echocardiography. A Society of Cardiovascular Anesthesiologists Monograph*. Philadelphia: JB Lippincott Co; 1991: 59–75.
22 Nessly ML, Basheln G, Detmer PR, Graham, MM, Kao R, Martin RW. Left ventricular ejection fraction: single-plane and multiplanar transesophageal echocardiography versus equilibrium gated-pool scintigraphy. *J Cardiothorac Vasc Anesth* 1991; **5**: 40–5.

23 Cahalan MK, Ionescu, P, Melton HE Jr, Adler S, Kee LL, Schiller NB. Automated real-time analysis of intraoperative transesophageal echocardiograms. *Anesthesiology* 1993; **78**: 477–85.

24 Lindower PD, Rath L, Preslar J, Burns TL, Rezai K, Vandenberg BF. Quantification of left ventricular function with an automated border detection system and comparison with radionuclide ventriculography. *Am J Cardiol* 1994; **73**: 195–9.

25 Mirsky I. Elastic properties of the myocardium: a quantitative approach with physiological and clinical applications. In: Berne RM, ed, *Handbook of physiology*, *Section 2, Cardiovascular system, The Heart*, Volume 1. Bethesda: American Physiological Society, 1979: 407–32.

26 Nichols WW, Pepine CJ. Left ventricular after load and aortic input impedance: implications of pulsatile blood flow. *Prog Cardiovasc Dis* 1982; **XXIV**: 293–305.

27 Pasipoularides A. Clinical assessment of ventricular ejection dynamics with and without outflow obstruction. *J Am Coll Cardiol* 1990; **15**: 859–82.

28 Noble MIM. Left ventricular load, arterial impedance and their interrelationship. *Cardiovasc Res* 1979; **13**: 183–98.

29 Covell JW, Pouleur H, Ross J Jr. Left ventricular wall stress and aortic input impedance. *Fed Proc* 1980; **39**: 202–7.

30 Merillon JP, Fontenier GJ, Lerallut JF, *et al.* Aortic input impedance in normal man and arterial hypertension: its modification during changes in aortic pressure. *Cardiovasc Res* 1982; **16**: 646–56.

31 O'Rourke MF, Kelly RP. Wave reflection in the systemic circulation and its implications in ventricular function. *J Hypertens* 1993; **11**: 327–37.

32 Pouleur H, Covell JW, Ross J Jr. Effects of alterations in aortic input impedance on the force–velocity–length relationship in the intact canine heart. *Circ Res* 1979; **45**: 126–36.

33 Yin FCP. Ventricular wall stress. *Circ Res* 1981; **49**: 829–42.

34 Arts T, Prinzen FW, Reneman RS. Mechanics of the wall of the left ventricle. In: Strackee J, Westerhof N, eds, *The physics of heart and circulation*. Bristol: Institute of Physics, 1993: 153–74.

35 Sunagawa K, Sagawa K, Maughan ML. Ventricular interaction with the vascular system in terms of pressure–volume relationships. In: Yin FCP, Ed. *Ventricular/Vascular coupling*. New York: Springer Verlag, 1987: 210–39.

36 Kass DA, Maughan WL, Guo ZM, Kono A, Sunagawa K, Sagawa K. Comparative influence of load versus inotropic states on indexes of ventricular contractility: experimental and theoretical analysis based on pressure–volume relationships. *Circulation* 1987; **76**: 1422–36.

37 Suga H, Sagawa K, Shoukas AA. Load independence of the instantaneous pressure–volume relation of the canine left ventricle and the effects of epinephrine and heart rate on the ratio. *Circ Res* 1973; **32**: 314–22.

38 Grossman W, Braunwald E, Mann T, McLaurin LP, Green LH. Contractile state of the left ventricle in man as evaluated from end-systolic pressure–volume relations. *Circulation* 1977; **56**: 845–52.

39 Kass DA, Maughan WL. From "Emax" to pressure–volume relations: a broader view. *Circulation* 1988; **77**: 1203–12.

40 Mehmel HC, Stockins B, Ruffmann K, van Olshausen K, Schuler G, Kübler W. The linearity of the end-systolic pressure–volume relationship in man and its sensitivity for assessment of left ventricular function. *Circulation* 1981; **63**: 1216–22.

41 Van Der Velde ET, Van Dijk AD, Steendijk P, *et al.* Nonlinearity and afterload sensitivity of the end-systolic pressure–volume relation of the canine left ventricle in vivo. *Circulation* 1991; **83**: 315–27.

42 Kass DA. Clinical evaluation of left heart function by conductance catheter technique. *Eur Heart J* 1992; **13**(suppl E): 57–64.

43 Asanoi H, Shigetake S, Kameyama T. Ventriculoarterial coupling in normal and failing heart in humans. *Circ Res* 1989; **65**: 483–93.

44 Schreuder JJ, Biervliet JD, van der Velde ET, *et al.* Systolic and diastolic pressure–volume relationships during cardiac surgery. *J Cardiothorac Vasc Anesth* 1991; **5**: 539–45.

45 Sasayama S. Matching of ventricular properties with arterial load under normal and variably depressed cardiac states. In: Lewis BS, Kimchi A, eds, *Heart failure mechanisms and management*. Berlin: Springer-Verlag, 1991: 59–67.

46 Gorcsan J III, Romand JA, Mandarino WA, Deneault LG, Pinsky MR. Assessment of left ventricular performance by on-line pressure–area relations using echocardiographic automated border detection. *J Am Coll Cardiol* 1994; **23**: 242–52.

47 Gorcsan J III, Gasior TA, Mandarino WA, Deneault LG, Hattler BG, Pinsky MR. Assessment of the immediate effects of cardiopulmonary bypass on left ventricular performance by on-line pressure–area relations. *Circulation* 1994; **89**: 180–90.

48 O'Kelly BF, Tubau JF, Knight AA, *et al*. Measurement of left ventricular contractility using transesophageal echocardiography in patients undergoing coronary artery bypass grafting. *Am Heart J* 1991; **122**: 1041–9.

49 Dahlgren G, Veintemilla F, Settergren G, Liska J. Left ventricular end-systolic pressure estimated from measurements in a peripheral artery. *J Cardiothorac Vasc Anesth* 1991; **5**: 551–3.

50 Carabello BA, Spann JF. The uses and limitations of end-systolic indexes of left ventricular function. *Circulation* 1984; **69**: 1058–64.

51 Carabello BA. Ratio of end-systolic stress to end-systolic volume: is it a useful clinical tool? *J Am Coll Cardiol* 1989; **14**: 496–8.

52 Glower DD, Spratt JA, Snow ND, *et al*. Linearity of the Frank–Starling relationship in the intact heart: the concept of preload recruitable stroke work. *Circulation* 1985; **71**: 994–1009.

53 Feneley MP, Skelton TN, Kisslo KB, Davis JW, Bashore TM, Rankin JS. Comparison of preload recruitable stroke work, end-systolic pressure-volume and dP/dt_{max}-end-diastolic volume relations as indexes of left ventricular contractile performance in patients undergoing routine cardiac catheterization. *J Am Coll Cardiol* 1992; **19**: 1522–30.

54 Takeuchi M, Odake M, Takaoka H, Hayashi Y, Yokoyama M. Comparison between preload recruitable stroke work and the end-systolic pressure–volume relationship in man. *Eur Heart J* 1992; **13**(suppl E): 80–4.

55 Lang RM, Briller RA, Neumann A, Borow KM. Assessment of global and regional left ventricular mechanics: applications to myocardial ischemia. In: Kerber RE, ed, *Echocardiography in coronary artery disease*. Mount Kisco, NY: Futura, 1988: 221–57.

56 Seed WA, Walker JM. Relation between beat interval and force of the heartbeat and its clinical implications. *Cardiovasc Res* 1988; **22**: 303–14.

57 Erdmann E, Beuckelmann D, Boehm M, Schwinger HG. Klinische Gesichtspunkte der medikamentoesen Differentialtherapie der chronischen Herzinsuffizienz. *Z Kardiol* 1992; **81**(suppl) 4): 97–103.

58 Freeman GL, Little WC, O'Rourke RA. Influence of heart rate on left ventricular performance in conscious dogs. *Circ Res* 1987; **61**: 455–64.

59 DePauw M, Bao SM, Heyndrikx GR. Reversible left ventricular dysfunction induced by short term (48 hrs) rapid pacing in conscious dogs: non-ischemic myocardial stunning (abstract). *Circulation* 1993; **88** (part 2): I29.

60 Sunagawa K, Maughan WL, Burkhoff D, Sagawa K. Left ventricular interaction with arterial load studied in isolated canine ventricle. *Am J Physiol* 1983; **245**: H773–80.

61 Burkhoff D, Sagawa K. Ventricular efficiency predicted by an analytical model. *Am J Physiol* 1986; **250**: R1021–7.

62 Starling MR. Left ventricular-arterial coupling relations in the normal human heart. *Am Heart J* 1993; **125**: 1659–66.

63 Suga H. Ventricular energetics. *Am J Physiol* 1990; **70**: 247–77.

64 Nozawa T, Yasumura Y, Futaki S, *et al*. Relation between oxygen consumption and pressure–volume area of in situ dog heart. *Am J Physiol* 1987; **253**: H31–40.

65 Nozawa T, Cheng C-P, Noda T, Little WC. Relation between left ventricular oxygen consumption and pressure–volume area in conscious dogs. *Circulation* 1994; **89**: 810–7.

66 Takaoka H, Takeuchi M, Odake M, Yokoyama M. Assessment of myocardial oxygen consumption (VO_2) and systolic pressure–volume area (PVA) in human hearts. *Eur Heart J* 1992; **13**(suppl E): 85–90.

67 Vanoverschelde J-LJ, Wijns W, Essamri B, *et al*. Hemodynamic and mechanical determinants of myocardial O_2 consumption in normal heart: effects of dobutamine. *Am J Physiol* 1993; **265**: H1884–92.

68 Guyton AC, Jones CE, Coleman TG. *Circulatory physiology: Cardiac output and its regulation*. Philadelphia: WB Saunders, 1973: 137–252.

69 Elzinga G. "Starling's law of the heart" a historical misinterpretation. *Basic Res Cardiol* 1989; **84**: 1–4.
70 Melbin J, Detweiler DK, Riffle RA, Noordergraaf A. Coherence of cardiac output with rate changes. *Am J Physiol* 1982; **243**: H499–504.
71 Jacob R, Dierberger B, Kissling G. Functional significance of the Frank–Starling mechanism under physiological and pathophysiological conditions. *Eur Heart J* 1992; **13**(suppl E): 7–14.
72 Plotnick GD, Becker LC, Fisher ML, *et al.* Use of the Frank–Starling mechanism during submaximal versus maximal upright exercise. *Am J Physiol* 1986; **251**: H1101–5.
73 Parker JO, Case RB. Normal left ventricular function. *Circulation* 1979; **60**: 4–11.
74 Lee J-D, Tajimi T, Patritti J, Ross J Jr. Preload reserve and mechanisms of afterload mismatch in normal conscious dog. *Am J Physiol* 1986; **250**: H464–73.
75 Ross J Jr. Afterload mismatch and preload reserve: a conceptual framework for the analysis of ventricular function. *Prog Cardiovasc Dis* 1976; **28**: 255–63.
76 Nishimura RA, Abel MD, Hatle LK, Tajik AJ. Assessment of diastolic function of the heart: background and current applications of Doppler echocardiography. Part II. Clinical studies. *Mayo Clin Proc* 1989; **64**: 181–204.
77 Mirsky I, Pasipoularides A. Clinical assessment of diastolic function. *Prog Cardiovasc Dis* 1990; **XXXII**: 291–318.
78 Little WC, Downes TR. Clinical evaluation of left ventricular diastolic performance. *Prog Cardiovasc Dis* 1990; **XXXII**: 273–90.
79 Brutsaert DL, Sys SU. Relaxation and diastole of the heart. *Physiol Rev* 1989; **69**: 1228–1315.
80 Brutsaert DL, Sys SU, Gillebert TC. Diastolic dysfunction in post-cardiac surgical management. *J Cardiothorac Vasc Anesth* 1993; 7(suppl 1): 18–20.
81 Gillebert TC, Sys SU. Physiologic control of relaxation in isolated cardiac muscle and intact left ventricle. In: Gaasch WH, LeWinter MM, Eds. *Left ventricular diastolic dysfunction and heart failure*. Philadelphia: Lea & Febiger, 1994: 25–42.
82 Bruitsaert DL, Sys SU, Gillebert TC. Diastolic failure: pathophysiology and therapeutic implications. *J Am Coll Cardiol* 1993; **22**: 318–25.
83 Moon MR, Ingels NB Jr, Daughters GT, Stinson EB, Hansen DE, Miller DC. Alterations in left ventricular twist mechanics with inotropic stimulation and volume loading in human subjects. *Circulation* 1994; **89**: 142–50.
84 Gaasch WH, Quinones MA, Waisser E, Thiel HG, Alexander JK. Diastolic compliance of the left ventricle in man. *Am J Cardiol* 1975; **36**: 193–201.
85 Gaasch WH. Passive elastic properties of the left ventricle. In: Gaasch WH, LeWinter MM, eds, *Left ventricular diastolic dysfunction and heart failure*. Philadelphia: Lea & Febiger, 1994: 143–9.
86 March HW, Ross JK, Lower RR. Observations on the behavior of the right ventricular outflow tract, with reference to its developmental origins. *Am J Med* 1962; **32**: 835–45.
87 Morris JJ III, Wechsler AS. Right ventricular function: the assessment of contractile performance. In: Fisk RL, ed, *The right heart*. Philadelphia: FA Davis, 1987: 3–18.
88 Furey SA III, Zieske HA, Levy MN. The essential function of the right ventricle. *Am Heart J* 1984; **107**: 404–10.
89 Hurford WE, Zapol WM. The right ventricle and critical illness: a review of anatomy, physiology, and clinical evaluation of its function. *Intensive Care Med* 1988; **14**: 448–57.
90 Piene H. Matching between right ventricle and pulmonary bed. In: Yin FCP, ed, *Ventricular/Vascular coupling*. New York: Springer-Verlag, 1987: 180–202.
91 Pouleur H, Lefevre J, van Eyll C, Jaumin PM, Charlier AA. Significance of pulmonary input impedance in right ventricular performance. *Cardiovasc Res* 1978; **12**: 617–29.
92 Ghignone M, Girling L, Prewitt RM. Effect of increased pulmonary vascular resistance on right ventricular systolic performance in dogs. *Am J Physiol* 1984; **246**: H339–43.
93 Bove A, Santamore WP. Ventricular interdependence. *Prog Cardiovasc Dis* 1981; **23**: 365–88.
94 Olsen CO, Tyson GS, Maier GW, Spratt JA, Davis JW, Rankin JS. Dynamic ventricular interaction in the conscious dog. *Circ Res* 1983; **52**: 85–104.
95 Weber KT, Janicky JS, Schroff S, Fishman AP. Contractile mechanics and interaction of the right and left ventricles. *Am J Cardiol* 1981; **47**: 686–95.

96 Beyar R, Dong S-J, Smith ER, Belenkie I, Tyberg JV. Ventricular interaction and septal deformation: a model compared with experimental data. *Am J Physiol* 1993; **265**: H2044–56.
97 Clyne CA, Alpert JS, Benotti JR. Interdependence of the left and right ventricles in health and disease. *Am Heart J* 1989; **117**: 1366–73.
98 Jones DL, Guiraudon GM, Klein GJ. Total disconnection of the right ventricular free wall: physiological consequences in the dog. *Am Heart J* 1984; **107**: 1169–77.

3: Cardiac electrophysiology

JOHN L ATLEE III

The heart's primary function is to generate contractile forces for the distribution of adequate amounts of blood to the lungs and systemic tissues. To accomplish this in an effective manner requires properly synchronised atrial and ventricular contractions. Ventricular contractions are accomplished by the heart's specialised conducting system, whereby tiny electrical impulses, termed "action potentials" (APs), are generated and propagated to excite cardiac muscle to contract. Cardiac electrophysiology is the study of normal and abnormal mechanisms for generation and propagation of cardiac APs; it provides the basis for understanding normal sinus rhythm as well as cardiac arrhythmias.

Normal cardiac electrophysiology

Transmembrane and action potentials

Cardiac cell membrane

The cell membrane or sarcolemma is a phospholipid bilayer, with a non-polar (hydrophobic) core and polar (hydrophilic) surface. The sarcolemma provides a high resistance cellular enclosure which exhibits selective permeability to biological anions and cations. Movement of these ions across the sarcolemma is through ion specific, voltage gated, protein channels within the membrane, which span the lipid bilayer.[1] In addition to membrane ion channels, other sarcolemmal protein complexes serve as receptors for hormones or neurotransmitters, or as supplementary active or passive ion transport systems (pumps).

Terminology

Cardiac transmembrane potentials (TMPs) are recorded by inserting a glass capillary microelectrode (tip diameter $= 0.5$ μm) into a single cell. Two types of TMPs can be recorded:

1 This is the TMP during electrical quiescence or diastole, characteristic of working atrial and ventricular muscle, and most Purkinje fibres. This TMP is termed the "resting membrane potential" (RMP). Fibres with a stable RMP require a propagating AP or some external source of electrical stimulation for excitation.

Terms

Cardiac transmembrane potentials (TMPs)	Electrical potential across cell membrane
Resting membrane potential (RMP)	Electrical potential across cell membrane during diastole
Action potentials (APs)	Change in TMP following excitation of cell
Automaticity	Spontaneous depolarisation pacemaker fibres
Maximum diastolic potential (MDP)	Maximum (most negative) TMP during diastole in automatic fibres

2 The TMP that can be recorded in excited cardiac fibres is the action potential. The AP describes the changes in TMP that occur when the cell has been brought to threshold for regenerative excitation. How the cell is brought to threshold differs for various cardiac fibre types.

As noted, working myocardial and most Purkinje fibres require a propagating AP or some external stimulus. In contrast, pacemaker fibres, found in the sinoatrial (SA) node and remote sites of latent (also subsidiary or secondary) pacemakers, will spontaneously depolarise during diastole towards threshold for regenerative excitation—a property termed "automaticity." Normally, latent pacemakers are overdriven by the faster discharge rate of the SA node, that is, overdrive suppression of automaticity. As automatic cells do not really have an RMP, the corresponding term is "maximum diastolic potential" (MDP), the maximum TMP reached during diastole. APs for representative quiescent and automatic cardiac fibre types are shown in fig 3.1, and a comparison of transmembrane potential characteristics for these fibre types

Abbreviations

AP	action potential	MDP	maximum diastolic potential
AV	atrioventricular	RMP	resting membrane potential
DAD	delayed afterdepolarisation	SA	sinoatrial
EAD	early afterdepolarisation	TMP	transmembrane potential
LMP	loss of membrane potential		

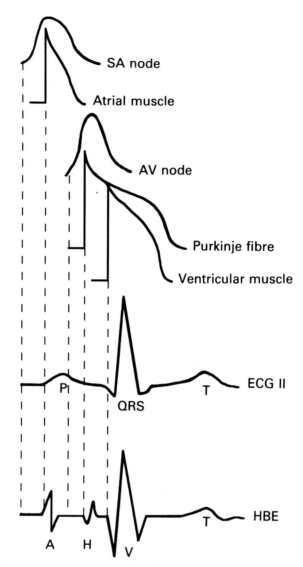

Fig 3.1 Schematic representation of cardiac action potentials (AP) from various cardiac fibre types. Approximate timing of action potentials in relationship to events of surface ECG lead II and His bundle ECG (HBE) within a single cardiac cycle is shown. Note that SA and AV nodal activation is electrically silent in both ECG II and HBE.

in table 3.1. Finally, TMPs at any given time may be depolarised, repolarised, or hyperpolarised with respect to a reference or immediately preceding level of TMP (fig 3.2)

Table 3.1 Comparison of transmembrane potentials and other action potential characteristics from various cardiac fibre types★

	SA node	Atrial	AV node	Purkinje	Ventricular
RMP or MDP (mV)	− 50 to − 60	− 80 to − 90	− 60 to − 70	− 90 to − 95	− 80 to − 90
Amplitude (mV)	60–70	110–120	70–80	120	110–120
Overshoot (mV)	0–10	30	5–15	30	30
Duration (ms)	100–300	100–300	100–300	300–500	200–300
Upstroke (V/s)	1–10	100–200	5–15	500–700	100–200
Conduction (m/s)	<0·05	0·3–0·4	0·1	2–3	0·3–0·4

★ Data from Sperelakis.[2] SA, sinoatrial; AV, atrioventricular; RMP or MDP, resting membrane potential (quiescent fibres) or maximum diastolic potential (automatic fibres); Upstroke, maximum upstroke velocity.

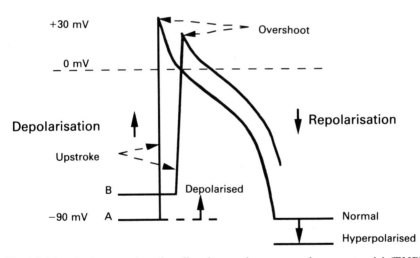

Fig 3.2 Terminology used to describe changes in transmembrane potential (TMP) during cardiac action potential (AP). Depolarisation is towards a more positive (lower) level of TMP, and repolarisation towards a more negative (higher) level of TMP. Membrane potential is said to be depolarised when, compared with the norm, it is at a lower level of potential, and hyperpolarised when, compared with the norm, it is at a higher level of potential. Note that action potential "B" arises from a depolarised membrane potential compared with action potential "A." As a result, action potential "B" has a slower rate of rise and less overshoot compared with action potential "A." See text for further discussion.

Action potential phases

The action potential of a quiescent Purkinje fibre has five distinct phases:

1 *Phase 0*—upstroke or rapid depolarisation phase.
2 *Phase 1*—early rapid repolarisation.
3 *Phase 2*—plateau phase.
4 *Phase 3*—final rapid repolarisation.
5 *Phase 4*—resting membrane potential (diastolic potential in automatic fibres).

That portion of phase 0 when the transmembrane potential is positive to 0 mV is termed the AP overshoot. Cardiac AP phases, major ionic currents responsible for generation of the APs, and ion exchange pumps that help to restore ion gradients during phase 4 are depicted in fig 3.3. Brief description of these is given below, although more detailed discussion can be found elsewhere.[1-6]

Resting membrane potential (phase 4)

Intracellular and extracellular ion concentrations that determine the RMP for cardiac fibres are given in table 3.2. Potassium is the major ion determining RMP, because during phase 4 the cell membrane is quite permeable for K^+ but relatively or virtually impermeable to other ions. A cell membrane bound, Na^+/K^+ exchange pump (fig 3.3), which depends on energy supplied by the hydrolysis of adenosine triphosphate (ATP), transports three Na^+ out of the cell for two K^+ into the cell during phase 4. This pump is electrogenic because it generates a net outward movement of positive charges. As a result, the intracellular Na^+ and K^+ concentrations are kept high and low, respectively, and the inside of the cell is negative with respect to the outside. In fact, in most cardiac cell types, RMP (see table 3.1) approaches the electrochemical equilibrium potential for a K^+ electrode (table 3.2). Also, depending on the TMP and Na^+ and Ca^{2+} concentrations inside and outside the cell, a non-energy dependent Na^+/Ca^{2+} exchanger can run in the forward or reverse modes to move Na^+ or Ca^{2+} into or out of cells (fig 3.3). Finally, in parallel with the Na^+/Ca^{2+} exchanger, an ATP dependent Ca^{2+} transport system (fig 3.3) also exists in the cardiac cell membrane.

Upstroke—rapid depolarisation (phase 0)

The depolarising stimulus (usually the propagating AP) must be of sufficient strength to reduce the level of TMPs to threshold potential (fig 3.3). The threshold potential is about -65 mV in normal Purkinje fibres. Once the threshold potential has been reached, an "all-or-nothing" AP response occurs, which can propagate to excite adjacent tissue. Smaller depolarising stimuli, which do not bring the cell to the threshold potential, result in non-propagated APs (local or "electrotonic effects"). Such "electro-

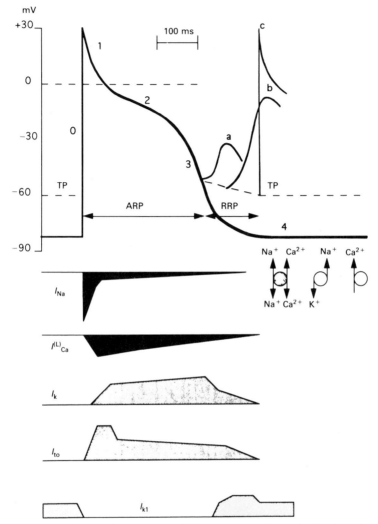

Fig 3.3 Phases of the action potential (AP—quiescent Purkinje fibre), major ionic currents responsible for generation of the AP, ion exchange pumps that help to restore ion gradients during phase 4, and refractory periods during inscription of the AP. Inward ion movements are shown in black, whereas outward movements are hatched. Ion exchange pumps that operate during phase 4 are shown as circles, with the direction of ion movement denoted by arrows (out = ↑; in = ↓). Pumps denoted by open circles require energy in the form of ATP. During the absolute refractory period (ARP), the fibre cannot be excited. During the relative refractory period (RRP), excitation produces AP with reduced amplitude, slower upstrokes, and no overshoot (that is, action potentials "a" and "b"). Such APs either fail to propagate or do so slowly. Following the RRP, threshold potential (TP) for a fully regenerative AP has returned to normal, and a normal AP occurs with excitation. See text for further discussion.

Table 3.2 *Ion concentrations and equilibrium potentials in cardiac fibres*

	Na$^+$	K$^+$	Cl$^-$	Ca^{2+}
Extracellular (mmol/l)	145	4	120	2
Intracellular (mmol/l)	15	150	5	0·0001
Ratio (E/I)	9·7	0·027	24	20 000
E_i (mV)	+60	−94	−83	+129

* Data from Sperelakis.[2] E, extracellular; I, intracellular; E_i, equilibrium potential.

tonic effects" may, however, impair conduction of subsequent propagating APs. The ionic basis for the upstroke of the APs depends on the fibre type. Two types of fibres are distinguished:

1 In fast response fibres, namely atrial and ventricular muscle or Purkinje fibres with high RMP, rapid upstrokes, and pronounced overshoots (see fig 3.1 and table 3.1), the AP upstroke results from the rapid (>1–2 ms) influx of Na$^+$ through ion specific, membrane bound, protein channels—the Na$^+$ inward current (I_{Na}).
2 In slow response fibres, namely SA node and atrioventricular (AV) node cells with lower RMP, slower upstrokes, and little or no overshoot (see fig 3.1 and table 3.1), depolarisation during phase 0 is dependent primarily on the slow inward current carried predominantly by Ca^{2+} (I_{Ca}).

This current passes through protein membrane channels that are selective for Ca^{2+}. Two types of Ca^{2+} inward current exist in cardiac fibres:

1 A slowly inactivating, high threshold, dihydropyridine sensitive current (that is, long lasting, large, or "L type").
2 A rapidly inactivating, low threshold, dihydropyridine insensitive current (transient, tiny, or "T type").

The L type Ca^{2+} channel is the major type in cardiac fibres. Both Na$^+$ and Ca^{2+} channels in cardiac fibres exhibit time and voltage dependent gating characterisics. The Ca^{2+} channel has, however, slower activation and inactivation gating kinetics than the Na$^+$ channel.

Repolarisation and plateau (phases 1–3)
Several different K$^+$ currents, the Na$^+$ "window" current, and the Ca^{2+} current contribute to phase 1 (early rapid) and phase 3 (final rapid) repolarisation, and the AP plateau—phase 2 (see fig 3.3). A transient outward K$^+$ current (I_{to}), together with rapid inactivation of I_{Na} and slowly inactivating I_{Ca}, is responsible for early rapid repolarisation (phase 1). Inward

Table 3.3 Potassium currents involved in repolarisation of cardiac action potential under special circumstances

Current	Function
Ca^{2+} activated	Accelerates repolarisation in Ca^{2+} overloaded myocardium
Na^+ activated	Promotes repolarisation in Na^+ overloaded myocardium
ATP sensitive	Normally inhibited by ATP, but which opens up with depletion of energy stores
ACh activated	Activates in response to cholinergic stimulation and hyperpolarises RMP
AA activated	Activated by arachidonic acid and other fatty acids, especially at low pH

ATP, adenosine triphosphate; ACh, acetylcholine; RMP, resting membrane potential; AA, arachidonic acid.

movement of Cl^- through a Cl^- channel may also contribute to this phase.[6] During the plateau (phase 2), when membrane conductance for all ions is reduced, several currents contribute to help maintain the TMP at or around 0 mV:

1 The Na^+ "window" current (possibly the result of different Na^+ channel populations with different kinetics of activation/inactivation).
2 Slowly inactivating I_{Ca}.
3 Cl^- current.
4 Inward ("anomalous") rectifying K^+ current (I_{K1}).

Also, both electrogenic Na^+/K^+ and Na^+/Ca^{2+} exchange help to maintain the AP plateau. Both inward (I_{K1}) and outward (I_K) rectifying K^+ currents are responsible for final rapid repolarisation (phase 3), along with lesser contributions by time dependent inactivation of I_{Ca} and outward current generated by the Na^+/K^+ exchange pump. Other K^+ currents may be involved in repolarisation under special circumstances,[13] and are listed in table 3.3. Concerning K^+ repolarisation currents, as the TMP becomes more negative during repolarisation, K^+ conductance increases as a result of "inward going rectification" (caused by the K^+ current), Inward going rectification enhances the outward movement of K^+ during repolarisation, thereby accelerating repolarisation by further increasing K^+ conductance. This regenerative increase in K^+ conductance partly explains all-or-none repolarisation. Therefore, towards the end of the plateau phase, a large repolarising current will result in full repolarisation to a normal RMP, or maximum diastolic potential in the case of automatic cells (these gradually depolarise during diastole, phase 4, so that there can be no stable level of RMP). In contrast, a smaller subthreshold repolarising current will return the AP to the plateau level of the TMP.

Automaticity

Specialised cardiac fibres that exhibit automaticity (that is, pacemaker fibres) do not have a stable or "resting" level of TMPs during electrical diastole (phase 4). Instead, they gradually depolarise over 0·3–2·0 s during phase 4. The highest (most negative) TMP reached just before phase 4 depolarisation in pacemaker fibres is termed the "maximum diastolic potential" (MDP). MDP and mechanisms for slowing or increasing the rate of automaticity are illustrated in fig 3.4. Under the right circumstances, pacemaker fibres will depolarise to threshold potential for a regenerative AP—one that can propagate successfully to the rest of the heart. However, occasionally a pacemaker fibre will depolarise only to some lower, but stable, level of membrane potential.

Ionic mechanism for automaticity
Automaticity must result from a net reduction in the outward movement of

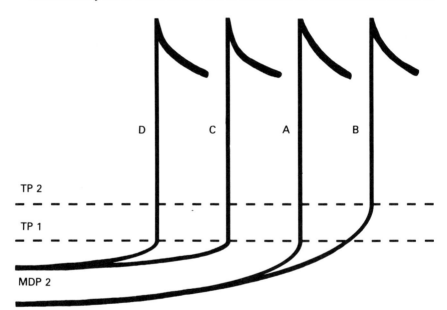

Fig 3.4 Maximum diastolic potential (MDP) and mechanisms for slowing or increasing the rate of automaticity. Schematic of a Purkinje fibre exhibiting automaticity. (A) Normal MDP (MDP 1): rate of spontaneous phase 3 depolarisation and threshold potential (TP 1). (B) Rate of phase 4 depolarisation remains the same, but TP is now reduced (TP 2) to slow the rate of automaticity. (C) MDP has been reduced to MDP 2, but the rate of phase 4 depolarisation and TP (TP 1) remain as in (A). As a result, TP is reached sooner and the rate of automaticity increases. (D) MDP remains reduced (MDP 2) and TP remains the same (TP 1), but the rate of phase 4 depolarisation has increased. Therefore, the rate of automaticity must increase.

positive charges. Although there are controversies concerning the ionic mechanisms for automaticity, there is general agreement on several points:

1 In SA node fibres, the excitatory inward current is subserved primarily by L type Ca^{2+} channels.
2 In Purkinje fibres, the pacemaker process is determined mostly by the "pacemaker current" (I_f), a time dependent inward current activated by hyperpolarisation of the membrane. I_f is carried by both Na^+ and Ca^{2+}.
3 Most SA node cells also have I_f, which passes through the same membrane protein channels as I_f in Purkinje fibres.
4 Ion exchange pumps (see fig 3.3) are not required for phase 4 depolarisation, but may modify the depolarisation rate.
5 I_{K1} (inward rectifying or "anomalous" K^+ current) is small or absent in SA node fibres, increasing instability of TMP during phase 4.[3]

The pacemaker process could involve the interaction of four or more currents.[3] For example, in the presence of a background outward current, either a rising I_f or a declining I_K (outward rectifying K^+ current) could bring the cell membrane to threshold potential for regenerative depolarisation and a propagated AP. Mathematical models for the pacemaker process in SA node or Purkinje fibres, based on results of voltage clamp studies, are given below.

Sinoatrial node

The model of Rasmusson *et al* simulates pacemaker behaviour in normal frog sinus venosus cells, which lack I_f.[7] These investigators combined measurements of I_K and I_{Ca} with estimates of background currents, currents generated by the Na^+/K^+ and Na^+/Ca^{2+} exchange pumps, and intracellular buffering systems for Ca^{2+}. The key conclusions of this model are:

1 Automaticity does not arise from one current, but rather from the interaction of I_K, background currents, the intracellular Ca^{2+} concentration, and the absence of I_{K1}.
2 Inward Na^+/Ca^{2+} exchange current immediately after repolarisation is small because of Ca^{2+} buffering, and it declines as the intracellular Ca^{2+} concentration is reduced by the Na^+/Ca^{2+} exchange pump. Also, the Na^+/K^+ exchange pump current is time invariant and small. Neither of these pump currents alone or in combination is sufficient to generate the pacemaker potential, but they are both large enough to influence it.
3 Accumulation or depletion of ions just beneath the surface of the cell membrane plays no significant role in the pacemaker process.
4 Results would be the same with I_f included (as it is in mammalian SA node cells), provided that voltage dependent activation of I_f was very small at the voltage range of the SA node pacemaker potential. Further, I_f might contribute if SA node cells were hyperpolarised by activation of other K^+ channel currents, as with vagal stimulation (table 3.3).

71

Purkinje fibres

The model of DiFrancesco and Noble[8] model for the pacemaker process in Purkinje fibres divides the pacemaker potential into three phases:

1 MDP and *initial* depolarisation rate during phase 4 depends on the deactivation of I_K.
2 The *middle* phase is dominated by a rising I_f, combined with little or no rise in outward K^+ current because the I_{K1} channels show inward rectification.
3 The *final* phase shows accelerating depolarisation because of low grade activation of the fast inward current (I_{Na}), and possibly also the slow inward current (I_{Ca}) through the T type Ca^{2+} channels.

Other latent pacemakers

Latent pacemakers include the AV junctional and subsidiary atrial pacemakers, which are located inferior to the SA node along the sulcus terminalis, in Bachmann's bundle, at the coronary sinus, and in the AV valve leaflets.[9] The pacemaker potential in latent pacemaker fibres may have an ionic basis intermediate between that for SA node and that for Purkinje fibres. The actual mechanism would depend at least in part on the MDP reached in a particular fibre.

Refractoriness

In contrast to nerve, cardiac fibres exhibit prolonged refractoriness following excitation. During the AP plateau (phase 2), fibres cannot be re-excited regardless of stimulus intensity, that is, they are absolutely refractory (see fig 3.3). The reason for this is that Na^+ channels are inactivated during phase 2, and are therefore unable to generate current for the AP upstroke. Ca^{2+} channels also cannot supply current for the AP upstroke, because these too are inactivated or remain open to maintain the plateau level of membrane potential. Repolarisation must occur before Na^+ channels can reopen. In fast response fibres, restoration of the normal RMP is usually sufficient for full recovery of excitation (see fig 3.3). With partial repolarisation during phase 3, the fibre again becomes excitable, but incompletely so. This defines the end of the absolute refractory period and the start of the relative refractory period (see fig 3.3). During the relative refractory period the stimulus required for excitation is larger than normal. Resulting APs will vary in morphology depending on the degree of recovery towards the normal RMP, and they will be either too small to propagate or do so more slowly than normal. In slow response fibres, and also depressed fast response fibres (above), the relative refractory period may extend several hundred milliseconds beyond full phase 3 repolarisation.

Conduction

Sources, sinks, and AP propagation

Factors that are important to the success of AP propagation (conduction) are considered as active generator properties and passive membrane properties.[3] The generator is inward Na^+ or Ca^{2+} current during the AP upstroke phase. This inward current provides the source of energy needed for conduction. In turn, because the passive membrane merely absorbs energy introduced by the source, it is considered to be the sink. Interaction of the source with the sink determines the characteristics of cardiac conduction.

Source—Most experimental studies of cardiac conduction have concerned properties of the source.[3] Thus, indirect measurements of the source, such as maximum rate of AP upstroke rise (V_{max}, phase 0), are often considered as a measure or even a determinant of conduction velocity. However, V_{max}, phase 0 can be only an approximation of conduction velocity, one that applies most to normal fast response fibres. Greatest non-linearity between V_{max}, phase 0 and conduction velocity is observed in depressed fast response or slow response fibres.

Sink—Cable analysis has been found useful for describing properties of the sink.[3] A biological cable (for example, free running strands of Purkinje fibres) consists of a low resistance intracellular core surrounded by the relatively high resistance cell membrane. In turn, the membrane is surrounded by low resistance extracellular fluid. As a result, the coordination of electrical activity, conduction, and aspects of both normal and abnormal cardiac excitability is influenced by the cable properties of the fibre strand. This is because current communicated from one cell to the next depends on characteristics of the sarcolemma, myoplasm, and intercellular connections. However, there are limitations to cable analysis of cardiac conduction. Varying structural complexities of cardiac cells, including a number of low resistance gap junctions[10] and variations in fibre geometry,[11] must play an important role in determining the speed of conduction. For example, cable theory would not predict a dependence of conduction velocity on the direction of conduction, as has been shown by several investigators.[12 14] Basically, the degree of intercellular coupling through low resistance gap junctions varies with the specific geometry of cellular connections and fibre orientation, such that conduction is two to three times faster in the longitudinal compared with the transverse direction. Also, a number of factors can lead to cellular uncoupling, thereby increasing resistance to current flow and lowering conduction velocity. Among these are myocardial ischaemia, hypoxia, acidosis, and Ca^{2+} overload.

Safety factor of conduction

The relationship between the current source and sink will determine whether electrotonic effects (small, local responses incapable of being

73

propagated—that is, AP "a" in fig 3.3) or successful impulse propagation will occur. Simply put, the safety factor of conduction is the excess of the current source over the sink. For example, excitation of adjacent fast response fibres with high RMP, upstroke velocities, and overshoots (such as atrial and ventricular muscle, and Purkinje fibres) is likely to result in successful impulse transmission. Consequently, fast response fibres are said to have a high safety factor of conduction. In contrast, excitation of adjacent slow response or depressed fast response fibres (above) is less likely to result in successful impulse propagation as a result of lower RMP, upstroke velocities, and overshoots. In these fibres, either conduction is slow or only electrotonic effects occur; hence, the safety factor of conduction is said to be low.

Abnormal cardiac electrophysiology

Abnormal cardiac electrophysiological phenomena include uneven conduction and refractoriness associated with the depressed fast response, abnormal automaticity, early or delayed afterdepolarisations with triggered activity, and re-entry of excitation. Such abnormal phenomena result from disruption of normal cardiac electrophysiological processes, either by disease or altered physiological states. Altered states are extremely common in anaesthetised or critically ill patients, and can have a multiplicity of causes (see box).

Common causes for acutely altered physiological states

Autonomic imbalance	Drug interactions
Electrolyte imbalance	Myocardial ischaemia
Metabolic imbalance	Too light anaesthesia
Acid–base imbalance	Too deep anaesthesia
Temperature extremes	Hypo- or hypercapnia
Adverse drug effects	Cerebral hypoxia

Loss of membrane potential

Some abnormal electrophysiological processes may be caused by loss of membrane potential (LMP)—that is, partial depolarisation of fast response fibres.[3 5 6] Consequent to LMP in fast response fibres, there is reduced Na^+ channel availability, less Na^+ current is generated, and conduction is slower. In fact, measured values for AP upstroke velocity, amplitude, and overshoot in fast response fibres with LMP may be similar to those in slow response fibres (see table 3.1).[2] LMP also affects AP repolarisation, and may extend

AP duration. In fibres with LMP, similar to slow response fibres, refractoriness may extend beyond restoration of RMP.

Depressed fast response

Fast response fibres with LMP are termed "depressed fast response fibres." As altered states responsible for LMP are often non-uniform processes, depression of the fast response throughout the heart is probably heterogeneous.[3 5 6] Therefore, depending on Na^+ channel availability, conduction velocity in depressed fast response fibres may be only slightly reducd from normal or more nearly similar to values reported for slow response fibres (see table 3.1). Similarly, there may be uneven prolongation of refractoriness. Thus, altered conduction and refractoriness in depressed fast response fibres create a substrate favourable for re-entry (see below). LMP in fast response fibres may also contribute to early or delayed afterdepolarisations with triggering or to abnormal automaticity.

Altered normal automaticity

The term "altered normal automaticity" means that the ionic mechanisms for automaticity in a fibre which normally exhibits automaticity (either SA node or latent pacemaker fibres) remain unchanged, although the kinetics or magnitude of currents responsible for automaticity are altered.[6] Therefore, the rate of pacemaker discharge is changed, but still appropriate for that pacemaker. For example, automaticity of latent pacemakers is normally suppressed resulting either from overdrive suppression by the SA node or from electrotonic depression from contiguous fibres. Latent pacemakers may emerge as a result of either default of the SA node (that is, with sinus bradycardia, arrest, or pause, or sinoatrial block) or their rate increasing sufficiently so that they can usurp control of the heart from the sinus node.

Abnormal automaticity

Abnormal automaticity is the result of an ionic mechanism that is substantially different from that for normal automaticity in the same fibre type (for example, Purkinje fibres), or it occurs in fibres that do not normally exhibit automaticity (for example, atrial or ventricular muscle fibres).[3 5 6 9] Depolarisation of Purkinje, atrial, or ventricular muscle fibres by disease or other interventions can induce automaticity in previously quiescent fibres, hence, the term "depolarisation induced automaticity," sometimes used in place of abnormal automaticity. Abnormal automaticity has been observed in Purkinje fibres removed from dogs subjected to experimental myocardial infarction, adrenaline damaged rat myocardium, diseased human atrium, and ventricular myocardium from patients having aneurysectomy or endocardial resection for ventricular tachyarrhythmias.[6] The ionic basis for abnormal automaticity has not been established, and probably varies depending on the fibre type, amount of membrane depolarisation, and the condition that initiated automaticity. That the slow inward current may be involved is suggested by suppression of automaticity by verapamil, but not lignocaine (lidocaine), in partially depolarised Purkinje fibres.[15] In contrast, lignocaine (not verapamil) suppresses normal automaticity in non-depolarised Purkinje fibres.[15]

Afterdepolarisations and triggering

Afterdepolarisations (also called "afterpotentials") are oscillations in the TMP which follow the AP upstroke.[3 5 6 16] Afterdepolarisations may or may not trigger sustained rhythmic activity. Such triggered activity is distinguished from automaticity, which results from spontaneous diastolic depolarisation and is not critically dependent on preceding afterdepolarisations. Afterdepolarisations, with or without triggered activity, may occur at virtually any level of TMP.[3] Afterdepolarisations may be early or delayed. Early afterdepolarisations (EADs) occur before and delayed afterdepolarisations (DADs) after full repolarisation of the AP (fig 3.5). DADs are frequently preceded by afterhyperpolarisations (fig 3.5). When EADs or DADs are large enough to achieve threshold for regenerative depolarisation, the resulting APs are referred to as triggered. If this process continues, it is referred to as *triggered* (as opposed to automatic) *sustained rhythmic activity*. The key characteristic of a triggered as opposed to automatic rhythm is that the automatic can arise *de novo*, without any prior electrical activity.[3]

Delayed afterdepolarisations

DADs with triggered rhythmic activity usually occur under circumstances in which there is a large increase in intracellular Ca^{2+}, termed "Ca^{2+} overload."[3] DADs and triggered activity are caused by an oscillatory membrane current, the transient inward current, which is distinct from the pacemaker currents discussed earlier. The transient inward current is a manifestation of what Tsien et al[17] have referred to as an "internal oscillator," the result of oscillatory release and reuptake of Ca^{2+} from an overloaded sarcoplasmic reticulum. Fabiato[18] has suggested that the oscillatory increase in myoplasmic Ca^{2+} is the result of Ca^{2+} induced Ca^{2+} release. Regardless of the mechanism for an oscillatory increase in myoplasmic Ca^{2+}, how this increase produces transient inward current is uncertain. The two possibilities are:

1 Increased myoplasmic Ca^{2+} gives rise to the inward movement of (mainly) Na^+ current.
2 Increased myoplasmic Ca^{2+} gives rise to inward current through electrogenic Na^+/Ca^{2+} exchange.[3]

DADs and triggered rhythmic activity have been observed experimentally in all fast response fibre types. Digitalis excess is a well known cause, possibly by inhibition of the Na^+/K^+ exchange pump. Such inhibition leads to accumulation of Na^+ inside the cell, which reduces the driving force for Na^+ extrusion across the sarcolemma. In turn, increased intracellular Na^+ reduces Ca^{2+} extrusion by the Na^+/Ca^{2+} exchange pump. Catecholamines, by increasing L type Ca^{2+} current, may also produce the required increase in intracellular Ca^{2+} for DADs and triggered rhythmic activity to occur. Myocardial ischaemia and reperfusion injury are also causes for DADs and triggered rhythms.[3-5] Finally, in contrast to EADs, DADs increase in amplitude or increase the likelihood that they will trigger sustained rhythmic activity with faster heart rates or increasing prematurity of prior impulses.

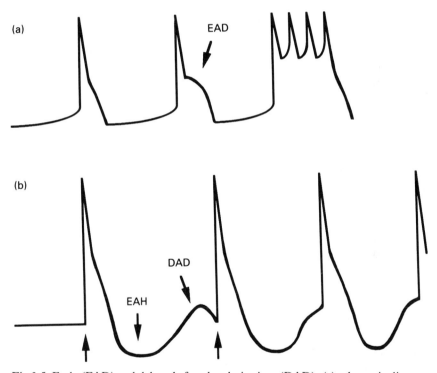

Fig 3.5 Early (EAD) and delayed after depolarisations (DAD): (a) schematic diagram of action potentials (AP) from an automatic Purkinje fibre. The first AP is normal. An EAD occurs before full repolarisation during the plateau phase of the second AP, but triggers three beats of rhythmic activity with the third AP. (b) Schematic diagram of AP from a driven Purkinje fibre. The first AP driven (upright arrow) is followed by an early afterhyperpolarisation (EAH), and this is followed in turn by a delayed afterdepolarisation (DAD). The DAD fails to trigger an AP, so that the second AP is also driven (upright arrow). The DAD following the second and third APs, however, does trigger non-driven or spontaneous APs (that is, triggered activity). See text for further discussion.

Some experimental interventions or drugs that have been associated with early afterdepolarisations and triggered rhythmic activity

Ionic imbalance	Catecholamines
Hypercapnia	Electrotonus†
Veratridine	Acidosis
Fibre stretch/injury	Caesium
Hypoxia	Quinidine*
Aconite (aconitine)	BAY K8644‡

* Class 1 antiarrhythmics that prong AP duration. † Electronic interactions between fibres. ‡ Experimental Ca^{2+} channel agonist.

Early afterdepolarisations

EADs are oscillations of TMPs that occur during repolarisation of an AP that has arisen from a high level of membrane potential (> -75 mV).[3] They may appear as oscillations at the plateau level of TMP or occur during phase 3 repolarisation. Under certain conditions, EADs can lead to what Cranefield referred to as "second upstrokes"[16] or APs. The second AP occurring during repolarisation is triggered in the sense that it is evoked by an EAD, which in turn was induced by a prior AP. This second AP may be followed by additional APs (triggered rhythmic activity), all occurring at the low level of membrane potential characteristic of the plateau phase (as depicted in fig 3.5). Such rhythmic activity may continue for a variable number of beats, but terminates when repolarisation of the initiating AP returns the membrane potential to a high level (fig 3.5). EADs and triggered rhythmic activity have been produced in studies on isolated heart tissue with a variety of experimental interventions and drugs (see box).[3-5] Little is known of the ionic basis for EADs, although they are believed to result from abnormalities involving repolarising currents. Normally, a net outward current causes the TMP to shift progressively in a more negative direction during phase 3 repolarisation.[3] However, an EAD might occur if there was a shift in the current–voltage relationship so as to cause a region of net inward current (for example, a Na^+ "window" current[19]) during the AP plateau range of TMPs. This would retard or prevent repolarisation, and might lead to EADs during the plateau or phase 3 repolarisation if a regenerative inward current was activated. Then, the current responsible for APs with extrasystoles or sustained rhythmic activity triggered by EADs is determined by the level of TMP at which the APs arise. Triggered APs during the AP plateau and early during phase 3, when most Na^+ channels are inactivated, would flow through the L type Ca^{2+} channels. At higher TMPs, progressively more current would flow through reactivated Na$^+$ channels. Finally, in contrast to DADs, EADs increase in amplitude and increase the likelihood of triggering rhythmic activity as the heart rate slows.

Re-entry of excitation

Under normal circumstances, the propagating AP will die out following sequential activation of the atria and ventricles. Either the propagating AP becomes surrounded by refractory tissue that it has just excited or it encounters the inexcitable fibrous annulus.[3] Under abnormal circumstances, however, the propagating AP may not die out. Instead, it somehow persists to re-excite non-refractory atrial or ventricular tissue as extrasystoles or tachycardia. This process is termed "re-entry of excitation" (also, circus movement, reciprocation, and reciprocal or echo beats). The basic criteria for ascribing abnormal beats or rhythm to re-entry were first formulated by Mines:[20 21]

1 There must be an area of unidirectional conduction block.
2 The re-entrant pathway must be defined—namely, the movement of the excitatory wavefront should be observed to progress through the pathway, return to its point of origin, and then return to re-excite the same pathway.
3 It must be possible to terminate re-entry by interrupting the circuit at some point to rule out a focal origin (that is, automatic, triggered).

Basic requirements for re-entry (slow conduction, unidirectional conduction block) and various types of re-entry (with anatomical obstacle, functional) are discussed below. Also discussed are the SA and AV nodes as preferential re-entry sites.

Slow conduction

It has long been recognised that a basic requirement for re-entry was sufficient delay of the propagating impulse in an alternative pathway to permit tissue proximal to the site of unidirectional block to recover from refractoriness. Therefore, re-entry would be facilitated by conduction that was slower than normal. In fast response fibres, the speed of conduction is largely dependent on the magnitude of the Na$^+$ current during phase 0 of the AP, and the rapidity with which this current reaches its maximum. This will depend on the number of available (open) Na$^+$ channels, in turn dependent on the level of TMP at a given moment in time. In addition, time is required for Na$^+$ channels to regain excitability following inactivation. If so, conduction of a premature AP (for example, stimulated or spontaneous—from a protected automatic focus, or triggered by a DAD or EAD) might be slowed in distal tissue as a result of the reduced Na$^+$ channel availability or incomplete recovery from inactivation. The amplitude and upstroke velocities of premature AP initiated during repolarisation are reduced (see fig 3.3);

consequently, their speed of propagation is also reduced. Re-entry may occur during propagation of a premature AP in a region with different AP durations, because of slow conduction and unidirectional conduction block (see below). Re-entry may also occur in fibres with persistent low levels of membrane potential (that is, slow response or depressed fast response fibres), resulting from slow conduction and refractoriness which extends beyond full repolarisation. Finally, coupling resistance between adjacent cells is another factor that may influence the speed of conduction. As coupling resistance increases, conduction velocity decreases. Increased intracellular Ca^{2+} and acidosis are two factors that may increase coupling resistance.[3]

Unidirectional conduction block

Unidirectional block of conduction may occur as a result of non-uniform recovery of excitability, geometric factors, or of asymmetrical depression of conduction and excitability.[3]

Non-uniform recovery of excitability—When an impulse propagates through tissue with regional differences in refractoriness, conduction may fail in regions with the longest refractory periods. The regions will, however, be available for re-excitation, provided that the propagating impulse can somehow return to the site of former block. This is unlikely in normal working myocardium, even at fast heart rates, because there is still substantial time during diastole when excitability is normal (that is, tissue is non-refractory). Re-entry induced by premature beats may, however, be facilitated because refractory periods shorten with short cycle lengths (for example, resulting from increased prematurity or faster heart rates). It follows that the pathways over which the impulse must propagate are shortened as well. The amount of refractory period non-uniformity required for unidirectional conduction block following a premature impulse may be quite small. Minimal differences of about 10 and 40 ms have been reported for atrial and ventricular fibres, respectively.[3]

Geometric factors—When a thin bundle of fibres inserts into a relatively large muscle mass—for example, the Purkinje fibre–ventricular muscle junction ("junction")—the insertion point can be the site for unidirectional block.[3] Although such a block has not been observed in normal fibres, nevertheless anterograde conduction delay at the junction may be longer than that in the retrograde direction. With reduced Na^+ channel availability, however, anterograde block at the junction may occur whereas retrograde conduction remains possible.[22] More recent studies indicate that the Purkinje fibre–muscle junction is better represented by a three dimensional model of overlying two dimensional sheets of fibres, rather than terminal Purkinje fibres inserting into a three dimensional ventricular muscle mass.[23] If so, activation of the ventricular muscle layer occurs only at specific junctional sites; otherwise, a considerable resistive barrier exists between the two cell layers. It follows that reasons for unidirectional block between Purkinje and ventricular fibres include differences in excitability and fibre thickness between the two layers, and increased coupling resistance at sites of unidirectional conduction block.[24] Additionally, sites where the cross sectional area of interconnected cells suddenly increases may be sites for unidirectional block (for example, insertion of accessory AV connections in patients with the Wolff–Parkinson–White syndrome), as well as sites of fibre branching and junctions of separate muscle bundles.[3] Finally, the way in which myocardial cells are connected to one another influences the speed of conduction, with longitudinal conduction velocity being about three times transverse conduction velocity.[3]

Asymmetrical depression of conduction and excitability—Asymmetry of conduction in a region of depressed excitability can also result in unidirectional conduction block (fig 3.6),[3] first suggested by Schmitt and Erlanger.[25] A number of experimental interventions have been used to produce local depression of excitability, including high potassium, cold, and depolarising current.[3]

Re-entry with an anatomical obstacle

The simplest model of re-entry in cardiac tissue involves a fixed anatomical obstacle (fig 3.7a), and was first proposed by Mines in 1913.[20] Mines believed that re-entry could occur in an anatomically defined cardiac tissue circuit, if conduction velocity was sufficiently slowed in conjunction with shortened refractoriness. An important feature of Mines' model of re-entry was

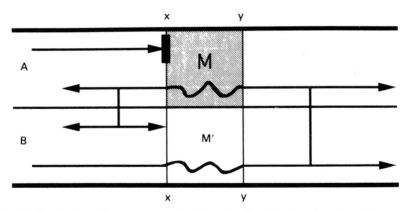

Fig 3.6 Depiction of linear re-entry in a fibre bundle with a local region of depressed excitability (M), similar to that first proposed by Schmitt and Erlanger.[25] Region M is also the zone of unidirectional conduction block. The impulse propagates in fibre A from left to right, and blocks at x—the proximal border of M. However, in adjacent fibre B excitability is less depressed (M'); therefore, the impulse conducts slowly beyond the more depressed region (M) in fibre A. It continues to propagate in fibre B, and also crosses back to distal fibre A via lateral connections. In fibre A it propagates distally as well as slowly back through the former site of block (that is, y to x in M) to re-excite proximal fibre A, before it is excited by another impulse arriving from above.

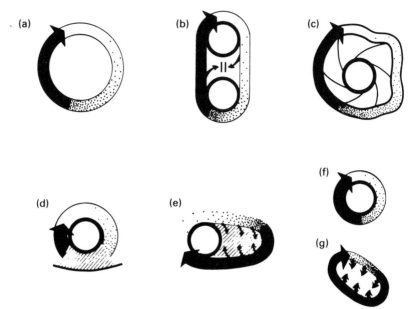

Fig 3.7 Schematic depiction of various types of re-entry. The arrows represent the crest of the circulating wave front, and in its wake are areas of absolute refractoriness (black areas) and relative refractoriness (stippled areas). White areas represent excitable tissue, that is, "excitable gap" (see fig 3.8). (a) Circus movement around a gross anatomical obstacle, as envisioned by Mines. (b) Circus movement around the vena caval orifices, separated by a zone of bidirectional block. This was suggested by Lewis to be the mechanism for atrial flutter. (c) Model of circus movement introduced by Moe and co-workers, in which the impulse is thought to circulate in a loop composed of bundles having a greater conduction velocity than the tissue around it. (d, e) Types of circus movement based on a combination of an anatomical obstacle and an adjacent area of diseased tissue exhibiting depressed conduction (hatched areas). (f) Circus movement around a relatively small obstacle has become possible because of a shortening of the refractory period and a decrease in conduction velocity, resulting in a shortening of the wavelength of the impulse. (g) Circus movement without involvement of an anatomical obstacle—the leading circle model of re-entry proposed by Allessie and co-workers. (Reproduced from Allessie *et al*[26], with permission.)

presence of an *excitable* gap (figs 3.7 and 3.8). The excitable gap implies that an impulse originating outside the re-entry circuit can penetrate the circuit and influence the rhythm.[3] As normal pacemakers of the heart are, however, usually suppressed (that is, overdriven) during re-entrant tachycardia, impulses that can penetrate the circuit must come from external sources (extrastimulation, burst pacing, chest thump, etc). There are several variations on re-entry involving a fixed anatomical obstacle.[3 26] Lewis and co-workers used rapid atrial pacing or alternating current to initiate re-entrant tachycardia (that is, atrial flutter) around the caval orifices in dogs (fig 3.7b),[27] but the question remained whether such natural obstacles were large enough for sustained re-entry to occur.

Moe's group suggested that *anisotropic conduction* within the atria would remove the need for a large anatomical obstacle (fig 3.7c).[28] It was believed that anatomically distinct, interatrial or intranodal preferential conducting

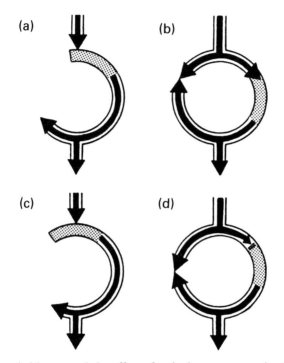

Fig 3.8 The excitable gap and the effect of a single premature stimulus to reset or terminate re-entrant tachycardia. The re-entry circuit is similar to that proposed by Mines (fig 3.7a). The arrows represent the crest of the circulating wavefront, and the black tails absolutely refractory portions of the re-entry circuit. Relative refractoriness (stippling) within the excitable gap decreases with increasing distance from the tail of the advancing wavefront. In (a), a premature impulse reaches the tachycardia re-entry circuit fairly late, when tissue behind the advancing wave front of tachycardia has almost regained full excitability (no longer refractory). In (b), a moment later, the premature impulse wavefront has invaded the re-entry circuit in two directions. In the left or retrograde limb of the re-entry circuit, the premature impulse blocks as it encounters the advancing wave front of tachycardia. In the right or anterograde limb of the re-entry circuit, the premature impulse advances normally, and changes the phase of (or "resets") tachycardia. In (c), the premature impulse reaches the tachycardia re-entry circuit earlier, when tissue behind the advancing wave front of tachycardia is only partially excitable (relatively refractory). In (d), the premature impulse blocks not only in the retrograde limb as it encounters the advancing wavefront of tachycardia, but also in the anterograde limb as a result of relative refractoriness. Thus, rather than resetting tachycardia, a single premature stimulus earlier within the excitable gap is able to terminate re-entrant tachycardia. (Reproduced from Janse *et al*[29] with permission.)

pathways, with faster conduction velocities than surrounding atrial myocardium, could form the loops required for re-entry.[28]

It is now believed that anatomically distinct preferential conducting pathways do not exist, but that preferential interatrial or intranodal conduction may still occur because of geometric fibre arrangements within the atrial myocardium, or differing electrophysiological properties among fibres.[3 5] Further, as mentioned earlier, fibre orientation may affect conduction velocity, with conduction fastest in the longitudinal direction.[3 12–14] Directional differences might provide the anisotropy required for re-entry.[3] Allessie and co-workers proposed that an anatomical obstacle along with an adjacent area of depressed conduction would facilitate re-entry (fig 3.7d,e).[26] Finally, changes in the electrophysiological properties of fibres (that is, slowed conduction, decreased refractoriness) may reduce the size of the anatomical obstacle needed for re-entry (fig 3.7f).[3]

Functional re-entry

Re-entry may be possible based on the entirely functional properties of the tissue(s) involved, and not require an anatomical obstacle. Examples of functional re-entry include leading circle and anisotropic re-entry, and reflection. Allessie and colleagues used extrastimulation to induce re-entrant tachycardia in small pieces of left atria from rabbit heart.[30] In this preparation, no anatomical obstacles were present, and the re-entry circuit was entirely defined by electrophysiological properties of the tissue involved.

This was termed "leading circle re-entry" (fig 3.7g); the leading circle was the smallest pathway in which the impulse continued to circulate, and in which the stimulating efficacy of the wavefront was just sufficient to excite the tissue ahead—this tissue still being relatively refractory.[30] In contrast to re-entry involving an anatomical obstacle, where the circuit length is defined by the perimeter of the anatomical obstable, conduction velocity and refractory periods define the circuit length with leading circle re-entry. Also there is no gap of fully excitable tissue with leading circle re-entry (that is, a premature stimulus cannot penetrate the re-entry circuit).

Anisotropic re-entry is also functional in the sense that no gross anatomical obstacle is present. In contrast to leading circle re-entry, however, anisotropic re-entry is characterised by the presence of a distinct excitable gap. This excitable gap is produced by changes in propagated AP duration at pivotal points within the re-entry circuit.[3]

Finally, *reflection* is a form of re-entry occurring in a one dimensional structure, in which the impulse is conducted to and fro over the same pathway.[3] Reflection can be observed experimentally when a linear bundle of tissue with two excitable ends is separated by an area of depressed conduction (the "inexcitable gap"—sometimes produced by a high K^+ solution[31]). Under clinical circumstances, the inexcitable gap may be produced by regional ischaemia, which can be associated with locally high extracellular K^+

concentrations.[32] Regardless of the cause, it is most important that conduction across a zone of depressed conduction is discontinuous, with resulting delays of up to several hundred milliseconds—the time required for proximal cells to recover and regain full excitability.

SA and AV node re-entry

As a result of slow conduction and prolonged refractoriness, the SA and AV nodes are preferential sites for re-entry.[3] Although it has not been possible to produce sustained *SA node re-entry* tachycardia in animal models, it has been possible to demonstrate SA node re-entry as echo beats.[33] [34] Nevertheless, in patients, SA node re-entry may account for up to 10% of cases of paroxysmal (sudden onset) supraventricular tachycardia (PSVT), and is suspected whenever P waves with PSVT are morphologically similar to those with sinus rhythm.[35]

The *AV node* may participate in re-entry tachycardia (that is, PSVT) in one of two ways:

1 The first requires participation of other tissues, so that the AV node is only part of a larger pathway.
2 The second requires only the AV node, which is functionally dissociated into fast and slow conducting pathways.

Patients with accessory ventricular connections (accessory pathways) and ventricular pre-excitation (that is, the Wolff–Parkinson–White syndrome) may have a type of PSVT known as AV reciprocating tachycardia. PSVT in these patients is initiated by properly timed atrial or ventricular premature beats which block either in the accessory pathway or in the AV node. Then, with AV reciprocating PSVT, the re-entrant pathway includes the atria, AV node, accessory pathway, and ventricles. For PSVT resulting from AV node re-entry, the re-entry circuit is confined to the AV node or its inputs.

Experiments of Mendez and Moe provided the first direct evidence that the upper AV node is functionally and spatially dissociated into slow (α) and fast (β) conducting pathways.[36] In the lower AV node, these pathways come together to form the final common pathway, which connects to the common (His) bundle. Fast–slow pathway dissociation within the AV node may produce re-entry as atrial echo beats or PSVT (fig 3.9). Such dissociation is presumed to be more on a functional (that is, dissimilar refractoriness of α and β pathways) as opposed to an anatomical basis.[3] The AV node does, however, have two atrial inputs, one via the crista terminalis and the other via the interatrial septum, which could serve as the α and β pathways.[3]

Correlation of mechanisms with clinical arrhythmias

Clinical arrhythmias most certainly result from the cellular phenomena discussed above. Criteria used by cardiac electrophysiologists to establish

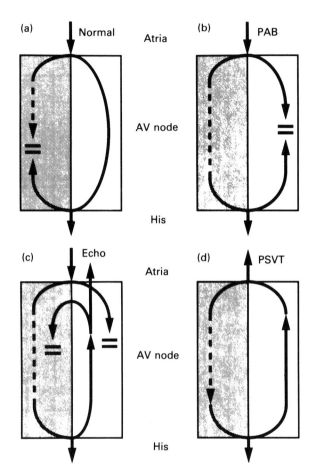

Fig 3.9 AV node re-entry resulting from functional dissociation into fast (white) and slow (hatched) conducting pathways. (a) Normal beats: a sinus or atrial beat preferentially proceeds downwards (anterograde direction) through the AV node to engage the His bundle via the fast pathway. However, the impulse blocks in both directions (anterograde and retrograde) in the slow pathway. (b) Premature atrial beats (PABs): because of longer refractoriness of the fast pathway, PABs block within it, but reach the His bundle via the slow pathway. The PABs may then penetrate the fast pathway in the retrograde direction, but block there. (c) Atrial echo beats: on the other hand, the same PABs as in (b) may not undergo retrograde block in the fast pathway. Instead, if tissue ahead has recovered excitability, the impulse may return to produce a single atrial echo beat. The echo beat then blocks in the anterograde direction in the slow pathway. (d) Paroxysmal supraventricular tachycardia (PSVT): the process in (c) can also perpetuate itself as PSVT caused by AV node re-entry if the returning echo beat (c) does not block in the anterograde direction in the slow pathway.

Postulated mechanisms for clinical arrhythmias

Altered normal automaticity

Sinus bradycardia	AV junctional rhythm
Sinus tachycardia	Idioventricular rhythm
Sinus arrhythmia	Wandering atrial pacemaker

Abnormal automaticity

Slow monomorphic VT (AMI)	Accelerated AV junctional rhythm
Some ectopic atrial tachycardia	Accelerated idioventricular rhythm

Triggered rhythmic activity

Reperfusion VT (DAD)★	Ectopic atrial tachycardia (DAD)†
Catecholamine VT (DAD)‡	Polymorphic VT/Torsades (EAD)¶

Re-entrant excitation

Atrial flutter	AV reciprocating tachycardia (WPW)
Atrial fibrillation§	Paroxysmal supraventricular tachycardia
Some VT with MI	Ventricular fibrillation§

AMI, acute myocardial infarction; AV, atrioventricular; VT, ventricular tachycardia; DAD, delayed afterdepolarisation; EAD, early afterdepolarisation; Torsades, torsade de pointes; WPW, Wolff–Parkinson–White syndrome; MI, myocardial ischaemia and/or infarction.
★ Reperfusion of ischaemic myocardium.
† With digitalis toxicity and/or (maybe) hypokalaemia.
‡ Catecholamine mediated VT without organic heart disease.
¶ Associated with long Q–T interval.
§ Maybe, but probably together with other mechanisms.

---

which of the possible cellular mechanisms is responsible for clinical arrhythmias are discussed elsewhere.[3–6][35] Involvement of particular cellular mechanisms in a specific arrhythmia can, however, never be certain, because in vitro cardiac electrophysiological studies only tell us what might occur, not necessarily what does occur in intact heart. This is especially true for patients undergoing anaesthesia and surgery, because in vitro electrophysiological processes may be affected in mostly unknown ways by multiple drugs, neurohumoral factors, disease, and physiological imbalance. With these reservations, postulated cellular mechanisms for clinical arrhythmias are given in the box.

Anaesthetic drugs and cardiac electrophysiology: arrhythmic potential of anaesthetic drugs

None of the contemporary anaesthetic drugs is arrhythmogenic in the sense that they are known to cause serious forms of cardiac arrhythmias.

87

Older anaesthetic drugs such as chloroform, halopropane, and cyclopropane did have such potential.[37] Even so, contemporary anaesthetic drugs do have effects on cardiac electrophysiological parameters which might predispose to or aggravate arrhythmias in susceptible patients. On the other hand, the same anaesthetic drug might have actions on other electrophysiological properties that are definitely antiarrhythmic.[38 39] However, before we consider anaesthetic arrhythmic potential in terms of reported effects on normal or abnormal cardiac electrophysiology, it is first necessary to elaborate on what is included by the term "arrhythmia."

Arrhythmias in the context of anaesthesia

Most anaesthetists would not include "lesser" arrhythmias—for example, inappropriate sinus bradycardia or tachycardia, sinus pause, wandering atrial pacemaker, escape beats, etc—in their definition of arrhythmia, because these are considered rather inconsequential in terms of outcome. However, it is increasingly recognised that "lesser" arrhythmias can have an adverse circulatory impact, perhaps subtle, in patients with compromised cardiac function.[40] Whether this imbalance affects patient outcomes during anaesthesia and surgery must be determined. With this in mind, most reported studies of the incidence of anaesthesia arrhythmia with continuous electrocardiographic monitoring include only ectopic atrial, AV junctional, or ventricular rhythm disturbance in the definition of arrhythmia.[41] By this definition, arrhythmias are expected in 60% or more of patients.[41] If, however, "lesser" arrhythmias (above) which could impact adversely on circulatory dynamics are also included, then the incidence of arrhythmias might well approach 80–90%. It is with this "broader" definition in mind of what constitutes an arrhythmia (that is, emphasis on functional versus morphological significance) that the potential for anaesthetic arrhythmia is considered below. Known anaesthetic effects on arrhythmias and electrophysiology are only summarised briefly here. The interested reader can consult Katz and Bigger[37] or Atlee and Bosnjak[39] for more detail concerning older or contemporary agents, respectively. Reports that have appeared since 1988 are cited below, and earlier work elsewhere.[37 39]

Normal cardiac electrophysiology

Nothing has been published to date concerning the effects of desflurane or sevoflurane on normal cardiac electrophysiology.

SA node automaticity

Enflurane, halothane; and isoflurane slow the rate of phase 4 depolarisation, and depress sinus rate in isolated heart or intact heart with autonomic blockade.[39] This direct effect of contemporary volatile anaesthetic agents on

SA node automaticity may be countered by autonomic compensatory mechanisms in patients. For example, anaesthetic agents that appear less depressant of the baroreflex arc (that is, isoflurane) may increase sinus rate in patients.

Latent pacemakers

Wandering atrial pacemaker and AV junctional rhythm (also termed "isorhythmic AV dissociation") are common in patients anaesthetised with any of the volatile anaesthetic agents. If so, it is possible that anaesthetic drugs interact with increased adrenergic tone or circulating catecholamines to enhance automaticity of latent pacemakers relative to that of the SA node. Results of experiments with halothane or isoflurane and adrenaline or noradrenaline in the perfused, canine, right atrial preparation support this hypothesis.[42 43] In the intact canine heart, pacemaker shifts to subsidiary atrial, AV junctional, or ventricular pacemakers caused by enflurane, halothane, or isoflurane during exposure to adrenaline result partly from baroreflex enhanced vagal tone (muscarinic blockade opposes shifts).[44 45] Then, assuming that automaticity of the SA node and latent pacemakers is similarly enhanced by adrenaline, latent pacemakers must have less suppression by the vagus than the SA node. Further with regard to anaesthetic drugs and automaticity of latent pacemakers, enflurane, halothane, and isoflurane increase the spontaneous discharge rate of normal Purkinje fibres exposed to adrenaline,[46] although only enflurane enhanced recovery from overdrive suppression of automaticity.[46] There are no available reports of anaesthetic drug effects on automaticity of AV junctional pacemakers. Thus, provided the evidence to date, none of the volatile anaesthetic drugs is expected to slow the rate of escape rhythms in patients with complete heart block or sinus arrest.

Specialised AV conduction times and refractory periods

Enflurane, halothane, and isoflurane shorten AP duration and refractoriness in normal Purkinje fibres.[39 47] With halothane and isoflurane, shortening of AP duration may be the result of inhibition of the Na^+ "window" current (see earlier) during AP phases 1 and 2.[48 49]

Enflurane, halothane, and isoflurane increase His–Purkinje and ventricular conduction times, but only halothane has been shown to increase ventricular refractoriness.[39] These same anaesthetic drugs also increase AV node conduction time and refractoriness, with enflurane and halothane having the most pronounced effects.[39] None of these effects appears to be of sufficient magnitude to cause advanced AV heart block in normal hearts, although Wenckebach second degree AV block could be observed at heart rates over 120 beats/min with high concentrations of enflurane or halothane. Depressant effects of enflurane, halothane, or isoflurane on AV node conduction time and refractoriness are enhanced by similar effects of diltiazem or verapamil.[39][50] However, occurrences of "apparent" complete AV heart block in patients receiving diltiazem or verapamil and volatile anaesthetics,[39] appear more likely to be the result of sinoatrial block or sinus arrest than of AV heart block.[50] Finally, enflurane, halothane, and isoflurane tend to increase atrial effective and functional refractoriness, and this is more a direct effect of any of these agents.[39]

Abnormal cardiac electrophysiology

Nothing has been published to date concerning the effects of desflurane or sevoflurane on abnormal cardiac electrophysiology. Other anaesthetic drugs can have antiarrhythmic or proarrhythmic actions to the altered normal or abnormal electrophysiological mechanisms believed responsible for arrhythmias. "Proarrhythmic" means that a drug can aggravate existing arrhythmias, or cause new or worse ones.

Anaesthetic sensitisation

Electrophysiological mechanisms—The cellular electrophysiological mechanisms responsible for anaesthetic–catecholamine arrhythmias are unknown. Although a large body of evidence supports re-entry as the mechanism for ventricular extrasystoles and tachycardia, DAD triggered rhythmic activity and altered normal automaticity are also possible.[37][39] In support of re-entry, a recent report demonstrates that catecholamines potentiate the modest slowing of conduction produced by halothane or isoflurane in Purkinje fibres, and that this effect is more pronounced with halothane compared with the less sensitising isoflurane.[51] Slow conduction is a basic requirement for re-entry (above). With regard to DAD triggered activity, catecholamines increase the slow inward and pacemaker currents, intracellular Ca^{2+}, and transient inward current associated with DAD triggered activity.[52] It must, however, be shown that anaesthetic agents differentially increase these parameters according to their sensitising potential. Finally, as discussed earlier, recent evidence suggests that the altered relationship between automaticity of the SA node and latent pacemakers may explain some arrhythmias (for example, atrial ectopy, AV junctional rhythm) seen during the course of sensitisation.[42-46]

Sensitising potential—Regardless of the mechanism for sensitisation arrhythmias, the contemporary volatile anaesthetic drugs vary greatly in their ability to sensitise the heart to catecholamines. Halothane appears most and desflurane, isoflurane, and sevoflurane least (all about equally so) likely to potentiate sensitisation.[39][53][54] Further, at least in dogs, thiopentone (thiopental) causes an approximately twofold reduction in the dose of adrenaline required for ventricular arrhythmias with enflurane, halothane, or isoflurane.[39]

Arrhythmias in patients with coronary artery disease

Most ventricular arrhythmias with myocardial ischaemia or infarction are probably caused by re-entry, whereas those associated with reperfusion of ischaemic myocardium may be triggered.[52 55]

Myocardial ischaemia and infarction—Actions of anaesthetic drugs on re-entry are sometimes studied in Purkinje fibres derived from 24 hour old infarcted canine hearts. Ischaemic fibres from such hearts exhibit abnormal electrophysiological phenomena conducive to re-entry, including loss of membrane potential, reduction in AP amplitude and overshoot, reduced AP upstroke velocity, and prolonged AP duration.[52 56] Enflurane, halothane, and isoflurane increase disparity between repolarisation times of ischaemic and those of non-ischaemic Purkinje fibres, as well as increasing the conduction time of premature impulses into the infarcted zone—changes that are conducive to re-entry.[47] As for facilitating re-entry in the infarcted canine heart preparation, both halothane and isoflurane increase the likelihood that a stimulated premature beat will initiate re-entry (from 33% to 69% versus 25% to 37% incidence, respectively).[57] Halothane also widens the zone of re-entry (that is, range of stimulated premature beat cycle lengths that will induce re-entry), whereas isoflurane shortens the re-entry zone but has no effect on its width.[57] Halothane's increased "pro-re-entry" potential compared with isoflurane appeared related to its more depressant effect on conduction time of stimulated premature beats.[57] In contrast to these results, halothane suppresses induction of re-entrant ventricular tachycardia in intact heart several days to weeks following experimental infarction.[39 58 59] Aside from autonomic and neurohumoral influences, the apparent discrepancy between in vitro and in vivo results may in part be explained by normalisation of abnormal Purkinje fibre AP characteristics 2–3 days after infarction.[55] Also, the substrate that supports re-entry in chronic infarction models may be less dependent on abnormal AP characteristics of depressed fibres (that is, results from loss of membrane potential) as compared with differences in fibre geometry.[55] For example, recent studies suggest that in vivo re-entry in chronic models of infarction may be of the leading circle type (see earlier), involving fibres that exhibit striking directional differences in conduction velocity and cell to cell coupling.[60]

Reperfusion of ischaemic myocardium—Although the mechanisms for myocardial cell injury following reperfusion of ischaemic myocardium are complex and poorly understood, excessive influx of Ca^{2+} and intracellular accumulation appear important to the genesis of arrhythmias.[52] Intracellular Ca^{2+} may increase for several reasons:

- increased Ca^{2+} influx
- enhanced release of Ca^{2+} from sarcoplasmic reticulum (SR)
- reduced Ca^{2+} binding to SR
- impaired Na^+/Ca^{2+} exchange.

91

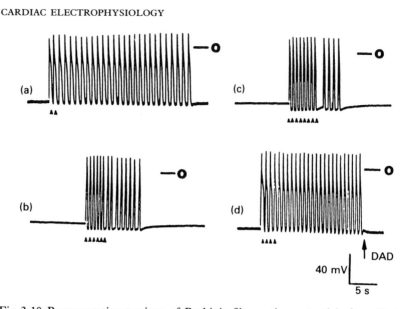

Fig 3.10 Representative tracings of Purkinje fibre action potentials from 24 hour infarcted canine heart, illustrating the effects of anaesthetic drugs on triggered rhythmic activity. (a) Triggered rhythmic activity (26 beats) is initiated by two driven beats (arrows) in the absence of anesthetic drugs. (b) With 1·5% halothane, six driven beats are required for eight beats of triggered rhythmic activity; (c) with 3·5% enflurane, triggered activity requires eight driven beats; (d) with 2% isoflurane, triggered activity (21 beats) requires four driven beats and is followed by a delayed afterdepolarisation (DAD) (large arrow). 0 = zero transmembrane potential (mV). (Reproduced from Laszlo et al[61] with permission.)

Regardless of the mechanism for the increase, it does facilitate arrhythmias resulting from abnormal automaticity or DAD triggered activity. Older reports indicate that anaesthetic drugs oppose coronary ventricular fibrillation induced by occlusion–reperfusion.[39] Recently, Laszlo and co-workers examined the effects of enflurane, halothane, and isoflurane on abnormal automaticity and DAD triggered activity in Purkinje fibres from day old infarcted hearts.[61] No anaesthetic agent affected abnormal automaticity, but all three (enflurane the most) opposed induction of triggered activity (fig 3.10). Anaesthetic drugs probably oppose DAD triggered activity by reducing intracellular Ca^{2+} accumulation, either by decreasing Ca^{2+} influx or affecting Ca^{2+} release from the SR.[52]

Arrhythmic potential of anaesthetics

It is reasonably certain that none of the contemporary anaesthetics acts alone to cause life threatening cardiac arrhythmias. They do, however, have the potential to interact with other drugs, underlying pathology, neuro-humoral factors, or a physiological imbalance to promote arrhythmias. They also have recognised potential to affect existing arrhythmias. Either they can cause more disturbing ones (a proarrhythmic action) or they will suppress or terminate them (an antiarrhythmic action). The mechanisms for either of these actions are incompletely understood, in part because causes and contributing factors to perioperative arrhythmias are multifactorial and usually difficult to identify.[62] Nevertheless, progress has been made over the past few decades to further our understanding of anaesthetic effects on normal and abnormal cardiac electrophysiological mechanisms and this has been summarised in this chapter. It is hoped that more complete knowledge of mechanisms for arrhythmias and anaesthetic effects will lead to improved patient outcomes, particularly, as anaesthetists and critical care specialists increasingly must care for patients at the extremes of life or with major systemic illness and susceptibility to serious arrhythmias.

1 Katz AM. Cardiac ion channels. *N Engl J Med* 1993; **328**: 1244–51.
2 Sperelakis N. Origin of the cardiac resting potential. In Berne RM, ed, *Handbook of physiology, Section 2, The cardiovascular system. The heart*, Vol 1, Bethesda: American Physiological Society, 1979: 187–267.
3 Fozzard HA, Haber E, Jennings RB, *et al*, eds, *The heart and cardiovascular system: Scientific foundations*, 2nd edn. New York: Raven Press, 1991: 63–98, 863–1169, 2021–193.
4 Zipes DP, Jalife J, eds, *Cardiac electrophysiology: From cell to bedside*. Philadelphia: WB Saunders Co., 1990.
5 Atlee JL III. *Perioperative cardiac dysrhythmias*, 2nd edn. Chicago: Year Book Medical Publishers, 1990: 14–118.
6 Zipes DP. Genesis of cardiac arrhythmias: Electrophysiological considerations. In Braunwald E, ed, *Heart disease*, 4th edn. Philadelphia: WB Saunders, 1992: 588–627.
7 Rasmusson RL, Clark JW, Giles WR, *et al*. A mathematical model of a bullfrog cardiac pacemaker cell. *Am J Physiol* 1990; **259**: H352–69.
8 DiFrancesco D, Noble D. A model of cardiac electrical activity incorporating ionic pumps and concentration changes *Philosophical Trans R Soc Lond B: Biol Sci* 1985; **307**: 353–98.
9 Gilmour RF Jr, Zipes DP. Abnormal automaticity and related phenomena. In Fozzard HA, Haber E, Jennings RB, *et al*, eds, *The heart and cardiovascular system: Scientific foundations*. New York: Raven Press, 1986: 1239–57.
10 Gros D, Jongsma HJ. The cardiac connection. *News in Physiological Sciences* 1991; **6**: 34–40.
11 Goldstein SS, Rall W. Changes in action potential shape and velocity for changing core conductor geometry. *Biophys J* 1974; **14**: 731–57.
12 Sano T, Takayama N, Shimamoto T. Directional difference of conduction velocity in cardiac ventricular syncytium studied by microelectrodes. *Circ Res* 1959; **7**: 262–7.
13 Spach MS, Miller WT, Geselowitz DB, *et al*. The discontinuous nature of propagation in normal canine cardiac muscle. Evidence for recurrent discontinuities of intracellular resistance that affect membrane currents. *Circ Res* 1981; **48**: 39–54.
14 Spach MS, Miller WT, Dolber PC, *et al*. The functional role of structural complexities in the propagation of depolarization in the atrium of a dog. Cardiac conduction disturbances due to discontinuities of effective axial resistivity. *Circ Res* 1982; **50**: 175–91.
15 Elharrar V, Zipes DP. Voltage modulation of automaticity in cardiac Purkinje fibres. In Zipes DP, Bailey JC, Elharrar V, Eds, *The slow inward current and cardiac arrhythmias*. The Hague: Martinus Nijhoff, 1980: 357–73.
16 Cranefield PF. Action potentials, afterpotentials, and arrhythmias. *Circ Res* 1977; **41**: 415–23.
17 Tsien RW, Kass RS, Weingart R. Cellular and subcellular mechanisms of cardiac paacemaker oscillations. *J Exp Biol* 1979; **81**: 205–15.

18 Fabiato A. Calcium-induced release of calcium from the cardiac sarcoplasmic reticulum. *Am J Physiol* 1983; **245**: C1–14.

19 Attwell D, Cohen I, Eisner D, *et al.* The steady state TTX-sensitive ("window") sodium current in cardiac Purkinje fibres. *Pflüger's Arch* 1979; **379**: 137–42.

20 Mines GR. On dynamic equilibrium in the heart. *J Physiol (Lond)* 1913; **46**: 349–82.

21 Mines GR. On circulating excitations in heart muscles and their possible relation to tachycardia and fibrillation. *Transactions of the Royal Society of Canada*, Section IV, 1914; 43–52.

22 Mendez C, Mueller WJ, Urguiaga X. Propagation of impulses across the Purkinje fiber-muscle junctions in the dog heart. *Circ Res* 1970; **26**: 135–50.

23 Veenstra RD, Joyner RW, Rawling DA. Purkinje and ventricular activation sequences of canine papillary muscle: Effects of quinidine and calcium on Purkinje-ventricular conduction delay. *Circ Res* 1984; **54**: 500–15.

24 Joyner RW, Overhold ED, Ramza B, Veenstra RD. Propagation through electrically coupled cells: Two inhomogeneously coupled cardiac tissue layers. *Am J Physiol* 1984; **247**: H596–609.

25 Schmitt FO, Erlanger J. Directional differences in the conduction of the impulse through heart muscle and their possible relation to extrasystoles and fibrillary contractions. *Am J Physiol* 1929; **87**: 326–47.

26 Allessie MA, Lammers WJ, Bonke IM, Hollen J. Intra-atrial reentry as a mechanism for atrial flutter induced by acetylcholine and rapid atrial pacing in the dog. *Circulation* 1984; **70**: 123–35.

27 Lewis T, Feil HS, Stroud WD. Observations upon flutter and fibrillation. II. The nature of auricular flutter. *Heart* 1920; **7**: 191–346.

28 Pastelin G, Mendez R, Moe GK. Participation of atrial specialized conduction pathways in atrial flutter. *Circ Res* 1978; **42**: 386–93.

29 Janse MJ, Van Cappele FJ, Freud GE, Durrer D. Circus movement within the AV node on a basis for supraventricular tachycardia as shown by multiple microelectrode recording in the isolated rabbit heart. *Circ Res* 1971; **28**: 403–14.

30 Allessie MA, Bonke FI, Schapman FJ. Circus movement in rabbit atrial muscle as a mechanism of tachycardia. III. The "leading circle" concept: A new model of circus movement in cardiac tissue without the involvement of an anatomical obstacle. *Circ Res* 1977; **41**: 9–18.

31 Rozanski GJ, Jalife J, Moe GK. Reflected reentry in nonhomogeneous ventricular muscle as a mechanism of cardiac arrhythmias. *Circulation* 1984; **69**: 163–73.

32 Hill JL, Gettes LS. Effect of acute coronary artery occlusion on local myocardial extracellular K^+ activity in swine. *Circulation* 1980; **61**: 768–78.

33 Allessie MA, Bonke FIM. Direct demonstration of sinus node reentry in the rabbit heart. *Circ Res* 1979; **44**: 557–68.

34 Atlee JL III, Yeager TS. Electrophysiologic assessment of the effects of enflurane, halothane, and isoflurane on properties affecting supraventricular re-entry in chronically instrumented dogs. *Anesthesiology* 1989; **71**: 941–52.

35 Zipes DP. Specific arrhythmias: Diagnosis and treatment. In Braunwald E, ed, *Heart disease*, 4th edn. Philadelphia: WB Saunders, 1992: 667–725.

36 Mendez C, Moe GK. Demonstration of a dual A-V nodal conduction system in the isolated rabbit heart. *Circ Res* 1966; **19**: 378–93.

37 Katz RL, Bigger JT Jr. Cardiac arrhythmias during anesthesia and operation. *Anesthesiology* 1970; **33**: 193–213.

38 Atlee JL III. Halothane: Cause or cure for arrhythmias? *Anesthesiology* 1987; **67**: 617–18.

39 Atlee JL III, Bosnjak ZJ. Mechanisms for cardiac dysrhythmias during anesthesia. *Anesthesiology* 1990; **72**: 347–74.

40 Baig MW, Perrins EJ. The hemodynamics of cardiac pacing: Clinical and physiological aspects. *Prog Cardiovasc Dis* 1991; **33**: 283–98.

41 Atlee JL III. Perioperative cardiac dysrhythmias in perspective. In: Atlee JL III (Ed.) *Perioperative cardiac dysrhythmias*, 2nd edn. Chicago: Year Book Medical Publishers, 1990: 1–13.

42 Polic S, Atlee JL III, Laszlo A, Kampine JP, Bosnjak ZJ. Anesthetics and automaticity in latent pacemaker fibers. II. Effects of halothane and epinephrine or norepinephrine on

automaticity of dominant and subsidiary atrial pacemakers in the canine heart. *Anesthesiology* 1991; **75**: 298–304.

43 Boban M, Atlee JL III, Vicenzi M, Kampine JP, Bosnjak ZJ. Anesthetics and automaticity in latent pacemaker fibers. IV. Effects of isoflurane and epinephrine or norepinephrine on automaticity of dominant and subsidiary atrial pacemakers in the canine heart. *Anesthesiology* 1993; **79**: 555–62.

44 Woehlck HJ, Vicenzi MN, Bosnjak ZJ, Atlee JL III. Anesthetics and automaticity of dominant and latent pacemakers in chronically instrumented dogs. I. Methodology, conscious state and halothane anesthesia: Comparison with and without muscarinic blockade during exposure to epinephrine. *Anesthesiology* 1993; **79**: 1304–15.

45 Vicenzi MN, Woehlck HJ, Bosnjak ZJ, Atlee JL III. Anesthetics and automaticity of dominant and latent pacemakers in chronically instrumented dogs. II. Effects of enflurane and isoflurane during exposure to epinephrine with and without muscarinic blockade. *Anesthesiology* 1993; **79**: 1316–23.

46 Laszlo A, Polic S, Atlee JL III, Kampine JP, Bosnjak ZJ. Anesthetics and automaticity in latent pacemaker fibers. I. Effects of halothane and epinephrine or norepinephrine on automaticity and recovery of automaticity from overdrive suppression in Purkinje fibres derived from canine hearts. *Anesthesiology* 1991; **75**: 95–105.

47 Turner LA, Polic S, Hoffmann RG, *et al.* Actions of volatile anesthetics on ischemic and nonischemic Purkinje fibres in the canine heart: Regional action potential characteristics. *Anesth Anal* 1993; **76**: 726–33.

48 Turner LA, Marijic J, Kampine JP, Bosnjak ZJ. A comparison of the effects of halothane and tetrodotoxin on regional repolarization characteristics of canine Purkinje fibres. *Anesthesiology* 1990; **73**: 1158–68.

49 Eskinder H, Supan FD, Turner LA, *et al.* The effects of halothane and isoflurane on slowly inactivating sodium current in canine cardiac Purkinje cells. *Anesth Anal* 1993; **77**: 32–7.

50 Atlee JL III, Bosnjak ZJ, Yeager TS. Effects of diltiazem, verapamil, and inhalation anesthetics on electrophysiologic properties affecting reentrant supraventricular tachycardia in chronically instrumented dogs. *Anesthesiology* 1990; **72**: 889–901.

51 Vodanovic S, Turner LA, Hoffmann RG, *et al.* Transient negative dromotropic effects of catecholamines on canine Purkinje fibres exposed to halothane and isoflurane. *Anesth Anal* 1993; **76**: 592–7.

52 Bosnjak ZJ, Warltier DC. New aspects of cardiac electrophysiology and function: Effects of inhalational anesthetics. In: Conzen Z, Peter K, eds, *Baillière's clinical anaesthesiology*, Vol 7, *Inhalation Anaesthesia*. London: Baillière Tindall, 1993: 937–60.

53 Hayashi Y, Sumikawa K, Tashiro C, *et al.* Arrhythmogenic threshold of epinephrine during sevoflurane, isoflurane and enflurane anesthesia in dogs. *Anesthesiology* 1988; **69**: 145–7.

54 Weiskopf RB, Eger EI II, Holmes MA, *et al.* Epinephrine-induced premature ventricular contractions and changes in arterial blood pressure and heart rate during I-653, isoflurane, and halothane anesthesia in swine. *Anesthesiology* 1989; **70**: 293–8.

55 Janse MJ, Wit AL. Electrophysiological mechanisms of ventricular arrhythmias resulting from myocardial ischemia and infarction. *Physiol Rev* 1989; **69**: 1049–69.

56 Friedman PL, Stewart JR, Wit AL. Spontaneous and induced cardiac arrhythmias in subendocardial Purkinje fibers surviving extensive myocardial infarction in dogs. *Circ Res* 1973; **33**: 612–26.

57 Turner LA, Polic S, Hoffmann RS, *et al.* Action of halothane and isoflurane on Purkinje fibres in the infarcted canine heart: Conduction, regional refractoriness and reentry. *Anesth Anal* 1993; **76**: 718–25.

58 Deutsch N, Hantler CB, Tait AR, *et al.* Suppression of ventricular arrhythmias by volatile anesthetics in a canine model of chronic myocardial infarction. *Anesthesiology* 1990; **72**: 1012–21.

59 Gallagher JD, McClernan CA. The effects of halothane on ventricular tachycardia in intact dogs. *Anesthesiology* 1991; **75**: 866–75.

60 Weiss JN, Nademanee K, Stevenson WG, Singh B. Ventricular arrhythmias in ischemic heart disease. *Ann Intern Med* 1991; **114**: 784–97.

61 Laszlo A, Polic S, Kampine JP, *et al.* Halothane, enflurane and isoflurane on abnormal automaticity and triggered rhythmic activity of Purkinje fibres from 24-hour-old infarcted hearts. *Anesthesiology* 1991; **75**: 847–53.

62 Atlee JL III. Causes for perioperative cardiac dysrhythmias. In: Atlee JL III, ed, *Perioperative cardiac dysrhythmias*, 2nd edn. Chicago: Year Book Medical Publishers, 1990: 187–273.

4: Coronary physiology

HANS-JOACHIM PRIEBE

A thorough knowledge of normal coronary physiology is required to understand the mechanisms involved in coronary pathophysiology and, thus, for the optimal care of the patient with coronary artery disease. The heart, unlike any other organ, not only provides flow to the entire organism, but has to generate its own perfusion pressure. This poses an extraordinary metabolic load on the coronary circulation. Complicating matters further, unlike any other regional circulation, the coronary circulation is subjected to marked variations in extravascular compressive forces related to the cardiac cycle.

Such unique physiology requires a highly specialised circulation if metabolic requirements are to be met. Consequently, the coronary circulation is composed of different kinds of vessels each with distinct physiological, anatomical, and pharmacological characteristics.[1 2]

The myocardium is almost entirely dependent on aerobic metabolism. Thus, there is little capacity to accumulate an oxygen debt, and oxygen demand must be met on a beat by beat basis. As myocardial oxygen extraction is about 70% even at rest, increased myocardial oxygen consumption ($M\dot{V}_{O_2}$) is principally met by increases in coronary blood flow (CBF). This results in a linear relationship between CBF and $M\dot{V}_{O_2}$[3] (fig 4.1). As a consequence, coronary sinus O_2 tension (18–20 mm Hg or 2·4–2·7 kPa) and saturation (about 30%) remain remarkably constant, O_2 delivery in excess of demand (that is, "luxury" perfusion) is not usually observed, and inadequate O_2 supply in relation to demand will rapidly cause myocardial ischaemia.

Obviously, matching of O_2 delivery to O_2 demand is the essential task of the coronary circulation. In the following, the anatomical, physical, and biochemical factors responsible for this precise matching will be discussed. This will provide the basis for understanding the pathophysiology of the diseased coronary circulation.

Coronary anatomy

The right and left coronary arteries provide the entire blood supply to the myocardium. They arise from the coronary ostia in the sinuses of Valsalva located at the aortic root, above the anterior and left posterior cusps of the aortic valve. The anatomical arrangement between valve leaflets and coronary

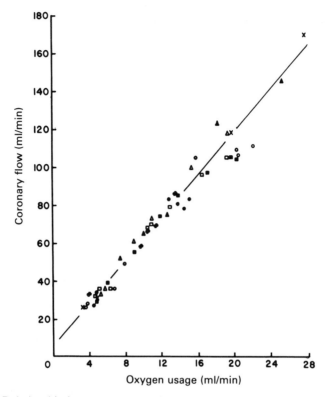

Fig 4.1 Relationship between coronary blood flow and myocardial oxygen consumption in conscious dogs. Each dog is represented by a separate symbol. A close correlation between the two variables over a wide range is evident. (Reproduced with permission from Khouri EM, Gregg DE, Rayford CR.[3] Effect of exercise on cardiac output, left coronary flow and myocardial metabolism in the unanesthetized dog. *Circ Res* 1965; **17**: 427–37.)

ostia ensures CBF even during systole. The two main coronary arteries run along their respective atrioventricular grooves where they branch repeatedly.

The left coronary artery divides into the anterior interventricular (also called left anterior descending) and the circumflex artery. Branches of the anterior interventricular artery supply the anterior walls of the left and right ventricles, part of the left lateral wall, and most of the interventricular septum. The circumflex artery supplies the left atrium, parts of the lateral and posterior left ventricular wall, and, in about 45% of hearts, the sinus node. It also perfuses the anterior papillary muscle of the left ventricle, whereas the posterior papillary muscle is perfused by branches of both right and left coronary arteries.

The right coronary artery supplies the remainder of the right ventricle and, in 90% of hearts, the atrioventricular node through its posterior interventricular branch. In about 55% of hearts, the sinus node artery originates from the right coronary artery. An extensive network of collateral and communicating vessels between branches of right and left coronary arteries encircles the epicardial surface of the heart. These vessels play an important role in maintaining some degree of regional perfusion when myocardial ischaemia develops.

The term "dominant" refers to that particular coronary artery from which the posterior interventricular artery originates, and which, therefore, will "dominantly" supply the myocardium. The vast majority of normal human hearts have a dominant right coronary system. When comparing results of different studies it is important to recall that significant species differences exist with regard to the dominant coronary system. Porcine hearts—like those of humans—have a dominant right coronary system,[4] whereas the canine heart has a dominant left coronary system.[5][6]

The myocardial wall is supplied by branches that arise from the large epicardial coronary arteries. These branches penetrate the ventricular wall in an almost perpendicular fashion. Within the myocardium there is further division of these branches into extensive networks of small arteries and arterioles which give rise to the myocardial capillary bed. Certain branches from the epicardial vessels arborise in the subepicardium whereas others plunge deep into the myocardial wall to form a dense subendocardial network of vessels. Control of vasomotor tone differs between these two types of vessels which enables changes in transmural flow distribution.

Most of the coronary vascular bed lies within the myocardial wall. As a result of easier accessibility, however, most of our knowledge of the coronary circulation is based on studies of the large epicardial vessels. Although they are the most frequent site of atherosclerotic alterations in coronary artery disease, they are not necessarily representative of coronary physiology in general.

After passage through the capillary beds, most of the venous blood returns to the right atrium through the coronary sinus. Of coronary sinus outflow 90–95% is derived from the left coronary artery. About 15% of the left coronary artery inflow not recovered from the coronary sinus drains into the left atrium and right ventricle. Most of the venous return from the right ventricle drains into the anterior cardiac veins which empty directly into the right atrium. A striking feature of the coronary venous system is the abundance of large anastomoses between all major veins[7] which may result in considerable fluctuations in coronary sinus outflow.

The adventitia, or outer layer, of small coronary arteries contains nerves. Although they do not penetrate the media, release of transmitter substances from nerve varicosities close to the smooth muscle layer is likely. Circumferentially arranged smooth muscle cells constitute the media. Layers of smooth muscle cells number between six in vessels of 300 μm diameter and

99

one in arterioles of 30–50 μm diameter. The smooth muscle cells behave electrically similar to a syncytium. The luminal surface of the coronary vessels is lined by endothelial cells which penetrate into the media. Through this contact with the smooth muscle cells, the vascular endothelium plays a key role in the control of coronary vasomotor tone.

Collateral circulation

Collateral vessels are accessory vascular channels which provide perfusion distal to an obstructed native coronary artery. Even in the normal myocardium, inter- and intracoronary collaterals exist at all levels of vessel size except the capillaries.[8] In certain species, such as humans and dogs, they are present even in the neonatal heart.[9] In the unstimulated state, collaterals are 40 μm in diameter and often only one cell layer thick. In the stimulated state, they may have diameters as large as 1 mm, and histologically they are similar to a myocardial arteriole.[9]

There are considerable species differences in localisation and extent of intercoronary collaterals which have to be taken into account when comparing results of different studies. The dog[10] and the guinea pig[11] have a relatively well-developed collateral circulation. Pigs (similar to humans without coronary artery disease) have practically no anatomically demonstrable collaterals.[10] Consequently, acute coronary occlusion leads very quickly to transmural infarction.

There are species differences not only in native (pre-existent) collaterals but also in transformed (developed) collaterals. In the human and porcine heart, collaterals develop predominantly in the subendocardium, and these have a histological resemblance to abnormally thin walled arteries. By contrast, collaterals in canine hearts develop only in a narrow subepicardial zone around the edge of the zone which is potentially ischaemic. These collaterals generally exhibit significantly higher resistance than that of the vessels they have replaced, although they are not nearly as flow limiting as the collaterals that develop in humans with ischaemia.

The factors that induce the transformation from the unstimulated to the stimulated state are largely unknown. Ischaemia seems to be a very powerful stimulus for the development of coronary collaterals.[12] Several experimental findings would, however, suggest that ischaemia of the cardiac myocyte may not necessarily be a prerequisite for the stimulation of collateral growth:[12 13]

1 Growing segments of collaterals are relatively far removed from areas of tissue hypoxia.
2 Progressive, ameroid induced, coronary artery stenosis leads to the development of collaterals in the surrounding subepicardium even though subepicardial perfusion is not necessarily impaired.
3 There are no defined time or spatial relationships between presumed ischaemia and collateral growth.

There is evidence that an inflammatory response may well be the primary stimulus for all types of collateral growth.[13] As a result of the lack of preformed arteriolar connections between superficial and deeper vascular territories in humans, a progressive stenosis of large epicardial vessels is likely to cause ischaemia-induced local micronecroses. The subsequent inflammatory response produces macrophage/monocyte mediated angiogenic mitogens which trigger collateral growth. Thus, in humans (unlike the dog but like the pig) development of subendocardial collateral plexus appears to be a result of true angiogenesis. Reduction in arterial inflow at rest may be the predominant trigger mechanism. Other factors such as coronary occlusion, anaemia, and hypoxaemia have also been shown to stimulate collateral growth.[14]

Although the protective role of coronary collaterals in humans has been debated in the past, prospectively collected data now provide evidence that the collateral circulation limits the degree of ischaemia, and improves survival during controlled intracoronary balloon occlusion, and following coronary artery spasm, acute myocardial infarction, and postcoronary artery bypass graft closure.[14] Thus, in humans the coronary collateral circulation appears to constitute an important alternative source of blood supply to "jeopardised" myocardium.

Vascular endothelium

The importance of the vascular endothelium in the control of vasomotor tone in health and disease is being increasingly recognised.[15-17] Various pharmacological agents (for example, acetylcholine, substance P, catecholamines) and physical stimuli (for example, blood flow, pulsatile flow, shear stress) can cause the release of endothelium dependent factors. The vascular endothelium of the coronary arteries is known to synthesise and secrete substances of various biological activity in response to certain hormonal, metabolic, and mechanical stimuli. Such substances include mitogens, prothrombogens, antithrombogens, and vasoactive substances.[16 17]

The net effect of various chemical and mechanical stimuli on coronary artery diameter and CBF is the result of (direct) smooth muscle-mediated and (indirect) endothelium-mediated actions. These actions are, in turn, modified by differences in the control mechanisms of diameter and flow, site specificity of action, concentration dependence of action, and presence of vascular disease.

In general, vasoactive stimuli tend to change arterial diameter and flow in the same direction. Different substances may, however, affect epicardial and resistance vessels to a different extent.[18] In addition, epicardial and resistance vessels interact with each other. Hyperaemia that is induced downstream causes flow-mediated epicardial vasodilatation, a response that is lost in the presence of abnormal endothelial function.[19]

101

As an example of site specificity, acetylcholine alters distal more than proximal vessel diameter in the presence of both normal and abnormal endothelial function.[20]

The net effect of a vasoactive stimulus on vessel diameter and flow tends to be extremely concentration dependent because the direct smooth muscle and the endothelium mediated effects may oppose each other.[18 20] For example, progressive increases in acetylcholine and serotonin concentrations result first in epicardial vasodilatation and subsequently in vasoconstriction.

Endothelial dysfunction appears very early in the development of coronary artery disease. Ischaemia mediated by endothelial dysfunction may well represent the pathogenesis of angina pectoris in some patients with normal coronary angiography.[21]

Endothelium derived relaxing factors (fig 4.2)

The first vasoactive substance derived from endothelium to be discovered was prostacyclin, or prostaglandin I_2 (PGI_2). Its production is stimulated by shear stress, pulsatile flow, hypoxaemia, and various vasoactive substances.[22]

Since the initial observation that an intact endothelium was necessary for acetylcholine-induced vasodilatation,[23] many physiological stimuli have been shown to cause vasodilatation by stimulating the release of a labile, diffusible, non-prostanoid molecule, the "endothelium derived relaxing factor" (EDRF). Nitric oxide (NO) has been shown to be a major endothelium derived relaxing factor[24] which is synthesised by the vascular endothelium from L-arginine.[25] The L-arginine analogue N_ω-monomethyl-L-arginine inhibits specifically the formation of NO from L-arginine,[26] and suppresses the vasodilatory effect of acetylcholine.[27] In addition, selective intravascular hypoxaemia causes dilatation only in the presence of an intact endothelium, and this dilatation is prevented by inhibition of NO release.[28]

Although the exact identity of EDRFs remains uncertain, it now seems probable that NO or a closely related compound represents at least one type of EDRF because both NO and EDRF display similar biological and pharmacological properties.[29] However, some studies have indicated that NO does not account for all the actions of EDRFs. Depending on the species and the vascular bed studied, and the mechanism of activation, there may be several types of EDRF.[30]

Coronary vasodilatation following intracoronary infusion of substances known to stimulate endothelial NO production (for example, acetylcholine,[20] substance P,[31] and serotonin[18]) have provided indirect evidence for a role of NO in the human coronary circulation. The degree of vasodilatation varies along the length of the epicardial coronary arteries, and at a given dose it is more marked in the distal than in the proximal segments. Such differences between proximal and distal vessel responsiveness may be non-specific and not confined to the NO system. Inhibition of NO synthesis blocks epicardial coronary artery dilatation of the distal segments induced by acetylcholine but not that of resistive vessels.[32] Furthermore, intracoronary acetylcholine may have both vasodilator and vasoconstrictor effects on the same angiographically normal coronary artery, depending on both the infusion concentration and the vessel segment being studied.[20]

There appears to be a small tonic release of NO under basal conditions.[32] Such continuous release of EDRF/NO may be the result of increased vascular wall stress following the cyclic increases in CBF induced by vasodilating

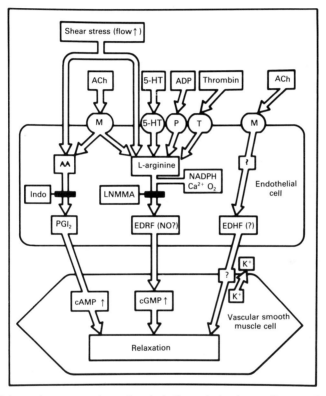

Fig 4.2 Schematic presentation of endothelium derived vasodilators. Prostacyclin (PGI$_2$) production via the cyclo-oxygenase pathway of arachidonic acid (AA) metabolism can be blocked by indomethacin (Indo) or aspirin. Endothelium derived relaxing factor (EDRF) is believed to be nitric oxide (NO) or a related substance. Its synthesis via action of NO synthase can be blocked by arginine analogues, such as L-NMMA (N_ω-monomethyl-L-arginine). Mechanism of action and characteristics of an endothelium derived hyperpolarising factor (EDHF) are not well defined. It possibly acts by activation of potassium (K$^+$) channels. ACh = acetylcholine; 5-HT = serotonin; ADP = adenosine diphosphate; M = muscarinic, P = purinergic, T = thrombin receptor. (Reproduced with permission from Rubanyi GM.[16] Endothelium, platelets, and coronary vasospasm. *Coronary Artery Disease* 1990; **1**: 645–53.)

metabolites or by a myogenic component. In the human coronary circulation, inhibition of NO synthesis causes a small increase in basal tone of the distal segments of the epicardial coronary arteries together with a small fall in basal CBF.[32] Inhibition of NO synthesis does not, however, universally affect resting CBF,[33-35] and it does not impair the normal coronary vasodilatation in response to exercise.[35] Overall evidence would suggest that NO formation may not be all that important in maintaining basal vasomotor tone in resistance and conductance vessels. It appears, however, to be responsible for mediating coronary vasodilatation in response to endothelium dependent agonists and to changes in flow pulse frequency.[36]

Endothelium derived contracting factors (fig 4.3)

Endogenous (for example, arachidonic acid, noradrenaline, thrombin) and pharmacological substances (calcium, nicotine, high potassium), and physio-chemical stimuli (shear stress, mechanical stress, hypoxia) can stimulate

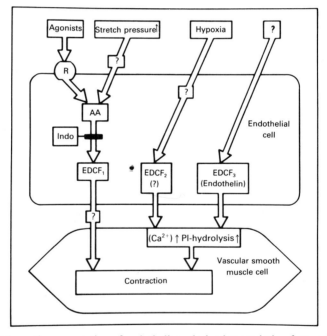

Fig 4.3 Schematic presentation of endothelium derived constricting factors (EDCFs). Production of $EDCF_1$ can be blocked by indomethacin (Indo). $EDCF_2$ is possibly released in response to hypoxia. The exact stimuli for the release of $EDCF_3$ are unknown. R = receptor; AA = arachidonic acid; PI = phosphatidylinositol. (Reproduced with permission from Rubanyi GM.[16] Endothelium, platelets, and coronary vasospasm. *Coronary Artery Disease* 1990; **1**: 645–53.)

endothelium dependent vasoconstriction.[16 17] Three different, endothelium derived contracting factors (EDCFs) have been described: $EDCF_1$, $EDCF_2$, and $EDCF_3$.

$EDCF_3$ exhibits potent coronary vascoconstrictor activity. Three closely related forms of $EDCF_3$ have been identified: endothelin-1, endothelin-2, and endothelin-3, the last being the most powerful known peptide vasoconstrictor; in pharmacological doses it can abolish CBF.[37] However, its exact role in the regulation of coronary vasomotor tone is not fully understood.[38] Other vasoconstrictors include thromboxane A_2 and angiotensin.[17]

EDRFs and EDCFs in coronary artery disease

Normal coronary arteries exhibit endothelium dependent dilatation in response to both local acetylcholine and increased flow. These physiological responses are lost in humans with advanced coronary artery disease.[39] Oxidised low density lipoproteins and hypoxia or anoxia inhibit the release of EDRFs, and ischaemia and reperfusion induce impairment in endothelium dependent relaxation to most EDRF/NO agonists.[40–42] Although such studies underscore the potential clinical relevance of impaired release of EDRFs/NO in ischaemic syndromes, a potentially important role for endothelin is also possible. Hypoxia[43] and decreased flow and shear stress[44] may induce endothelin gene expression and secretion. Following global myocardial ischaemia and reperfusion during cardiopulmonary bypass, there is not only impaired release of EDRFs in the coronary artery but the ischaemic event may also increase the production of an EDCF.[45]

The impaired release of EDRFs will suppress coronary vasodilatation in areas of endangered myocardium, and will facilitate platelet adhesion and aggregation as well as platelet induced coronary vasoconstriction. The stimulated release of endothelin resulting from vascular injury, reduced release of EDRFs, ischaemia, and decreased shear stress will, in turn, also promote vasoconstriction. The finding of augmented vasoconstrictor actions of endothelin with simultaneous inhibition of EDRF synthesis[46] supports the hypothesis that the endogenous EDRF system serves as a functionally important modulator of the vasoconstrictor actions of endothelin. When the delicate balance between endothelium mediated vasodilatation and vasoconstriction is disturbed in disease states associated with injured endothelium (for example, coronary atherosclerosis), the attenuated release of EDRFs and stimulated secretion of endothelin will facilitate vasoconstriction, thrombosis, and smooth muscle cell proliferation.

Non-vascular effects of endothelium

There is growing experimental evidence that locally released paracrine factors not only regulate CBF but also modify cardiac function.[47] For example, apart from being potent coronary vasoconstrictors endothelins also possess very potent positive inotropic properties.[48] Such modifying effects on myocardial function may help to explain the mechanism by which coronary flow rate per se acts as a determinant of cardiac contractile state.[49] Until recently, relative myocardial ischaemia at low flow rates and increased sarcomere length at high flow rates ("garden hose" effect) have been proposed as explanations for the finding of changes in contractility related to changes in CBF. Both mechanisms have, however, recently been excluded.[50] The possibility remains that the coronary microvascular endothelium releases paracrine acting mediators such as endothelin in response to changes in flow rates which, in turn, modify the myocardial contractile state.

All of the presented data indicate that the endothelial system can no longer be viewed as simply an inert lining of blood vessels, but must rather be regarded as a highly active endocrine organ which serves a wide variety of biological functions including synthesis, metabolism, and binding of various vasoactive and non-vasoactive substances. Impaired endothelial function probably contributes significantly to the pathophysiology of coronary artery disease and myocardial ischaemic syndromes.

Coronary physiology

Regulation of myocardial perfusion

Blood supply to the heart is affected by ventricular contraction and relaxation. Any myocardial stress is expected to alter underlying myocardial geometry and, in turn, geometry of intramyocardial vessels. This may affect vascular resistance and flow. Forces acting on a myocardial segment may include interactions of the following:

- myofibres and adjacent vessels
- intramyocardial tissue (fluid) pressure
- cavity pressure transmitted as radial stress
- myofibre force transmitted tangentially
- pericardial pressure.

Intramyocardial tissue pressure possibly constitutes a major component of coronary vascular resistance. It differs from the right to the left ventricular wall, the atrial to the ventricular chambers, the epicardial to the endocardial layers, and it varies with systole and diastole.

During systole the myocardial fibre bands which encircle both ventricles exert lateral shearing forces on the perpendicularly penetrating intramyocardial branches of the large epicardial vessels. This may entirely abolish flow to certain regions of the myocardium.[51] At the same time, however, those intramyocardial vessels running parallel to the muscle fibres are compressed during systole which propagates blood further downstream. This explains in part why coronary venous flow occurs almost entirely during systole.

Phasic myocardial perfusion

Intermittently high and low extravascular resistances during systole and diastole are responsible for the phasic pattern of coronary perfusion (fig 4.4). In the left ventricle, extravascular compression during systole is so great that normally only 20–30% of left coronary artery flow occurs during systole.[52] As a result of a considerably lower systolic and, thus, intramyocardial pressure generated by the thin walled right ventricle, right coronary arterial systolic flow constitutes a much greater proportion of total coronary inflow (30–50%) (fig 4.4). Systolic myocardial compression increases with rises in heart rate,

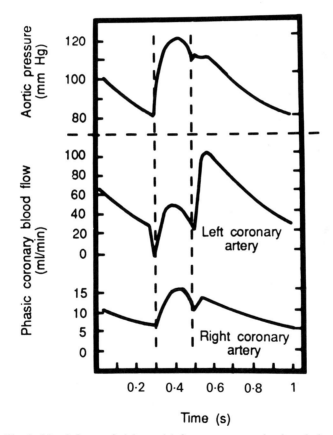

Fig 4.4 Phasic blood flows of right and left coronary arteries in relation to aortic pressure. Whereas right coronary artery flow exists throughout the cardiac cycle, left coronary flow is largely confined to diastole. (Reproduced with permission from Berne RM, Levy MP. *Cardiovascular physiology*, 5th edn. St Louis: CV Mosby, 1986: 200.)

107

afterload, preload, and contractility. The relative contribution of each of these factors to the regulation of myocardial perfusion remains controversial.[53]

The effects of contraction on phasic flow pattern seem to vary with the contractile state of the myocardium. During uniform global contraction local intramyocardial forces rather than transmitted forces (that is, cavity pressure) are primarily responsible for the phasic flow variations.[54] In a non-contracting region of myocardium, however, left ventricular pressure becomes a major determinant of phasic flow pattern.[54]

This dependence of flow characteristics on the contractile state may be explained by differences in myocardial behaviour during systole. During normal contraction the myocardium stiffens and then becomes resistant to deformation by externally transmitted stress such as cavitary pressure. When contraction is absent, however, the respective myocardial segment fails to stiffen, and the intramyocardial vessels are now prone to deformation by externally applied forces.

Normal intramyocardial and peripheral epicardial coronary arteries exhibit almost exclusive forward flow during diastole. Reverse flow is frequently observed during systole.[55] With coronary artery stenosis, systolic reverse flow increases whereas diastolic forward flow decreases.[56] Reduced back pressure to systolic reverse flow as a result of decreased poststenotic distal pressure, and increased coronary arterial capacitance caused by a pressure dependent capacitance change,[57] may both serve as explanations.

Transmural myocardial perfusion

During the cardiac cycle, transmural flow distribution is non-uniform. Normally, subendocardial flow exceeds subepicardial flow by about 10% resulting in an endo-/epicardial perfusion ratio of 1·1. As systolic intramyocardial compressive forces are greatest in the subendocardium, but low in the subepicardium, it was postulated that the subepicardium was perfused throughout the cardiac cycle whereas the subendocardium received blood only during diastole. However, findings of possibly very little flow to the subendocardium even during systole argue against such a mechanism.[58]

During normal contraction, primarily subendocardial vessels are compressed,[59] and a steep transmural gradient of intramyocardial pressure persists in an empty beating heart. When a beating heart is arrested, subendocardial flow has been shown to increase but subepicardial flow to decrease.[60] Thus, contraction appears to augment subepicardial perfusion. It has been proposed that during cardiac contraction blood is squeezed out of subendocardial vessels and translocated in a retrograde fashion to superficial layers of the myocardium. This way, the subepicardial vessels represent a low pressure and low resistance "sink" for any translocation of blood from deep to superficial layers. It is to be expected that the amount of retrograde flow will depend on the normal transmural pressure gradient. Consequently, absent global[60] or regional contraction[54] causes marked changes in phasic inflow to the myocardium and in transmural flow distribution, most probably by altering the transmural pressure gradient. When contraction is absent, left ventricular pressure becomes a powerful determinant of transmural flow distribution.[54] When regional contraction is abolished the subendocardial/subepicardial flow ratio more than doubles indicating favoured subendocardial perfusion.[54]

Thus, opposing factors such as wall stiffness, regional contractility, and cavity pressure influence phasic inflow and transmural flow distribution. The net result on myocardial perfusion will depend on their interactions during specific conditions. With changes in baseline conditions, the relative importance of each of the factors will also change. During uniform global contraction, local tissue–vessel interactions and/or intramyocardial fluid pressure caused by active contraction appear to play a dominant role in determining myocardial perfusion. When regional contraction is abolished, left ventricular pressure assumes a more prominent role. This, however, does not imply that the effects of intramyocardial forces resulting from contraction are simply removed when myocardial stiffness is low. Rather, changes in underlying conditions will result in complex changes in the spatial and temporal course of forces acting on intramyocardial vessels. Such considerations may help in understanding mechanisms that govern myocardial perfusion under clinical conditions of regional myocardial dysfunction (such as myocardial ischaemia and "stunned" myocardium).

Coronary vascular resistance
1 Traditionally, the coronary arterial bed has been considered as consisting of two compartments:

1 Large, conduit arteries which impose little resistance to flow.
2 Smaller, resistive vessels with a diameter between 250 μm and 10 μm.

It has been taught that arterioles of less than 50 μm in diameter are the major source of total coronary vascular resistance.[61] Recent studies, however, suggest that under resting conditions 45–50% of total coronary vascular resistance is caused by vessels larger than 100 μm in diameter.[62 63]

The border between the two vascular regions has not been defined precisely. In dogs a pressure drop of 5–15 mm Hg occurs, however, in distal epicardial vessels.[62] The principal functions of the resistive vessels are:

1 To match myocardial blood flow to $M\dot{V}o_2$ when metabolic demand varies.
2 To maintain myocardial perfusion (proportional to metabolic demand) when perfusion pressure varies.

Under pathological conditions, dilatation of the resistance vessels compensates for the increase in resistance of the conduit arteries caused by stenoses.

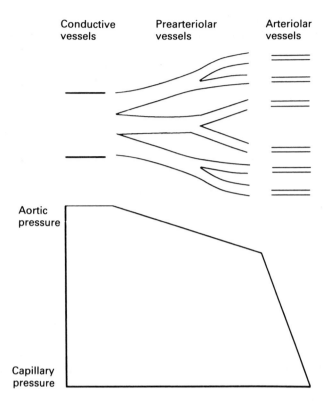

Fig 4.5 Schematic representation of pressure reduction from aorta to capillaries. Three components of the coronary circulation can be identified: (1) conductive vessels with negligible pressure drop; (2) prearteriolar vessels with moderate pressure drop; and (3) arteriolar vessels with greatest pressure drop. (Reproduced with permission from Maseri A, Crea F, Cianflone D.[64] Myocardial ischemia caused by distal coronary vasoconstriction. *Am J Cardiol* 1992; **70**: 1602–5.)

For a better understanding of vasomotor dysregulation which may lead to myocardial ischaemia it is helpful to distinguish functionally between two components within the resistive coronary vasculature that are arranged in series (fig 4.5):

1 More proximal, "prearteriolar" vessels in which vasomotor tone and flow are not metabolically regulated as a result of the epicardial position or thickness of the vessel wall.

2 More distal, "arteriolar" vessels in which major pressure reductions occur, and in which tone and flow are metabolically regulated.[64]

As no anatomical differentiation is possible between the two segments, functional differentiation is expected to be vague.[62]

110

The continuous matching of flow to demand by the resistive vessels is so precise that myocardial oxygen extraction remains practically constant over a wide range of metabolic demand and coronary perfusion pressure. The site of action and the mechanisms involved may, however, differ when flow is varied either in response to changes in metabolic demands at constant aortic pressure or when flow is maintained in the presence of changes in aortic pressure at constant metabolic demand.

Reduction of coronary perfusion pressure to 40 mm Hg causes dilatation of vessels less than 100 μm in diameter but constriction of larger vessels.[65]

Two possible explanations exist for such a heterogeneous response:

1 Large reductions in coronary perfusion pressure cause metabolically induced dilatation of arteriolar vessels but a passive, low, distending, pressure-induced reduction in prearteriolar vessel diameter.
2 Reduced flow mediated release of EDRF/NO causes prearteriolar constriction.

When CBF increases in response to metabolically mediated arteriolar vasodilatation, one would expect a proportional increase in pressure drop across the prearteriolar vessels unless they respond with compensatory flow mediated vasodilatation. If this does not occur (as with endothelial dysfunction in coronary artery disease), pressure at the origin of the maximally dilated arterioles may decrease to an extent that impairs subendocardial perfusion.[66] Thus, during metabolically induced arteriolar vasodilatation, adequate perfusion pressure at the origin of the arterioles can only be maintained if there is an appropriate change in vasomotor tone at the prearteriolar level. Flow mediated vasodilatation on the basis of a tonic release of endothelial NO[67] and/or other EDRFs[30] may be primarily involved in the adaptation of prearteriolar vessel size to changes in flow.

CBF varies little over a wide range of aortic pressures (see "Autoregulation"). This requires constant changes in coronary vasomotor tone and vascular resistance. Depending on the initiating stimulus the adaptive mechanisms maintaining CBF may differ. An increase in aortic pressure may primarily trigger prearteriolar constriction, thus maintaining optimal pressure at the origin of the arterioles. On the other hand, when aortic pressure decreases, metabolically induced arteriolar dilatation in addition to flow mediated prearteriolar dilatation may be required to maintain CBF.

It is the traditional view that myocardial ischaemia in coronary artery disease is caused by fixed or dynamic obstruction of large conduit coronary arteries, resulting in a critical reduction in perfusion pressure at the origin of fully dilated arterioles. Recent clinical studies, however, suggest that myocardial ischaemia can also result from constriction of small, distal, resistive coronary vessels.[68] Such small vessel constriction can result from dysfunction of either prearteriolar or arteriolar vessels. The mechanisms of the abnormal behaviour of the distal resistive vessels resulting in myocardial ischaemia can be multiple, and may involve different sites.[69][70]

The concept that coronary vascular resistance resides in large conduit arteries and, primarily, in small resistance vessels almost ignores the contribution of the venous system to total coronary vascular resistance. Whereas under control conditions only 7% of the total coronary vascular resistance resides in veins more than 150 μm in diameter, under conditions of vasodilatation with dipyridamole the total contribution of the venous component increased to 31%.[71] Thus, during coronary vasodilatation the coronary venous system may considerably modify myocardial perfusion. Furthermore, by affecting ventricular distensibility related to changes in myocardial blood volume,[72] alterations in venous reactivity may also have an impact on diastolic cardiac function.

Isolated coronary venules dilate in response to an increase in flow.[73] This flow-induced vasodilatation is endothelium dependent and mediated by the release of a nitrovasodilator. Endothelial disruption results in flow-induced constriction suggesting that shear stress may act directly on the vascular smooth muscle.[73] Whereas the additive effects of flow-induced dilatation and possibly myogenic relaxation of arterioles can maximise myocardial oxygen delivery during elevated $M\dot{V}_{O_2}$, the flow-induced venular dilatation may possibly contribute to a reduction in postcapillary resistance.

Pressure–flow relationships

Flow (F) across a resistance (R) is determined by the difference between pressures upstream and downstream of the resistance (ΔP), according to the equation

$$F = \Delta P/R.$$

The driving pressure, ΔP, is the coronary perfusion pressure. Whereas upstream pressure can clearly be defined as the pressure at the aortic root, definition of what constitutes downstream pressure remains controversial.[74][75] For fig 4.6, the downstream pressure is taken as the coronary sinus pressure or left ventricular end diastolic pressure, and the (apparent) coronary perfusion pressure is the difference between downstream and mean aortic diastolic pressure.

The normal pressure–flow relationship (A in fig 4.6) has three separate regions of interest:

1 A high pressure region, where flow increases with coronary perfusion pressure.
2 An intermediate pressure range, where flow changes little with changes in coronary perfusion pressure (referred to as "autoregulation").
3 A low pressure region, where flow decreases with decreasing coronary perfusion pressure.

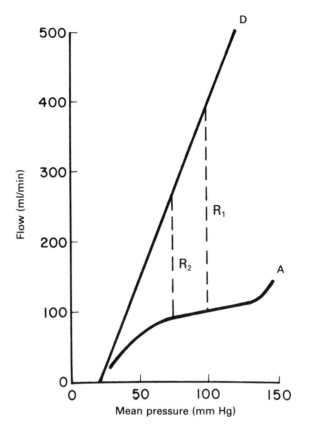

Fig 4.6 Schematic presentation of coronary pressure–flow relationships in the normal left ventricle during autoregulated flow (A), and during maximal vasodilatation (D). R_1 and R_2 denote coronary vascular reserves at mean coronary perfusion pressures of 100 (R_1) and 75 mm Hg (R_2). (Reproduced with permission from Hoffman JIE. Maximal coronary flow and the concept of coronary vascular reserve. *Circulation* 1984; **70**: 153–9.)

The controversy surrounding the downstream value for coronary perfusion pressure centres around the extrapolation of the low pressure region to zero flow (fig 4.7). It is accepted that the coronary pressure–flow relationship always has a positive intercept.[74-77] It had been suggested that myocardial perfusion stopped at pressures considerably higher than coronary sinus pressure.[78] The pressure at which flow stopped was termed "critical closing pressure" or "zero-flow pressure" (P_{zf} or $P_{f=0}$) (fig 4.7). This would imply that the effective downstream pressure for the calculation of coronary vascular resistance would be P_{zf} rather than the much lower coronary sinus or left ventricular end diastolic pressure. Results were, however, obtained on the basis of measurements on large proximal epicardial vessels, and it now

113

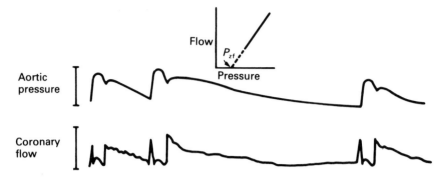

Fig 4.7 Graphic presentation of the concept of critical closing pressure (P_{zf}). During a long diastole, pressure in aortic root or coronary artery and flow through an epicardial coronary artery are recorded simultaneously (——). The pressure at which flow through the (epicardial) coronary artery is zero (P_{zf}) is either determined directly or derived by linear extrapolation (– – –). (Reproduced with permission from Sethna DH, Moffitt EA. An appreciation of the coronary circulation. *Anesth Analg* 1986; **65**: 294–305.)

seems that flow through intramural coronary vessels actually continues after large superficial vessel flow has already ceased.[61] Furthermore, it has been shown that forward movement of red blood cells in arterioles of 20 μm diameter continues until perfusion pressure is only a few millimetres of mercury higher than coronary sinus pressure.[79] Thus, the initial findings of considerably higher P_{zf} than coronary sinus pressure can probably be explained on the basis of arterial collateral flow[80] and coronary capacitance.[81]

An increase in coronary sinus pressure can shift the entire pressure–flow relationship to a higher P_{zf} without affecting its slope.[76 77] This way, coronary sinus pressure may become a determinant of CBF and transmural flow distribution. There appear to be regional differences in the response of the pressure–flow relationship to an increase in coronary sinus pressure: whereas the subepicardial pressure–flow relationship behaves as the total relationship, in the subendocardium neither pressure–flow relationship nor intramyocardial tissue pressures changed in response to high coronary sinus pressure.[77] Such transmural differences in intramyocardial pressures and P_{zf} support the existence of a vascular waterfall mechanism in the myocardium.[82]

Although the concept of P_{zf} remains controversial, the clinical relevance of changes in P_{zf} in response to interventions remains questionable. For clinical purposes, coronary perfusion pressure in normal coronary arteries can be defined as the difference between (mean) aortic diastolic and coronary sinus or left ventricular end diastolic (or even right atrial) pressures.

Autoregulation

Autoregulation has been defined as[83]

"the intrinsic tendency of an organ to maintain constant blood flow despite changes in arterial perfusion pressure."

Using a more operational definition, autoregulation is a proportional change in vascular resistance in response to a change in perfusion pressure.[84] This active change in vascular resistance constitutes an intrinsic mechanism that is independent of extrinsic neurohumoral factors.

Such a mechanism requires immediate adjustment of vasomotor tone in response to alterations in perfusion pressure. Autoregulatory changes in coronary vasomotor tone behave in a dynamic fashion. If metabolic demand is kept constant, a sudden change in coronary perfusion pressure results in an immediate directionally identical change in CBF which returns to normal over 10–30 s[85] (fig 4.8). The primary site of autoregulation resides in smaller coronary arterioles (≤ 100 μm).[86] As the coronary vasculature at rest appears to be under greater vasoconstrictor tone than other vascular beds,[87] this greater vasodilatory reserve provides the capacity to increase flow remarkably.

The definition of autoregulation assumes that organ metabolism and venous pressure do not change as arterial perfusion pressure is altered. As aortic pressure is a major determinant of left ventricular afterload, and developed left ventricular systolic pressure correlates with left ventricular $M\dot{V}_{O_2}$,[88] it is impossible to study coronary autoregulation simply by changing

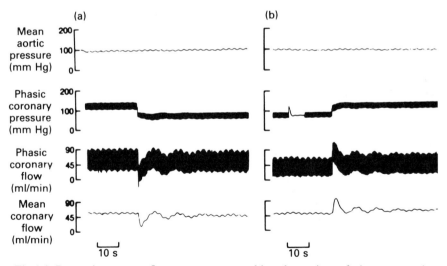

Fig 4.8 Dynamic coronary flow response to a sudden change in perfusion pressure in the left circumflex artery in the dog. (a) Flow response to a step decrease in pressure; (b) response to a step increase in pressure. (Reproduced with permission from Dole WP. Autoregulation of the coronary circulation. *Progr Cardiovasc Dis* 1987; **29**: 293–323.)

115

aortic pressure because this would lead to marked changes in myocardial metabolism. This problem can be overcome by cannulating a coronary artery and perfusing it with a pump. Nevertheless, low perfusion pressures may cause myocardial ischaemia with subsequent decreases in myocardial metabolism and increases in venous pressures. On the other hand, higher than normal perfusion may elicit the "Gregg effect."

When CBF is increased above the normal autoregulated level, cardiac contractility and myocardial metabolism increase as well. Doubling resting CBF may increase the strength of cardiac contraction by 15%.[89] This phenomenon is referred to as the "Gregg effect," after the person who discovered it.[49] Increasing CBF either by increasing cannulated coronary artery pressure or by pharmacological vasodilatation at constant coronary perfusion pressure will elicit this effect, so changing myocardial metabolism simultaneously. The common variable involved in both interventions appears to be an increase in intramyocardial blood volume. It has been proposed that the Gregg phenomenon is based on a "garden hose" effect, whereby engorgement of the coronary vasculature elongates myocardial sarcomere length during diastole and, subsequently, increases contractility via the Frank–Starling mechanism.[90] However, as mentioned earlier this mechanism has been excluded.[50] As autoregulation constitutes a flow response to changes in CBF, a Gregg effect will always be involved in autoregulatory investigations. Such simultaneous changes in $M\dot{V}O_2$ will complicate the interpretation of acquired data on autoregulation.

Left ventricular autoregulation

With stable myocardial metabolism, in anaesthetised animals CBF remains rather constant over a pressure range of 60–160 mm Hg.[91 92] Increasing myocardial metabolism results in an upward shift of the autoregulatory curves.[93]

Autoregulatory capacity of the subendocardium is considerably less than that of the subepicardium. Whereas in the awake animal subepicardial autoregulation was preserved until perfusion pressure reached 25 mm Hg, subendocardial autoregulation was impaired at a pressure of 40 mm Hg.[94] Such reduced subendocardial vasodilator reserve explains the well known greater vulnerability of the left ventricular subendocardium to ischaemia when compared with the subepicardium.[95]

Experimental conditions and extent of cardiac work influence the lower limits of autoregulation. At a heart rate of 100 beats/min perfusion pressure can decrease to 38 mm Hg before subendocardial ischaemia develops, although ischaemia develops at 61 mm Hg if heart rate is 200 beats/min.[96] Even during tachycardia and at pressures as low as 33 mm Hg subepicardial flow was maintained.

What could the explanation be for the lower subendocardial vasodilator reserve? The pressure–flow relationship during a long diastole would suggest that pressure at zero flow (P_{zf}) is higher in the subendocardium than in the subepicardium.[78] However, P_{zf} is unlikely to be high in any myocardial layer, and unlikely to be higher in the subendocardium by more than 2–3 mm Hg.[58] This excludes the possibility that different diastolic, myocardial, compressive forces account for the differences in regional vasodilator reserve.

During systole compressive forces are greatest in the subendocardium resulting in higher vascular resistance. With the start of diastole, flow follows first the way of lowest vascular resistance, that is, the large subepicardial vessels, before reaching the higher resistance subendocardial vessels. This hypothesis of an interaction between systole and diastole has been proposed as a possible explanation for the lower subendocardial vasodilator reserve.[58]

Right ventricular autoregulation

Autoregulation is present in the right ventricle although, at first glance, less distinct than in the left ventricle.[97-99] However, when correcting for changes in $M\dot{V}o_2$ caused by an exaggerated Gregg effect in the right ventricle, autoregulatory responses in right and left ventricles appear to be comparable.[97 100] Probably related to low right ventricular systolic pressures, inner and outer layers of the right ventricle have similar lower limits of autoregulation.[97]

Mechanism

The precise mechanism(s) responsible for maintaining CBF in the presence of decreasing coronary perfusion pressure remain(s) controversial.[85 100] As matching of O_2 supply to metabolic demands remains almost unaffected when neurohumoral factors are eliminated[101] there is general agreement that CBF is metabolically regulated.[102 103] Alterations in the level of myocardial energy use,[104] or in the balance of O_2 supply to demand, cause production of vasodilator substances which restore the supply/demand balance and, thus, maintain myocardial function.

Despite extensive research in this area the exact mediators of this highly effective metabolic regulation are still unknown; O_2, CO_2, H^+, K^+, Ca^{2+}, prostacyclin, EDRF/NO, as well as other substances, have been investigated in this context.[85] However, changes in their concentrations in the perivascular space are small, and their significance in controlling steady state coronary vascular resistance has been questioned.[105]

Adenosine

The exact role of adenosine in this context remains inconclusive. Data exist supporting[103 106-109] as well as rejecting the hypothesis[110-112] that adenosine is the major metabolite regulating CBF. According to this hypothesis, adenosine is released from myocardial cells as cellular O_2 tension decreases. It traverses the interstitial space and acts on coronary vascular smooth muscle to

117

cause vasodilatation. Subsequent increase in CBF restores myocardial O_2 tension.

Physiological and pathological conditions as diverse as resting CBF,[113] exercise induced coronary dilatation,[114] autoregulation,[108] and reactive hyperaemia[106] are largely unrelated to the release of adenosine. Furthermore, intracoronary infusion of adenosine deaminase or adenosine receptor antagonists that blunt reactive hyperaemia did not affect coronary autoregulation,[105 108 111 113] and interstitial levels of adenosine did not change with decreases in coronary perfusion pressure within the autoregulatory range.[105] These data would suggest that adenosine plays at best a minor role in coronary autoregulation.

On the other hand, uncoupling of increases in CBF from increases in myocardial metabolism has recently been demonstrated. Blockade of adenosine receptors almost abolished the hyperaemia associated with dobutamine-induced increases in cardiac work, and it dramatically exaggerated the reduction in CBF associated with intracoronary vasopressin infusion.[115] These findings would suggest a role for adenosine as a mediator of CBF changes.

Overall, evidence would suggest that adenosine is probably involved to some extent in the metabolic control of myocardial perfusion. It does not, however, appear to be the primary mediator of the close coupling between flow and metabolism.

Oxygen and carbon dioxide tension

Changes in myocardial O_2 and CO_2 tensions may mediate coronary autoregulation.[92 93] There appears to be a strong inverse correlation between coronary venous O_2 tension and coronary autoregulation. Good autoregulation was observed when coronary venous O_2 tension was 25 mm Hg (3·3 kPa) or less, and autoregulation was lost when venous O_2 tension was more than 32 mm Hg (4·3 kPa).[93] This, again, would indicate that the dominant mechanism of coronary autoregulation is metabolic. The normal resting coronary sinus Po_2 of 15–20 mm Hg (2·0–2·7 kPa) indicates a tight coupling between $M\dot{V}o_2$ and myocardial O_2 delivery.

Although possibly involved in the phenomenon of autoregulation, the effect of CO_2 tension is probably small at venous O_2 tension (Pvo_2) of more than 20 mm Hg (2·7 kPa).[92] It remains unclear whether coronary autoregulation is mediated directly by changes in tissue O_2 tension or by some mediating factors, such as ATP-sensitive K^+ channels (K^+_{ATP} channels).

ATP sensitive K^+ channels

Several studies suggest that K^+_{ATP} channels may be involved in the control of CBF.[116–119] Glibenclamide, a putative blocker of K^+_{ATP} channels, prevents hypoxic or ischaemic vasodilatation of coronary arteries,[120] prevents coronary epicardial microvascular dilatation associated with proximal coronary artery stenosis,[117] and abolishes autoregulation in the canine heart perfused with blood *in situ.*[119] Infusion of pinacidil, a K^+_{ATP} channel opener, induces coronary vasodilatation comparable to that observed during the peak reactive flow response.[121]

The mechanism by which a decrease in coronary perfusion pressure facilitates opening of K^+_{ATP} channels is unknown. It is, however, known that K^+_{ATP} channels open when intracellular ATP concentration falls in myocardial and vascular smooth muscle cells.[118 120 122] It has recently been suggested that a decrease in myocardial tissue O_2 tension may be sensed by the vascular smooth muscle cell; by regulation of the generation of ATP, this may subsequently lead to an opening of K^+_{ATP} channels in vascular smooth muscle cells.[118] This is consistent with the previous finding that coronary autoregulation is coupled strongly to tissue O_2 tension rather than $M\dot{V}o_2$.[93] It is, however, also conceivable that other tissue factors modify coronary autoregulation because K^+_{ATP} channel activity is also affected by tissue concentrations of ADP, lactate, and extracellular cations.[123] It is interesting to note that adenosine-induced coronary vasodilatation is in part mediated by K^+_{ATP} channels.[116 120]

EDRF/NO

Endothelium dependent production of NO in coronary vessels appears to be an important mechanism in the regulation of myocardial perfusion during hypoperfusion.[34] Inhibiting NO synthesis with the arginine analogue N_ω-nitro-L-arginine methyl ester (L-NAME) increased the critical pressure at which myocardial ischaemia began (lower autoregulatory break point) from 45 ± 3 mm Hg under control conditions to 61 ± 2 mm Hg after L-NAME (fig 4.9). In addition, both the slope of the coronary pressure–flow relation below the autoregulatory point and the peak reactive hyperaemic flow response were reduced, reflecting impaired capability to minimise coronary vascular resistance. On the other hand, flow recruitment in response to increased metabolic demand (that is, a twofold increase in heart rate) was not affected by L-NAME. These findings would suggest that both initial autoregulatory adjustments to decreases in coronary perfusion pressure and flow recruitment in response to increased metabolic demand are probably mediated by metabolic factors independent of NO production. During hypoperfusion, however, endothelium dependent production of NO has an important role in minimising coronary vascular resistance.

Myogenic effects

Studies in isolated coronary resistance arterioles that are uncoupled from metabolic mediators of vascular tone have shown that endothelium dependent mechanisms that are both myogenic and flow mediated may be involved in local blood flow regulation throughout much of the coronary microcirculation.[124] In this regard, transmural differences in the potential for

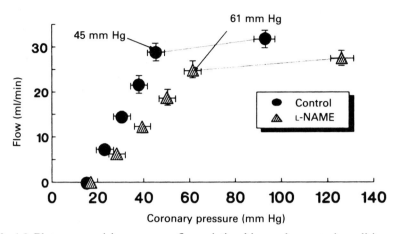

Fig 4.9 Plots summarising pressure–flow relationships under control conditions (●) and following inhibition of nitric oxide synthesis by N_ω-nitro-L-arginine (L-NAME) (hatched triangles). L-NAME had no significant effect on flow regulation over the autoregulatory plateau. However, the lower autoregulatory breakpoint (arrows) as well as the pressure–flow relationship during ischaemia were shifted to the right after inhibition of nitric oxide production. (Reproduced with permission from Smith TP, Canty JM Jr. Modulation of coronary autoregulatory responses by nitric oxide. *Circ Res* 1993; **73**: 232–40.)

myogenic dilatation seem to exist. In subendocardial arterioles, myogenic dilatation was maximal at pressures of 60 cm H_2O, whereas in subepicardial arterioles myogenic dilatation was present up to pressures as low as 40 cm H_2O.[125] The changes in vessel diameter over the pressure range studied were, however, only modest (<10% of resting values). In contrast, flow dependent influences on coronary vasomotor tone increased arteriolar diameter by up to 25% of resting value.[124]

Thus, although myogenic responses have been observed in isolated coronary vessels, their demonstration in vivo has been difficult, probably because of the predominance of the metabolic control of CBF. Although some argument can be made for a myogenic component in coronary reactive hyperaemia,[126] overall there is little experimental evidence for myogenic effects in the coronary circulation.

Conclusion

The exact mechanism(s) of coronary autoregulation remain(s) unclear. It is possible that O_2 tensions within a critical range may be the initial metabolic stimulus for coronary autoregulation. Although adenosine does not appear to be essential for autoregulation it is probably reasonable to speculate that compensatory mechanisms other than adenosine exist in the myocardium which gain importance once the action of adenosine is prevented. It is rather unlikely that a highly oxidative organ such as the heart depends on just one "host defence" mechanism to preserve the balance between supply and demand. Furthermore, the mechanisms involved in the control of coronary vasomotor tone may well be distributed in a way that either metabolic, flow dependent, or myogenic control mechanisms predominate in different classes of arteriolar vessel. Furthermore, each of the mediators may have differing physiological relevance under differing conditions.

Coronary flow reserve

The pressure–flow relationship during maximum coronary vasodilatation is almost straight (D in fig 4.6). Maximum flow at any given pressure is determined primarily by the cross sectional area of the resistance vessels. The difference between autoregulated (A in fig 4.6) and maximally dilated (D in fig 4.6) flow is the reserve capacity for vasodilatation, and this is called the coronary flow reserve.[87 127–129] As it varies with coronary perfusion pressure, it cannot be expressed as a single value.

Coronary flow reserve may be reduced principally by elevation of the autoregulatory line or depression of the line for maximally attainable flow. Anaemia, left ventricular hypertrophy, or increased $M\dot{V}o_2$ leads to higher resting CBF, thus elevating the autoregulation line (A_2 in fig 4.10). If the maximally attainable flow at any given pressure remains unchanged, coronary flow reserve will decrease ($R_1 - R_2$ in fig 4.10). Concomitant hypertension will, however, preserve coronary flow reserve (R_3 in fig 4.10).

Coronary artery disease, tachycardia, polycythaemia, and marked increases in left ventricular end diastolic pressure or contractility all decrease the slope of the line for maximally attainable flow (D in fig 4.10), so reducing the coronary flow reserve ($R_1 - R_2$ in fig 4.10). In the case of coronary artery disease, this reflects a decrease in total cross sectional area of the coronary vascular bed.[130]

Many studies have estimated coronary flow reserve from the reactive myocardial hyperaemia that follows transient total coronary occlusion.[131] If there is no hyperaemia, coronary vascular reserve is deemed to have been exhausted by having to compensate for a stenosis in the supply vessel, and the supply vessel is deemed to be "critically constricted."[132] Reactive hyperaemia is, however, the result of complex interactions of vasodilator metabolites, myogenic relaxation, and coronary capacitance.[133] It is difficult to standardise because it varies with the duration of occlusion, basal $M\dot{V}o_2$, coronary perfusion pressure, sympathetic tone, and reactivity of adenosine receptors.[133] Pharmacological vasodilators such as adenosine or dipyridamole may lower resistance much more than ischaemic stimuli[134] (fig 4.11). During maximal exercise in humans, CBF may increase by two or four times the control values, but, with dipyridamole, increases of three to five times the

121

control have been described.[135] Thus, endogenous (ischaemic) stimuli may not be as effective in revealing true (maximal) coronary flow reserve as potent pharmacological vasodilators (fig 4.11).

The overall evidence seems to indicate that the degree of coronary flow reserve provides potentially valid information on what might happen during maximal stress, provided that other factors which might modify maximally attainable and autoregulated flows are controlled (or accounted for if changes do occur during the study). Determination of coronary flow reserve using maximal pharmacological vasodilatation has been used to assess the physio-

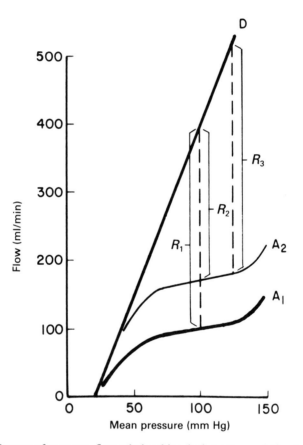

Fig 4.10 Diagram of pressure–flow relationships during autoregulation in the normal (A_1) and in the left ventricle with anaemia or increased contractility or hypertrophy (A_2). As pressure–flow relationships during maximal vasodilatation remain about the same (D), coronary vascular reserve will be lower in the abnormal (R_2) than in the normal left ventricle (R_1). Elevation of coronary perfusion pressure (as in hypertension) may restore or even increase absolute coronary vascular reserve (R_3). (Reproduced with permission from Hoffman JIE. Maximal coronary flow and the concept of coronary vascular reserve. *Circulation* 1984; **70**: 153–9.)

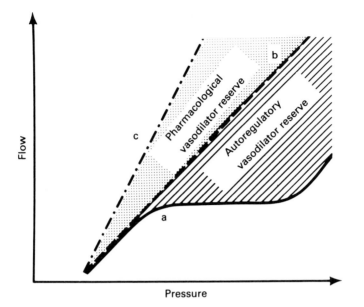

Fig 4.11 Autoregulation and coronary vasodilator reserve. Traditionally it was thought that the coronary pressure–flow relationship below the autoregulatory range (line a) was identical to the pressure–flow relationship in the maximally dilated bed (line b) indicating exhausted coronary vasodilator reserve. However, considerable flow reserve well below the autoregulatory range has been demonstrated in response to intracoronary application of vasodilatation (line c). Thus, pharmacological vasodilator reserve (c–a) may be preserved at times of exhausted (physiological) autoregulatory vasodilator reserve. (Reproduced with permission from Dole WP. Autoregulation of the coronary circulation. *Progr Cardiovac Dis* 1987; **29**: 293–323.)

logical significance of coronary stenoses, and the results of coronary angioplasty and coronary bypass surgery.

Neural control

Autonomic control

Superior, middle, and inferior cervical, and the first four sympathetic ganglia, supply the heart with sympathetic and the vagi with parasympathetic innervation. Sympathetic innervation is present at all coronary microvascular segments but the density of innervation may differ among various vascular levels.[61] Cholinergic stimulation consistently results in coronary dilatation.[136] Although in patients with angiographically normal coronary arteries, intracoronary acetylcholine causes dilatation,[137] it elicits constriction in atherosclerotic segments.[138] Intracoronary acetylcholine binds to endothelial muscarinic receptors and stimulates the release of EDRFs. Similarly,

123

coronary vasodilatation that normally follows parasympathetic stimulation may be dependent on the release of EDRFs.[139]

α-Adrenergic control

Both α_1- and α_2-adrenergic receptors exist throughout the coronary circulation. They are not, however, uniformly distributed.[140] α_1-Adrenergic receptors seem to predominate in large epicardial vessels, whereas α_2-adrenergic receptors predominate in vessels of less than 100 μm in diameter.[1 2]

Activation of either α_1- or α_2-adrenergic receptors produces coronary vasoconstriction.[2 141] In accordance with the non-uniform distribution of the receptor subtypes, the α-adrenergic responses of the coronary circulation to various physiological and pharmacological interventions seem to vary among vessel segments of different morphology and location. For example, sympathetic stimulation does little to epicardial vasomotor tone,[142] and mature coronary collaterals do not respond to α-receptor stimulation.[143]

During neurohumoral adrenergic stimulation, α-adrenergic stimulation competes with metabolic vasodilatation.[2 144 145] Although under physiological conditions the net result of α-adrenergic stimulations is always an increase in CBF, such stimulation, nevertheless, attenuates the increase in CBF by 20–30%.[145 146] Such attenuation in the presence of increased myocardial O_2 demand seems paradoxical, and the question remains whether α-vasoconstriction serves any physiological role.[147 148]

Extravascular compression restricts blood flow preferentially in the subendocardium.[58 149] It could be hypothesised that α-adrenergic coronary vasoconstriction occurs preferentially in the subepicardium and may, thus, counteract the enhanced extravascular compression in the subendocardium. It has been proposed that α-adrenergic coronary vasoconstriction "stiffens" intramural vessels and, subsequently, both reduces their compression during systole and facilitates their re-expansion during diastole. This may then result in improved diastolic flow to the subendocardium, particularly at high heart rates.[150]

Recent data would suggest that during neurohumoral adrenergic activation at baseline coronary vasomotor tone a physiological function of α-adrenergic coronary vasoconstriction does not exist.[151] Controversy continues, however, as to the importance of α-adrenergic receptor stimulation during myocardial hypoperfusion. In the presence of impaired vasodilator reserve, the coronary arterioles become sensitive to both α_1- and α_2-adrenergic agonists.[2] This would explain the increased vulnerability of patients with ischaemic heart disease to adrenergic vasoconstriction,[152] the simultaneously impaired myocardial contractile function,[153] and the improvement of subendocardial perfusion following α_2-adrenergic blockade during myocardial hypoperfusion.[154]

On the other hand, α-adrenergic mediated coronary constriction may have

124

beneficial effects on the transmural blood flow distribution.[150 151] α Blockade during myocardial hypoperfusion results in redistribution of CBF from the subendocardium to the subepicardium.[155] This would suggest that α-adrenergic receptor mediated vasoconstriction during hypoperfusion exhibits an "anti-steal" effect by limiting perfusion to the subepicardium and improving that to the subendocardium. A similar phenomenon has been observed in exercising animals in the presence of a coronary stenosis.[156]

The entire issue remains somewhat controversial. Overall, the impact of α-adrenergic coronary vasoconstriction on transmural blood flow distribution appears to be rather small, and its physiological significance remains uncertain.

β-Adrenergic control

Both β_1- and β_2-adrenergic receptors exist throughout the coronary circulation.[61] There appears to be a segmental distribution of β-adrenergic receptors, with a higher density of β receptors in resistance vessels than in large vessels.[157] The resistance vessels may contain both β_1 and β_2 receptor subtypes, whereas large epicardial vessels have predominantly β_1 receptors. Coronary vasodilatation mediated by β_1- and β_2-adrenergic receptors of both large and small coronary vessels,[101 158 159] and of mature canine collaterals,[160] has been demonstrated.

At first it would seem paradoxical that administration of noradrenaline causes simultaneous α-adrenergic receptor mediated coronary vasoconstriction and β-adrenergic receptor mediated vasodilatation.[159] These seemingly opposing effects may, however, be of benefit. α-Adrenergic receptor mediated vasoconstriction of large and medium sized coronary arteries possibly lessens the oscillation of flow from subendocardium to subepicardium during systole and diastole, thus preserving flow (see above).[60] On the other hand, direct β vasodilatation probably occurs mostly in small arteries, and serves to match blood flow and myocardial metabolism. It could therefore be postulated that α vasoconstriction serves to adjust phasic coronary impedance which preserves left ventricular subendocardial perfusion, whereas β vasodilatation prevents large decreases in myocardial tissue P_{O_2}.[159]

Inhibition of NO synthesis by L-NAME antagonises isoproterenol-induced coronary vasodilatation.[161] This would suggest that β-adrenergic mediated dilatation of resistance vessels involves an endothelium dependent mechanism which is linked to the L-arginine/NO pathway.

Peptidergic innervation

It is generally thought that the neural control depends primarily on the release of noradrenaline and acetylcholine from sympathetic and parasympathetic nerve terminals, respectively. It is now recognised, however, that in addition to the classic neurotransmitters, other putative transmitters including several vasoactive peptides may also be involved in regulating coronary vasomotor tone. Such peptides identified in nerves associated with coronary vessels include:[162]

- neuropeptide Y (NPY)
- vasoactive intestinal polypeptide (VIP)
- calcitonin gene related peptide (CGRP)
- tachykinins such as substance P and neuropeptide K.

Human epicardial coronary arteries are supplied by numerous perivascular nerve populations containing peptides.[162] The number of peptide-containing nerve fibres varies with vessel size, with the distal segments of epicardial coronary arteries more densely innervated than the proximal segments. NPY immunoreactive nerve fibres seem the most abundant of the peptide containing nerve populations identified in human epicardial coronary arteries. They appear to have a distribution pattern similar to that of nerves containing the catecholamine synthesising enzyme tyrosine hydroxylase.[162] Most NPY-containing nerves in the heart represent postganglionic sympathetic neurons originating in the stellate and other paravertebral ganglia. This supports the extracardiac origin of this neuropeptide.

NPY has generally been regarded as a vasoconstrictor peptide.[163] Its vasomotor activity appears, however, to vary with vessel size and location. NPY does not seem to elicit a vasoconstrictor response in epicardial coronary arteries but it induces some constriction of intramyocardial resistance vessels.[164] Its vasomotor action is possibly mediated by specific Y_1 and Y_2 receptors.[165] Although the functional significance of NPY in the regulation of coronary vasomotor tone has still to be defined, it may well play a role in modulating the effect of other vasoactive substances.[166]

Nerve fibres that are immunoreactive to CGRP and substance P are rare in the proximal region of epicardial coronary arteries and increase in number distally.[162] CGRP and substance P produce a marked relaxation of epicardial coronary arteries[167 168] but exert a weak vasodilatory effect on intramyocardial resistance vessels.[168 169]

VIP-containing nerve fibres have also been demonstrated in the adventitia of human epicardial coronary arteries.[162] Compared with other peptide-containing fibres, their density is, however, sparse. They presumably represent postganglionic parasympathetic or intrinsic cardiac neurons.[170] Their exact origin remains uncertain.

VIP induces coronary vasodilatation.[162] VIP specific receptors have been demonstrated in the coronary vasculature.[171] The vasodilatory effect appears to be endothelium independent. These data would suggest that VIP is involved in the regulation of CBF.

In summary, a network of neuropeptide-containing nerve fibres located in the adventitia and at the adventitial–medial border supplies human coronary arteries.[162] Neuropeptides appear to modify CBF either directly or indirectly by modifying the effects of other vasoactive substances.

Methods to determine CBF

Correct interpretation of coronary circulatory behaviour in response to a given intervention is critically dependent on reliable determination of CBF. Contradictory findings may at times reflect differences in methodology employed to measure flow. All methods of measuring CBF have technical limitations.[172]

Radioactive microsphere technique

This has become the standard technique for evaluation of transmural myocardial blood flow distribution in the experimental animal.[173] It is an extraction method that rests on the assumptions that microspheres injected into the blood stream are distributed in the same way as red blood cells, and that basically all microspheres are trapped in tissues on their first passage. Under such conditions, blood flow should be proportional to radioactivity per tissue mass.

Microspheres are denser and larger, and stream more centrally than red cells do. They are, therefore, not distributed in quite the same way as native blood. As subendocardial shunting (non-entrapment) of 9 μm spheres is somewhat greater than shunting of 15 μm spheres, endo-/epicardial flow ratios determined with 9 μm spheres tend to be lower than ratios determined with 15 μm spheres.[174] In general, endo-/epicardial values are lower in open chest preparations than in conscious dogs.[61] The necessity of obtaining multiple myocardial tissue samples requires sacrifice of the animal and prohibits its use in humans.

Inert gas clearance technique

By determining the arteriocoronary sinus difference in gas saturation, CBF can be calculated from equations originally developed by Kety and Schmidt.[175] For this technique to be accurate, several requirements must be fulfilled:[176]

1 The indicator must be physiologically inert.
2 Partition coefficients for the gas in myocardium, fat, red cells, and plasma must be known.
3 Venous blood from the entire myocardial region of interest must be sampled.

127

4 During the period of saturation and desaturation (5–20 min), CBF must be stable.

5 The entire washout curve must be analysed.

Principal disadvantages of the inert gas clearance technique (particularly when using non-radioactive tracers) include the following:

- poor spatial resolution
- length of time required for making measurements
- variations in venous drainage patterns distorting results
- inability to determine right ventricular and atrial flows because venous blood from those areas cannot be sampled.

Although the introduction of radioactive xenon-133 (^{133}Xe) has added spatial resolution to the inert gas clearance technique,[177] transmural blood distribution cannot be determined, the temporal resolution remains limited (requiring stable flow during measurements), only a limited number (two to five) of flow determinations is possible (resulting from the fact that the solubility of xenon is eight times greater in fat than in myocardium), and only flow rates below 200 ml/100 g can be measured with reasonable accuracy.[178] Therefore, determination of flow rates during maximal coronary vasodilatation is probably not possible.

Electromagnetic flow meters

The principle of this technique is based on Faraday's induction law which states that a conductor moving in a magnetic field generates electric current. When blood flows through the vessel, electrical voltage proportional to the rate of flow is generated, and this voltage is recorded by an appropriate flowmeter apparatus. Immediate, reliable determinations of blood flow have been made possible by the following:

- accurate, non-occlusive (electronic) zero, which can be used at any time and can be compared with occlusive (mechanical) zero
- automatic flow ranging (autoranging), which provides an instantaneous readout of blood volume flow
- precalibration during flow probe production, which eliminates the need for time consuming flow calibration.

Principal drawbacks of this technique include the relatively large flow probes (limiting its application to major epicardial vessels), its inability to determine transmural blood flow distribution, and its invasiveness (requiring thoracotomy and coronary artery dissection). Variability in contact between flow probe and vessel may result in major errors in measurement.

Ultrasonic Doppler flowmeter

This technique is based on the Doppler principle which states that when sound waves are reflected from a moving structure, the frequency of the reflected wave is shifted to a higher or lower frequency (Doppler shift). In the case of blood vessels, the Doppler shift is caused by ultrasonic waves which reflect off moving red blood cells.

The temporal resolution of this technique is ideal allowing continuous on line measurements of changes in velocity. The principal drawback of this technique is the fact that velocity rather than flow is measured. For the correct interpretation of results, precise knowledge of magnitude and direction of any change in coronary cross sectional area in response to a given intervention is crucial. Otherwise, statements regarding changes in absolute flow are not valid.

Recently developed small Doppler flowmeters can be placed directly into a coronary artery.[176] Among its limitations is some obstruction of the vessel by the catheter. A new intravascular Doppler guide wire appears, however, to provide accurate measurements of coronary artery flow velocity.[179]

Thermodilution technique

This technique is based on the principle that a change in temperature of a downstream fluid–blood mixture is proportional to blood flow. A fluid indicator (saline) with a known temperature (lower than that of blood) is infused (upstream) into the coronary sinus or great cardiac vein. The coronary sinus thermodilution is at present the most widely used clinical technique for the estimation of myocardial blood flow.[180] It has almost been forgotten that the initial studies validating this technique were performed in animals under the following very rigid conditions, which cannot be reproduced in humans:

- catheter tied into position in coronary sinus
- assurance of adequate mixing of blood and tracer
- normal coronary arteries and myocardium.

The technique has very crude spatial and only modest temporal resolution. Wide variations in coronary venous drainage patterns make direct comparisons of flow between patients impossible. Even slight variations in catheter position in the coronary sinus may have major effects on flow determination. This practical limitation makes the interpretation of results obtained during interventions that are likely to affect cardiac size difficult, and makes comparison of data gained on different occasions (even in the same patient) almost impossible.

As a result of both fundamental and practical deficiencies, thermodilution should only be used in very special circumstances. At present, only large changes (>30%) in coronary sinus or great cardiac vein flow in patients with no evidence of coronary artery disease should be accepted as semiquantitative indices of directional changes in CBF.[176]

Radioactive tracers

Myocardial perfusion can be assessed by myocardial distribution and uptake of radioactive tracers such as thallium. These techniques cannot, however, assess transmural flow distribution or acute changes in flow.

Quantitative digital subtraction angiography

This technique compares the density of a contrast medium that is power injected into a coronary artery with the contrast concentration, appearance time–density ratio, and myocardial washout time.[181] Absolute blood flow cannot be calculated.

Positron emission tomography

With this technique the essential features of myocardial perfusion, function, metabolism, and viability can be examined.[182] As with other methods, transmural flow distribution cannot, however, be determined.

Conclusion

All methods are invasive. They require either venous access or surgical dissection of vessels (electromagnetic flow probes), or they involve catheter manipulation in coronary arteries (intracoronary Doppler ultrasonography, xenon-133 clearance, videodensitometry). In addition, most methods expose the patient to ionising radiation. At present, no technique is available for clinical use that would allow determination of absolute myocardial perfusion with high temporal and spatial resolution.

In general, methods that use tracers have a poor temporal resolution because they require at least one circulation time for tracer distribution, or 5–20 minutes for inert gas saturation or desaturation to occur. In contrast, methods that assess arterial blood velocity or venous drainage have good temporal but poor spatial resolution. Newer techniques such as magnetic resonance imaging, contrast echocardiography, and ultrafast computed tomography have, in theory, a sufficient spatial resolution to distinguish variation in transmural perfusion.[172]

1 Chilian WM. Adrenergic vasomotion in the coronary microcirculation. *Basic Res Cardiol* 1990; **85** (suppl I): 111–20.
2 Chilian WM. Functional distribution of α_1- and α_2-adrenergic receptors in the coronary microcirculation. *Circulation* 1991; **84**: 2108–22.
3 Khouri EM, Gregg DE, Rayford CR. Effect of exercise on cardiac output, left coronary flow and myocardial metabolism in the unanesthetized dog. *Circ Res* 1965; **17**: 427–37.
4 Brooks J, Holland R, Al-Sadir J. Right ventricular performance during ischaemia: An anatomic and hemodynamic analysis. *Am J Physiol* 1977; **233**: H500–13.
5 Moore RA. The coronary arteries of the dog. *Am Heart J* 1930; **5**: 743–9.
6 Kazzaz D, Shanklin WM. The coronary vessels of the dog demonstrated by colored plastic (vinyl acetate) injections and corrosion. *Anat Rec* 1950; **107**: 43–59.
7 Hutchins GM, Moore GW, Hatton EV. Arterial–venous relationships in the human left ventricular myocardium. Anatomic basis for countercurrent regulation of blood flow. *Circulation* 1986; **74**: 1195–202.
8 Schaper W, Görge G, Winkler B, Schaper J. The collateral circulation of the heart. *Prog Cardiovasc Dis* 1988; **31**: 57–77.
9 Cohen MV. *Coronary collaterals: clinical and experimental observations.* Mount Kisco, NY: Futura, 1985.
10 Shaper W. *The collateral circulation.* Amsterdam: North Holland, 1971.
11 Rösen R, Marsen A, Klaus W. Local myocardial perfusion and epicardial NADH-fluorescence after coronary artery ligation in the isolated guinea pig heart. *Basic Res Cardiol* 1984; **79**: 59–67.
12 Cohen MV. Myocardial ischemia is not a prerequisite for the stimulation of coronary collateral development. *Am Heart J* 1993; **126**: 847–55.
13 Schaper W. New paradigms for collateral vessel growth (Editorial). *Basic Res Cardiol* 1993; **88**: 193–8.
14 Charney R, Cohen M. The role of the coronary circulation in limiting myocardial ischemia and infarct size. *Am Heart J* 1993; **126**: 937–45.
15 Bassenge E, Busse R. Endothelial modulation of coronary tone. *Prog Cardiovasc Dis* 1988; **30**: 349–80.
16 Rubanyi GM. Endothelium, platelets, and coronary vasospasm. *Coronary Artery Disease* 1990; **1**: 645–53.
17 Rubanyi GM. Endothelium-derived relaxing and constricting factors. *J Cell Biochem* 1991; **46**: 27–36.
18 Golino P, Piscione F, Willerson JT, *et al.* Divergent effects of serotonin on coronary–artery dimensions and blood flow in patients with coronary atherosclerosis and control patients. *N Engl J Med* 1991; **324**: 641–8.
19 Drexler H, Zeiher AM, Wollschläger H, Meinertz T, Just H, Bonzel T. Flow-dependent coronary artery dilatation in humans. *Circulation* 1989; **80**: 466–74.
20 Newman CM, Maseri A, Hackett DR, El-Tamini HM, Davies GJ. Response of angiographically normal and atherosclerotic left anterior descending coronary arteries to acetylcholine. *Am J Cardiol* 1990; **66**: 1070–6.
21 Motz W, Vogt M, Rabenau O, Scheler S, Lückhoff A, Strauer BE. Evidence of endothelial dysfunction in coronary resistance vessels in patients with angina pectoris and normal coronary angiograms. *Am J Cardiol* 1991; **68**: 996–1003.
22 Moncada S, Vane JR. Pharmacology and endogenous roles of prostaglandin, endoperoxides, thromboxane A_2, and prostacyclin. *Pharmacol Rev* 1978; **30**: 293–331.
23 Furchgott RF, Zawadzky JV. The obligatory role of endothelial cells in the relaxation of arterial smooth muscle by acetylcholine. *Nature* 1980; **288**: 373–6.
24 Palmer RMJ, Ferrige AG, Moncada S. Nitric oxide release accounts for the biological activity of endothelium-derived relaxing factor. *Nature* 1987; **327**: 524–6.
25 Palmer RMJ, Ashton DS, Moncada S. Vascular endothelial cells synthetize nitric oxide from L-arginine. *Nature* 1988; **333**: 664–6.
26 Rees DD, Palmer RMJ, Hodson HF, Moncada S. A specific inhibitor of nitric oxide

formation from L-arginine attenuates endothelium-dependent relaxation. *Br J Pharmacol* 1989; **96**: 418–24.

27 Yamabe H, Okumura K, Ishizaka H, Tsuchiya T, Yasue H. Role of endothelium-derived nitric oxide in myocardial reactive hyperemia. *Am J Physiol* 1992; **263**: H8–14.

28 Pohl U, Busse R. EDRF increases cyclic GMP in platelets during passage through the coronary vascular bed. *Circ Res* 1989; **65**: 1798–803.

29 Moncada S, Palmer RMJ, Higgs EA. Nitric oxide: physiology, pathophysiology, and pharmacology. *Pharmacol Rev* 1991; **43**: 109–42.

30 Boulanger C, Hendrickson H, Lorenz RR, Vanhoutte PM. Release of different relaxing factors by cultured porcine endothelial cells. *Circ Res* 1989; **64**: 1070–8.

31 Crossman DC, Larkin SW, Fuller RW, Davies GJ, Maseri A. Substance P dilates epicardial coronary arteries and increases coronary blood flow in humans. *Circulation* 1989; **80**: 475–84.

32 Lefroy DC, Crake T, Uren NG, Davies GJ, Maseri A. Effect of inhibition of nitric oxide synthesis on epicardial coronary artery caliber and coronary blood flow in humans. *Circulation* 1993; **88**: 43–54.

33 Parent R, Paré R, Lavallée M. Contribution of nitric oxide to dilation of resistance vessels in conscious dogs. *Am J Physiol* 1992; **262**: H10–16.

34 Smith TP Jr, Canty JM Jr. Modulation of coronary autoregulatory responses by nitric oxide. Evidence for flow-dependent resistance adjustments in conscious dogs. *Circulation* 1993; **73**: 232–40.

35 Altman JD, Kinn J, Duncker DJ, Bache RJ. Effect of inhibition of nitric oxide formation on coronary blood flow during exercise in the dog. *Cardiovasc Res* 1994; **28**: 119–24.

36 Canty JM, Schwartz JS. Nitric oxide mediates flow-dependent epicardial coronary vasodilatation to changes in pulse frequency but not mean flow in conscious dogs. *Circulation* 1994; **89**: 375–84.

37 Clozel J-P, Clozel M. Effects of endothelin on the coronary vascular bed in open-chest dogs. *Circ Res* 1989; **65**: 1193–200.

38 Kasuya Y, Ishikawa T, Yanagisawa M, Kimura S, Goto K, Masaki T. Mechanism of contraction to endothelin in isolated porcine coronary artery. *Am J Physiol* 1989; **257**: H1828–35.

39 Cox DA, Vita J, Treasure CB, Fish RD, Alexander RW, Ganz P, Selwyn AP. Atherosclerosis impairs flow-mediated dilation of coronary arteries in humans. *Circulation* 1989; **80**: 458–65.

40 Lüscher TF, Richard V, Tschdi M, Yang Z, Boulanger C. Endothelial control of vascular tone in large and small coronary arteries. *J Am Coll Cardiol* 1990; **15**: 519–27.

41 Lüscher TF, Richard V, Tanner FC. Endothelium-derived vasoactive factors and their role in the coronary circulation. *Trends Cardiovasc Med* 1991; **1**: 179–85.

42 Warren JB, Pons F, Brady AJB. Nitric oxide biology: implications for cardiovascular therapeutics. *Cardiovasc Res* 1994; **28**: 25–30.

43 Kourembanas S, Marsden PA, McQuillan LP, Faller DV. Hypoxia induces endothelin gene expression and secretion in cultured human endothelium. *J Clin Invest* 1991; **88**: 1054–7.

44 Sharefkin JB, Duamond SL, Eskin SG, McIntire LV, Dieffenbach CW. Fluid flow decreases preproendothelin I/mRNA levels and suppresses endothelin-1 peptide release in cultured human endothelial cells. *J Vasc Surg* 1991; **14**: 1–9.

45 Pearson PJ, Lin PJ, Schaff HV. Production of endothelium-derived contracting factor is enhanced after coronary reperfusion. *Ann Thorac Surg* 1991; **51**: 788–93.

46 Lerman A, Sandok EK, Hildebrand FL Jr, Burnett JC Jr. Inhibition of endothelium-derived relaxing factor enhances endothelin-mediated vasoconstriction. *Circulation* 1992; **85**: 1894–8.

47 Brutsaert DL, Sys SU. Ventricular function: Is the total more than the sum of the parts? *Circulation* 1991; **83**: 1444–9.

48 Ishikawa T, Yanagisawa M, Kimura S, Goto K, Masaki T. Positive inotropic action of a novel vasoconstrictor peptide endothelin on guinea pig atria. *Am J Physiol* 1988; **255**: H970–3.

49 Gregg DE. Effect of coronary perfusion pressure or coronary flow on oxygen usage of the myocardium. *Circ Res* 1963; **13**: 497–500.

50 Kitakaze M, Marban E. Cellular mechanism of the modulation of contractile function by coronary perfusion pressure in ferret hearts. *J Physiol* 1989; **414**: 455–72.

51 Downey JM, Kirk ES. Inhibition of coronary blood flow by a vascular waterfall mechanism. *Circ Res* 1975; **36**: 753–60.

52 Downey JM, Kirk ES. Distribution of the coronary blood flow across the canine heart wall during systole. *Circ Res* 1974; **34**: 251–7.

53 Westerhof N. Physiological hypotheses—intramyocardial pressure. A new concept, suggestions for measurement. *Basic Res Cardiol* 1990; **85**: 105–19.

54 Doucette JW, Goto M, Flynn AE, Austin RE Jr, Husseini WK, Hoffman JIE. Effects of cardiac contraction and cavity pressure on myocardial blood flow. *Am J Physiol* 1993; **265**: H1342–52.

55 Chilian WM, Marcus ML. Effects of coronary and extravascular pressure on intramyocardial and epicardial blood velocity. *Am J Physiol* 1985; **248**: H170–8.

56 Goto M, Flynn AE, Doucette JW, *et al.* Effect of intracoronary nitroglycerin administration on phasic pattern and transmural distribution of flow during coronary artery stenosis. *Circulation* 1992; **85**: 2296–304.

57 Canty JF, Klocke F, Mates RE. Pressure and tone dependence of coronary diastolic input impedance and capacitance. *Am J Physiol* 1985; **248**: H700–11.

58 Hoffman JIE. Transmural myocardial perfusion. In: Kajiya F, Klassen GA, Spaan JAE, Hoffman JIE, eds, *Coronary circulation—basic mechanism and clinical relevance.* Tokyo: Springer-Verlag, 1990: 141–52.

59 Goto M, Flynn AE, Doucette JW, *et al.* Cardiac contraction affects deep myocardial vessels predominantly. *Am J Physiol* 1991; **261**: H1417–29.

60 Flynn AE, Coggins DL, Goto M, *et al.* Does systolic subepicardial perfusion come from retrograde subendocardial flow? *Am J Physiol* 1992; **262**: H1759–69.

61 Feigl EO. Coronary physiology. *Physiol Rev* 1983; **63**: 1–206.

62 Marcus ML, Chilian WM, Kanatsuka H, Dellsperger KC, Eastham CL, Lamping KG. Understanding the coronary circulation through studies at the microvascular level. *Circulation* 1990; **82**: 1–7.

63 Mulvany MJ, Aalkjaer C. Structure and function of small arteries. *Physiol Rev* 1990; **70**: 921–61.

64 Maseri A, Crea F, Cianflone D. Myocardial ischemia caused by distal coronary vasoconstriction. *Am J Cardiol* 1992; **70**: 1602–5.

65 Chilian WM, Layne SM. Coronary microvascular responses to reductions in perfusion pressure: Evidence for persistent arteriolar vasomotor tone during coronary hypoperfusion. *Circ Res* 1990; **66**: 1227–38.

66 Hoffman JIE, Spaan JAE. Pressure–flow relations in coronary circulation. *Physiol Rev* 1990; **70**: 331–90.

67 Rees DD, Palmer RM, Moncada S. Role of endothelium-derived nitric oxide in the regulation of blood pressure. *Proc Natl Acad Sci USA* 1989; **86**: 3375–8.

68 Maseri A. Coronary vasoconstriction: visible and invisible. *N Engl J Med* 1991; **325**: 1579–80.

69 Maseri A, Crea F. Segmental control of vascular tone in the coronary circulation and pathophysiology of ischemic heart disease. *J Appl Cardiovasc Biol* 1991; **2**: 163–73.

70 Maseri A, Crea F, Kaski JC, Crake T. Mechanisms of angina pectoris in syndrome X. *J Am Coll Cardiol* 1991; **17**: 499–506.

71 Chilian WM, Layne SM, Klausner EC, Eastham CL, Marcus ML. Redistribution of coronary microvascular resistance produced by dipyridamole. *Am J Physiol* 1989; **256**: H383–90.

72 Watanabe J, Levine MJ, Bellotto F, Johnson RG, Grossman W. Effects of coronary venous pressure on left ventricular distensibility. *Circ Res* 1990; **67**: 923–32.

73 Kuo L, Arko F, Chilian WM, Davis MJ. Coronary venular responses to flow and pressure. *Circ Res* 1993; **72**: 607–15.

74 Spaan JAE. Coronary diastolic pressure–flow relation and zero-flow pressure explained on the basis of intramyocardial compliance. *Circ Res* 1985; **56**: 293–309.

75 Klocke FJ, Mates RE, Canty JM Jr, Ellis AK. Coronary pressure–flow relationships. Controversial issues and probable implications. *Circ Res* 1985; **56**: 310–23.

76 Bellamy RF, Lowessohn HS, Ehrlich W, Baer RW. Effect of coronary sinus occlusion on coronary pressure–flow relations. *Am J Physiol* 1980; **239**: H57–64.

77 Cantin B, Rouleau JR. Myocardial tissue pressure and blood flow during coronary sinus pressure modulation in anesthetized dogs. *J Appl Physiol* 1992; **73**: 2184–91.

78 Bellamy RF. Diastolic coronary artery pressure–flow relations in the dog. *Circ Res* 1978; **43**: 92–101.

79 Kanatsuka H, Ashikawa K, Suzuki T, Komaru T, Suzuki T, Takishima T. Diameter change and pressure-red blood cell velocity relations in coronary microvessels during long diastoles in the canine left ventricle. *Circ Res* 1990; **66**: 503–10.

80 Messina LM, Hanley FL, Uhlig PN, Baer RW, Grattan MT, Hoffman JIE. Effects of pressure gradients between branches of the left coronary artery on the pressure axis intercept and the shape of steady state circumflex pressure–flow relations in dogs. *Circ Res* 1985; **56**: 11–19.

81 Mates RE, Klocke FJ, Canty JM Jr. Coronary capacitance. *Prog Cardiovasc Dis* 1988; **31**: 1–15.

82 Fahri ER, Klocke FJ, Mates RE, *et al*. Tone-dependent waterfall behavior during venous pressure elevation in isolated canine hearts. *Circ Res* 1991; **68**: 392–401.

83 Johnson PC. Review of previous studies and current theories of autoregulation. *Circ Res* 1964; **15** (suppl 1): 2–9.

84 Norris CP, Barnes GE, Smith EE, Granger HJ. Autoregulation of superior mesenteric flow in fasted and fed dogs. *Am J Physiol* 1979; **237**: H174–7.

85 Dole WP. Autoregulation of the coronary circulation. *Prog Cardiovasc Dis* 1987; **29**: 293–323.

86 Kanatsuka H, Lamping KG, Eastham CL, Marcus ML. Heterogeneous changes in epimyocardial microvascular size during graded coronary stenosis: Evidence of the microvascular site for autoregulation. *Circ Res* 1990; **66**: 389–96.

87 Hoffman JIE. Maximal coronary flow and the concept of coronary vascular reserve. *Circulation* 1984; **70**: 153–9.

88 Rooke GA, Feigl EO. Work as a correlate of canine left ventricular oxygen consumption, and the problem of catecholamine oxygen wasting. *Circ Res* 1982; **50**: 273–86.

89 Downey JM. Myocardial contractile force as a function of coronary blood flow. *Am J Physiol* 1976; **230**: 1–6.

90 Arnold G, Kosche F, Miessner E, Neitzert A, Lochner W. The importance of the perfusion pressure in the coronary arteries for the contractility and the oxygen consumption of the heart. *Pflügers Arch* 1968; **299**: 339–56.

91 Mosher P, Ross J Jr, McFate PA, Shaw FR. Control of coronary blood flow by an autoregulatory mechanism. *Circ Res* 1964; **14**: 250–9.

92 Broten TP, Feigl EO. Role of myocardial oxygen and carbon dioxide in coronary autoregulation. *Am J Physiol* 1992; **262**: H1231–7.

93 Dole WP, Nuno DW. Myocardial oxygen tension determines the degree and pressure range of coronary autoregulation. *Circ Res* 1986; **59**: 202–15.

94 Canty JM Jr. Coronary pressure–function and steady-state pressure–flow relations during autoregulation in the unanesthetized dog. *Circ Res* 1988; **63**: 821–36.

95 Hoffman JIE. Transmural myocardial perfusion. *Prog Cardiovasc Dis* 1987; **29**: 429–64.

96 Canty JM Jr, Giglia J, Kandath D. Effect of tachycardia on regional function and transmural myocardial perfusion during graded coronary pressure reduction in conscious dogs. *Circulation* 1990; **82**: 1815–25.

97 Yonekura S, Watanabe N, Caffrey JL, Gaugl JF, Downey HF. Mechanism of attenuated pressure–flow autoregulation in right coronary circulation of dogs. *Circ Res* 1987; **60**: 133–41.

98 Yonekura S, Watanabe N, Downey HF. Transmural variation in autoregulation of right ventricular blood flow. *Circ Res* 1988; **62**: 776–81.

99 Smolich JJ, Weissberg PL, Broughton A, Korner PI. Comparison of left and right ventricular blood flow responses during arterial pressure reduction in the autonomically blocked dog: evidence for right ventricular autoregulation. *Cardiovasc Res* 1988; **22**: 17–24.

100 Feigl EO. Coronary autoregulation. *J Hypertens* 1989; **7** (suppl 4): S55–8.

101 Bassenge E, Heusch G. Endothelial and neuro-humoral control of coronary blood flow in health and disease. *Rev Physiol Biochem Pharmacol* 1990; **116**: 77–165.

102 Berne RM. The role of adenosine in the regulation of coronary blood flow. *Circ Res* 1980; **47**: 807–13.

103 Bardenheuer H, Schrader J. Supply-to-demand ratio for oxygen determines formation of adenosine by the heart. *Am J Physiol* 1986; **250**: H173–80.

104 Olsson RA, Bünger R. Metabolic control of coronary blood flow. *Prog Cardiovasc Dis* 1987; **29**: 369–87.

105 Hanley F, Grattan MT, Stevens MB, Hoffman JIE. Role of adenosine in coronary autoregulation. *Am J Physiol* 1986; **250**: H558–66.

106 Saito D, Steinhart CR, Nixon DG, Ollson RA. Intracoronary adenosine deaminase reduces canine myocardial reactive hyperemia. *Circ Res* 1981; **49**: 1262–7.

107 Randall JR, Jones CE. Adenosine antagonist aminophylline attenuates pacing-induced coronary functional hyperemia. *Am J Physiol* 1985; **248**: H1–7.

108 Dole WP, Yamada N, Bishop VS, Olsson RA. Role of adenosine in coronary blood flow regulation after reductions in perfusion pressure. *Circ Res* 1985; **56**: 517–24.

109 Downey HF, Merrill GF, Yonekura S, Watanabe N, Jones CE. Adenosine deaminase attenuates norepinephrine-induced coronary functional hyperemia. *Am J Physiol* 1988; **254**: H417–24.

110 Jones CE, Hurst TW, Randall JR. Effect of aminophylline on coronary functional hyperemia and myocardial adenosine. *Am J Physiol* 1982; **243**: H480–7.

111 Gewirtz H, Olsson RA, Brautigan DL, Brown PR, Most AS. Adenosine's role in regulating basal coronary arteriolar tone. *Am J Physiol* 1986; **250**: H1030–6.

112 McKenzie JE, Steffen RP, Haddy FJ. Effects of theophylline on adenosine production in the canine myocardium. *Am J Physiol* 1987; **252**: H204–10.

113 Kroll K, Feigl EO. Adenosine is unimportant in controlling coronary blood flow in unstressed dogs hearts. *Am J Physiol* 1985; **249**: H1176–87.

114 Bache RJ, Dai X-Z, Schwartz JS, Homans DC. Role of adenosine in coronary vasodilation during exercise. *Circ Res* 1988; **62**: 846–53.

115 Martin SE, Lenhard SD, Schmarkey LS, Offenbacher S, Odle BM. Adenosine regulates coronary blood flow during increased work and decreased supply. *Am J Physiol* 1993; **264**: H1438–46.

116 Aversano T, Ouyang P, Silverman H. Blockade of ATP-sensitive potassium channel modulates reactive hyperemia in the canine coronary circulation. *Circ Res* 1991; **69**: 618–23.

117 Komaru T, Lamping KG, Eastham CL, Dellsperger KC. Role of ATP-sensitive potassium channels in coronary microvascular autoregulatory responses. *Circ Res* 1991; **69**: 1146–51.

118 Nichols CG, Lederer WJ. Adenosine triphosphate-sensitive potassium channels in the cardiovascular system. *Am J Physiol* 1991; **261**: H1675–86.

119 Narishige T, Egashira K, Akatsuka Y, *et al.* Glibenclamide, a putative ATP-sensitive K^+ channel blocker, inhibits coronary autoregulation in anesthetized dogs. *Circ Res* 1993; **73**: 771–6.

120 Daut J, Maier-Rudolph W, Von Beckerath N, Mehrke G, Günther K, Goedel-Meiner L. Hypoxic dilation of coronary arteries is mediated by ATP-sensitive potassium channels. *Science* 1990; **247**: 1341–4.

121 Imamura Y, Tomoike H, Narishige T, Takahashi T, Kasuya T, Takeshita T. Glibenclamide decreases basal coronary blood flow in anesthetized dogs. *Am J Physiol* 1992; **263**: H339–404.

122 Clapp LH, Gurney AM. ATP-sensitive K^+ channels regulate resting potential of pulmonary arterial smooth muscle cells. *Am J Physiol* 1992; **262**: H916–20.

123 Miyoshi Y, Nakaya Y, Wakatsuki T, *et al.* Endothelin blocks ATP-sensitive K^+ channels and depolarizes smooth muscle cells of porcine coronary artery. *Circ Res* 1992; **70**: 612–16.

124 Kuo L, Davis MJ, Chilian WM. Endothelium-dependent, flow-induced dilation of isolated coronary arterioles. *Am J Physiol* 1990; **259**: H1063–70.

125 Kuo L, Davis MJ, Chilian WM. Myogenic activity in isolated subepicardial and subendocardial coronary arterioles. *Am J Physiol* 1988; **255**: H1558–62.

126 McHale PA, Dube GP, Greenfield JC Jr. Evidence for myogenic vasomotor activity in the coronary circulation. *Prog Cardiovasc Dis* 1987; **30**: 139–46.

127 Hoffman JIE. A critical review of coronary reserve. *Circulation* 1987; **75** (suppl I): I-6-11.

128 Bradley AJ, Alpert JS. Coronary flow reserve. *Am J Cardiol* 1991; **122**: 1116–28.

129 Collins P. Coronary flow reserve. *Br Heart J* 1993; **69**: 279–81.

130 Gould KL, Lipscomb K. Effect of coronary stenoses on coronary flow reserve and resistance. *Am J Cardiol* 1974; **34**: 48–55.
131 Marcus ML, Wright C, Doty D, *et al.* Measurements of coronary velocity and reactive hyperemia in the coronary circulation of humans. *Circ Res* 1981; **49**: 877–91.
132 Gould KL, Lipscomb K, Hamilton GW. Physiologic basis for assessing critical coronary stenosis. *Am J Cardiol* 1974; **33**: 87–94.
133 Olsson RA, Bugni WJ. Coronary circulation. In: Fozzard HA, Haber E, Jennings RB, Katz AM, Morgan HE, eds, *The heart and cardiovascular system. Scientific Foundations*. New York: Raven Press, 1986: 987–1037.
134 Canty JM Jr, Klocke FJ. Reduced regional myocardial perfusion in the presence of pharmacological vasodilator reserve. *Circulation* 1985; **71**: 370–7.
135 Brown BG, Josephson MA, Peterson RB, *et al.* Intravenous dipyridamole combined with isometric handgrip for near maximal acute increase in coronary flow in patients with coronary artery disease. *Am J Cardiol* 1981; **48**: 1077–85.
136 Van Winkle DM, Feigl EO. Acetylcholine causes coronary vasodilation in dogs and baboons. *Circ Res* 1989; **65**: 1580–93.
137 Hodgson JMB, Marshall JJ. Direct vasoconstriction and endothelium-dependent vasodilation: Mechanisms of acetylcholine effects on coronary flow and arterial diameter in patients with nonstenotic coronary arteries. *Circulation* 1989; **79**: 1043–51.
138 Ludmer PL, Selwyn AP, Shook TL, *et al.* Paradoxical vasoconstriction induced by acetylcholine in atherosclerotic coronary arteries. *N Engl J Med* 1986; **315**: 1046–51.
139 Feigl EO. EDRF—a protective factor? *Nature* 1988; **331**: 490–1.
140 Chilian WM, Layne SM, Eastham CL, Marcus ML. Heterogeneous microvascular coronary alpha-adrenergic vasoconstriction. *Circ Res* 1989; **64**: 376–88.
141 Chen DG, Dai X-Z, Zimmermann BG, Bache RJ. Postsynaptic α_1- and α_2-adrenergic mechanisms in coronary vasoconstriction. *J Cardiovasc Pharmacol* 1988; **11**: 61–7.
142 Heusch G, Deussen A. Nifedipine prevents sympathetic vasoconstriction distal to severe coronary stenoses. *J Cardiovasc Pharmacol* 1984; **6**: 378–83.
143 Harrison DG, Sellke FW, Quillen JE. Neurohumoral regulation of coronary collateral vasomotor tone. *Basic Res Cardiol* 1990; **85** (suppl I): 121–9.
144 Feigl EO. Control of myocardial oxygen tension by sympathetic coronary vasoconstriction in the dog. *Circ Res* 1975; **37**: 88–95.
145 Mohrman DE, Feigl EO. Competition between sympathetic vasoconstriction and metabolic vasodilation in the canine coronary circulation. *Circ Res* 1978; **42**: 79–86.
146 Murray PA, Vatner SF. α-Adrenoceptor attenuation of coronary vascular response to severe exercise in the conscious dog. *Circ Res* 1979; **45**: 654–60.
147 Feigl EO. The paradox of adrenergic coronary vasoconstriction. *Circulation* 1987; **76**: 737–45.
148 Heusch G. α-Adrenergic mechanisms in myocardial ischemia. *Circulation* 1990; **81**: 1–13.
149 Ellis AK, Klocke FJ. Effects of preload on the transmural distribution of perfusion and pressure–flow relationships in the canine coronary vascular bed. *Circ Res* 1979; **46**: 68–77.
150 Huang AH, Feigl EO. Adrenergic coronary vasoconstriction helps maintain uniform transmural blood flow distribution during exercise. *Circ Res* 1988; **62**: 286–98.
151 Baumgart D, Ehring T, Kowallik P, Guth BD, Krajcar M, Heusch G. Impact of α-adrenergic coronary vasoconstriction on the transmural myocardial blood flow distribution during humoral and neuronal adrenergic activation. *Circ Res* 1993; **73**: 869–86.
152 Mudge GH, Grossman W, Mill RM Jr, Lesch M, Braunwald E. Reflex increase in coronary vascular resistance in patients with ischemic heart disease. *N Engl J Med* 1976; **295**: 1333–7.
153 Gwirtz PA, Dodd-O JM, Downey F, *et al.* Effects of a coronary α_1-constriction on transmural left ventricular flow and contractile function. *Am J Physiol* 1992; **262**: H965–72.
154 Seitelberger R, Guth BD, Heusch G, Lee J-D, Katayama K, Ross J Jr. Intracoronary α_2-adrenergic receptor blockade attenuates ischemia in conscious dogs during exercise. *Circ Res* 1988; **62**: 436–42.
155 Nathan HJM, Feigl EO. Adrenergic coronary vasoconstriction lessens transmural steal during coronary hypoperfusion. *Am J Physiol* 1986; **250**: H645–53.
156 Chilian WM, Ackell PH. Transmural differences in sympathetic coronary constriction during exercise in the presence of coronary stenosis. *Circ Res* 1988; **62**: 216–25.

157 Toda N. Response of isolated monkey coronary arteries to catecholamines and to transmural electrical stimulation. *Circ Res* 1981; **49**: 1228–36.

158 Trivella MG, Broten TP, Feigl EO. β-Receptor subtypes in the canine coronary circulation. *Am J Physiol* 1990; **259**: H1575–585.

159 Miyashiro JK, Feigl EO. Feedforward control of coronary blood flow via coronary β-receptor stimulation. *Circ Res* 1993; **73**: 252–63.

160 Feldman RD, Christy JP, Paul ST, Harrison DG. β-Adrenergic receptors on canine coronary collateral vessels: Characterization and function. *Am J Physiol* 1989; **257**: H1634–9.

161 Parent R, Al-Obaidi M, Lavallée M. Nitric oxide formation contributes to β-adrenergic dilation of resistance coronary vessels in conscious dogs. *Circ Res* 1993; **73**: 241–51.

162 Gulbenkian S, Opgaard OS, Ekman R, *et al*. Peptidergic innervation of human epicardial coronary arteries. *Circ Res* 1993; **73**: 579–88.

163 Tseng C-J, Robertson D, Light RT, Atkinson JR, Robertson RM. Neuropeptide Y is a vasoconstrictor of human coronary arteries. *Am J Med Sci* 1988; **296**: 11–16.

164 Clarke JG, Davies GJ, Kerwin R, *et al*. Coronary artery infusion of neuropeptide Y in patients with angina pectoris. *Lancet* 1987; **i**: 1057–59.

165 Sheikh SP, Håkanson R, Schwartz TW. Y_1 and Y_2 receptors for neuropeptide Y. *FEBS Lett* 1989; **245**: 209–14.

166 Gulbenkian S, Edvinsson L, Saetrum Opgaard O, Valença A, Wharton J, Polak JM. Neuropeptide Y modulates the action of vasodilator agents in guinea pig epicardial coronary arteries. *Regul Pept* 1992; **40**: 351–62.

167 Franco-Cereceda A. Calcitonin gene-related peptide and human epicardial coronary arteries: presence, release and vasodilator effects. *Br J Pharmacol* 1991; **102**: 506–610.

168 Yamamoto H, Yoshimura H, Noma M, Kai H, Kikuchi Y. Preservation of endothelium-dependent vasodilation in the spastic segment of the human epicardial coronary artery by substance P. *Am Heart J* 1992; **123**: 298–303.

169 Ludman PF, Maseri A, Clark P, Davies GJ. Effects of calcitonin gene-related peptide on normal and atheromatous vessels and on resistance vessels in the coronary circulation in humans. *Circulation* 1991; **84**: 1993–2000.

170 Wharton J, Gulbenkian S. Peptides in the mammalian cardiovascular system. *Experientia* 1987; **43**: 821–32.

171 Huang M, Roorstad OP. VIP receptors in mesenteric and coronary arteries: a radioligand binding study. *Peptides* 1987; **8**: 477–85.

172 Ludman PF, Poole-Wilson PA. Myocardial perfusion in humans: What can we measure? *Br Heart J* 1993; **70**: 307–14.

173 Domenech RJ, Hoffmann JIE, Nobel MIM, Saunders KB, Henson JR, Subijanto S. Total and regional coronary blood flow measured by radioactive microspheres in conscious and anesthetized dogs. *Circ Res* 1969; **25**: 581–96.

174 Marshall WG, Boatman GB, Dickerson G, Perlin A, Todd EP, Utley JR. Shunting, release, and distribution of nine and fifteen micron spheres in myocardium. *Surgery* 1976; **79**: 631–637.

175 Kety SS, Schmidt CF. The determination of cerebral blood flow in man by the use of nitrous oxide in low concentrations. *Am J Physiol* 1945; **143**: 53–66.

176 White CW, Wilson RF, Marcus ML. Methods of measuring myocardial blood flow in humans. *Prog Cardiovasc Dis* 1988; **31**: 79–94.

177 Cannon PJ, Dell RB, Dwyer EM Jr. Measurement of regional myocardial perfusion in man with 133 xenon and scintillation camera. *J Clin Invest* 1972; **51**: 964–77.

178 Morgan SM, Fisher JD, Horwitz LD. Validation of regional myocardial flow measurements with scintillation camera detection of xenon-133. *Invest Radiol* 1978; **13**: 132–7.

179 Doucette JW, Corl PD, Payne HM, *et al*. Validation of a Doppler guide wire for intravascular measurement of coronary artery flow velocity. *Circulation* 1992; **85**: 1899–911.

180 Ganz W, Tamura K, Marcus HS, Donoso R, Yoshida S, Swan HJ. Measurement of coronary sinus blood flow by continuous thermodilution in man. *Circulation* 1971; **44**: 181–95.

181 Vogel R, LeFree M, Bates E, *et al*. Application of digital techniques to selective coronary arteriography. *Am Heart J* 1984; **107**: 153–64.

182 Hutchins GD, Schwaiger M, Rosenspire KC, Krivokapich J, Schelbert H, Kuhl DE. Noninvasive quantification of regional blood flow in the human heart using N-13 ammonia and dynamic position emission tomographic imaging. *J Am Coll Cardiol* 1990; **15**: 1032–42.

5: The pulmonary circulation

KEITH SYKES

William Harvey reported the experiments which led him to conclude that blood must flow through the lungs in *De Motu Cordis* in 1628[1] but it was not until 1661 that Malpighi described the microscopic appearance of the pulmonary capillaries which provided the anatomical link between the right and left heart.[2] In 1894 Bradford and Dean[3] reported that the pulmonary artery pressure increased during hypoxia, but it was not until 1946 that von Euler and Liljestrand[4] concluded that this was the result of hypoxic pulmonary vasoconstriction, and suggested that this mechanism might improve the matching of perfusion to ventilation at the alveolar level. Nissel's subsequent demonstration of hypoxic vasoconstriction in the isolated perfused lung confirmed that this was a local response and not mediated by the autonomic system.[5] Meanwhile, the introduction of the cardiac catheter into clinical practice[6] in the 1940s had led to studies of the haemodynamics of the heart and lungs, and to the subsequent development of closed and, later, open heart surgery in the 1950s. The subsequent introduction of radio-isotope methods for measuring the distribution of ventilation and blood flow, and the development of practical methods of measuring gas and blood gas tensions, resulted in a vast increase in our understanding of the mechanisms governing gas exchange. Later studies have shown that the pulmonary circulation has three other important roles:

1 It has a regulatory function (for example, as part of the renin–angiotensin system)
2 It takes up or metabolises certain drugs (such as propranolol, lignocaine, and noradrenaline)
3 It filters out particulate matter (such as platelet or fat emboli).

The pulmonary circulation is also concerned with the generation of surfactant, which maintains alveolar stability, and with the exchange of water. As anaesthesia, mechanical ventilation, and surgery may produce major changes in the pulmonary circulation, it is important that the anaesthetist should have a clear understanding of the factors that govern the distribution of pulmonary blood flow. Readers interested in the pharmacological aspects of the lung are referred to a review by Bakhle.[7]

The mechanisms affecting the distribution of blood flow in the normal lung will be considered first. This will be followed by a discussion on the effects of posture, haemorrhage, mechanical ventilation, and lung disease. The methods of studying the pulmonary circulation will then be outlined, followed by a brief review of the way in which anaesthetic and related drugs may alter the distribution of blood flow, and so affect the efficiency of gas exchange. Finally, we shall consider the problem of pulmonary hypertension and the effects produced by pulmonary vasodilator drugs.

Anatomy and physiology

The pulmonary circulation extends from the right outflow tract to the left atrium. Blood from the right ventricle passes into the thin walled pulmonary artery which then branches repeatedly in parallel with the bronchi to supply the pulmonary capillary network surrounding the alveoli. The walls of the larger arteries contain more elastic tissue than smooth muscle, but smooth muscle predominates in arteries less than 1 mm in diameter. The pulmonary capillaries are 7–10 μm in diameter and form a dense network around the alveoli. They normally contain about 40% of the pulmonary blood volume, the volume contained in the pulmonary arteries, capillaries, and veins being about 120, 250, and 150 ml respectively, although these values are greatly influenced by the conditions of measurement. The blood from the capillaries is collected into the pulmonary veins which run alongside the arteries, bronchi, and lymphatics in the interstitial space, and finally drains into the left atrium. Although there is some autonomic control of the pulmonary circulation, it appears to be relatively unimportant.

There are three requirements for efficient gas exchange:

- the gas exchanging surface between the alveoli and pulmonary capillary blood must have a large area
- the alveolar–capillary membrane must be thin to ensure that there is little hindrance to diffusion
- there must be correct matching of ventilation to perfusion.

To achieve a perfect distribution of blood flow throughout the 30 cm height of the erect adult lung, it would be necessary to have a high pulmonary artery pressure and thick muscular arteries to overcome the effects of gravity. The lung is, however, unique in that it has to receive the whole of the cardiac output, and this may vary from 1–2 l/min in severe shock to 20–25 l/min in exercise. Furthermore, such changes in flow must be accommodated without imposing an undue load on the right heart. These constraints have led to the development of a low pressure, low resistance, pulmonary circulation in which distributon is relatively poorly controlled, but in which increases in flow are accommodated by the recruitment of extra vessels and the distension of vessels that are already open. The increase in flow thus increases the cross sectional area of the vascular bed and so decreases the total pulmonary vascular resistance. So effective is this mechanism that a doubling of flow can be accommodated with a rise of pulmonary artery pressure of only 2–5 mm Hg when the patient is in the erect position.

Gravity and the distribution of pulmonary blood flow

As there is a close anatomical relationship between the pulmonary vasculature and the alveoli, the dimensions of the vessels will be affected by the relationship between the vascular and alveolar pressures, and by changes in lung volume. The effects will depend on the location of the vessels. The large *extrapulmonary vessels* are situated outside the lung and within the mediastinum, and are thus affected by changes in pleural pressure, although these are probably modified by regional variations in pleural pressure and by local mechanical distortions around the hilum. The *intrapulmonary vessels* are situated within the lung but may be subdivided into three groups according to their anatomical location:

- the alveolar
- the extra-alveolar
- the corner vessels.

The alveolar vessels

The alveolar vessels are the pulmonary capillaries which are compressed when lung volume is increased by an increase in the transpulmonary pressure difference across the lung. Blood flow through these capillaries depends on the relationship of the alveolar pressure, the pulmonary artery pressure, and the pulmonary venous pressure, and so results in the gravitational distribution of blood flow described by West.[8] In the upright lung (with a height of 30 cm in the adult) three zones may be distinguished.

Zone 1 is the area in the non-dependent part of the lung in which alveolar pressure exceeds pulmonary artery pressure. This results in compression of the capillaries so that there is no blood flow or gas exchange. Continued ventilation of alveoli in this zone contributes to the alveolar dead space. In the supine position, however, the pulmonary artery pressure is usually greater than the vertical distance between the right atrium and the non-dependent part of the lung, so there is usually no zone 1 (fig 5.1).

In zone 2 pulmonary artery pressure is greater than alveolar pressure, which is, in turn, greater than pulmonary venous pressure, so capillary blood flow is present and increases linearly down the zone. The cause of the increase in flow is still debated, some workers suggesting that the capillaries behave like a Starling resistor, so that more vessels are recruited in the lower parts of the zone, whereas others claim that the increase in flow down the zone is the result of increased distension of the vessels. It has also been suggested that there are critical opening pressures, as there are in the systemic circulation, and that these must be overcome before blood flow

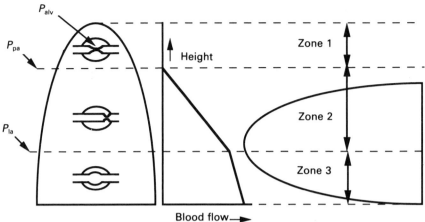

Fig 5.1 The three zone model of the lung. Left: upright lung. Centre: blood flow versus lung height. Right: supine lung. In zone 1 alveolar pressure (P_{alv}) exceeds both pulmonary artery pressure (P_{pa}) and left atrial pressure (P_{la}) so the capillaries are collapsed and there is no blood flow. In zone 2 pulmonary artery pressure is greater than alveolar pressure, but the alveolar pressure is greater than left atrial pressure, so that the capillaries behave as Starling resistors. In zone 3 both P_{pa} and P_{la} exceed P_{alv}. All the capillaries are open so that the small increase in flow down the zone is due to further distension. As the height of the supine lung is less than that of the vertical lung, there is usually no zone 1.

occurs. Others have suggested that there are local control mechanisms which cause different capillary beds to open in sequence.

In zone 3 both pulmonary arterial and venous pressures exceed alveolar pressure. It is believed that all the capillaries are open, and that the small increase in flow down the zone results from further distension. A fourth zone of reduced flow in the most dependent parts of the lung has also been described. The presence of zone 4 was first noted in experimental perfusion preparations and was attributed to the formation of pulmonary oedema; this may well be the explanation for a reduced dependent zone flow in patients with left ventricular failure. Zone 4 has, however, also been demonstrated in normal patients, particularly at low lung volumes. The reduction in flow could be caused by narrowing of the extra-alveolar vessels resulting from a gravitationally induced decrease in lung volume in dependent zones or to hypoxic pulmonary vasoconstriction secondary to decreased ventilation caused by airway closure. It could also be caused by the increased vascular resistance resulting from the longer pathway from the hilum to the periphery of the lung. This theory is supported by the demonstration that, in the coronal plane, flow is less at the lung periphery than at the hilum.

The extra-alveolar vessels

The extra-alveolar vessels are the arteries and veins that connect the large extrapulmonary vessels to the alveolar–capillary network. They run parallel to the bronchi and are surrounded by an interstitial space which contains fluid, lymphatics, and the fibrous framework of the lung. The transmural pressure, which determines the diameter of these vessels, depends on the intravascular pressure and the interstitial pressure. The pressure in the interstitial space is generated by the elastic recoil of surrounding alveolar units and is believed to approximate to the subatmospheric pleural pressure. Both the intravascular pressure and the regional pleural pressure will be affected by the vertical height of the lung region and by the effects of gravity. There may also be regional variations in interstitial pressure caused by differences in regional lung expansion resulting from disease. For example, the reduction in lung volume resulting from an area of atelectasis causes the pleural pressure over that area to be more subatmospheric (that is, to have a lower absolute pressure) than the pressure in the remainder of the pleural space. The resulting increase in transmural pressure may increase the diameter of the extra-alveolar vessels and so decrease the effectiveness of hypoxic vasoconstriction.[9] In general, expansion of the lung will tend to reduce absolute interstitial pressure, so dilating the extra-alveolar vessels, whereas interstitial oedema will tend to increase absolute interstitial pressure and so will narrow them. This may account for the reduced basal blood flow in patients with mitral stenosis.

The corner vessels

The third type of intrapulmonary vessels are the corner vessels. These are small vessels situated at the junction of three alveoli. They are surrounded by an interstitial space, but it is not clear whether this is an extension of the space surrounding the extra-alveolar vessels. The importance of the corner vessels is that they appear to be shielded from the compressive effects of increased alveolar pressure and so permit some flow to occur in zone 1 conditions. It seems probable that this flow only occurs in systole and that it has little effect on gas exchange.

Effects of lung volume on pulmonary vascular resistance

The pulmonary vascular resistance is calculated by dividing the driving pressure (pulmonary artery minus left atrial pressure) by the flow, so it includes the resistance of all the vessels between the right and left heart. The importance of the differentiation between intra- and extra-alveolar vessels is that changes in lung volume exert opposing effects on the two sets of vessels. Expansion of the lung will occur when transpulmonary pressure is increased, whether this is produced by a reduction in absolute pleural pressure or an increase in alveolar pressure, and this will compress the intra-alveolar vessels and so *increase* their resistance to blood flow. These changes will also tend to increase the size of zone 1 and so to increase alveolar dead space. On the other

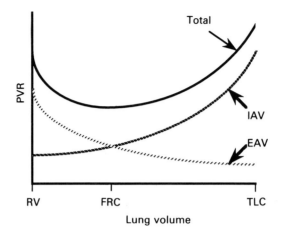

Fig 5.2 The contribution of the resistance of the intra-alveolar (IAV) and extra-alveolar (EAV) vessels to the total pulmonary vascular resistance (PVR) at different lung volumes. Total resistance is minimal at the functional residual capacity (FRC).

hand, expansion of the lung, by whatever means, will increase the diameter of extra-alveolar vessels and so *decrease* their resistance. The diameter of the extrapulmonary vessels will also tend to increase when absolute pleural pressure is decreased, but as these vessels are large the effects on resistance will be relatively small, and these effects may be offset by local distortions of the hilum associated with the expansion of the lung.

As the extra-alveolar vessels are narrow at low lung volumes but expanded at high lung volumes, whereas the pulmonary capillaries are compressed at high lung volumes and open at low lung volumes, the pressure–volume curve for the whole lung is U shaped, the resistance being minimal at the normal end expiratory position or functional residual capacity (fig 5.2). The different effects of lung volume changes on the intra- and extra-alveolar vessels also cause changes in the distribution of blood flow with lung volume, the increase in blood flow down the lung being completely abolished at residual volume.

Clinical implications

It has already been pointed out that effective gas exchange can only be maintained if ventilation and perfusion are evenly matched throughout the lung. Fortunately, the gravitationally induced increase in blood flow down the lung is normally matched by an increase in ventilation. This increase is generated by the interaction between the non-linear pressure–volume curve of the lung and the gravitationally induced gradient of pleural pressure (fig 5.3). When the lung is vertical (height 30 cm) the pressure in the pleural space is about -1 kPa (-10 cm H_2O) in the non-dependent areas and about -0.25 kPa (-2.5 cm H_2O) in dependent zones at the normal end expiratory

144

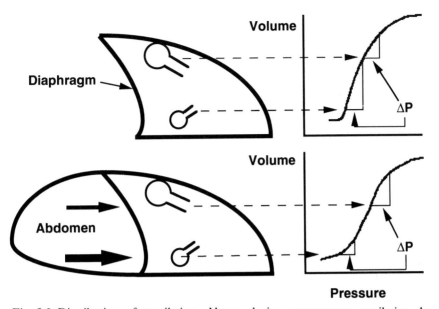

Fig 5.3 Distribution of ventilation. Above: during spontaneous ventilation the gravitationally induced gradient of pleural pressure causes the non-dependent alveoli to lie on the upper, curved part of the lung pressure–volume curve, whereas the dependent alveoli lie on the lower, steep portion. As a result the increase in transpulmonary pressure (ΔP) during inspiration causes more ventilation to enter the dependent zones of the lung. Below: the absence of diaphragmatic activity during controlled ventilation permits the hydrostatic pressure generated by the abdominal contents to influence distribution. The position of the alveoli on the pressure–volume curve of the total respiratory system (that is, lung plus chest wall) now causes ventilation to be preferentially distributed to the non-dependent zones. Note that changes in end expiratory lung volume may modify the distribution by moving the alveoli to different portions of the P/V curves.

lung volume. The resulting transpulmonary pressure of 1 kPa (10 cm H_2O) at the top of the lung and 0·25 kPa (2·5 cm H_2O) at the base causes the upper alveoli to have a larger resting volume than those at the base. When the transpulmonary pressure is increased by a reduction in absolute pleural pressure during inspiration, however, the lower alveoli will expand more than the upper because they lie on a steeper part of the pressure–volume curve. Thus, under normal conditions, the increase in ventilation down the lung (which is about half that of the increase in blood flow) minimises ventilation–perfusion inequalities (fig 5.4). If, however, there is dependent airway closure as a result of a loss of lung elastic recoil or of a reduction in functional residual capacity, there may be no ventilation to dependent zones during the early part of inspiration, so that these zones develop low ventilation–perfusion ratios and arterial P_{O_2} (P_{aO_2}) is reduced.

145

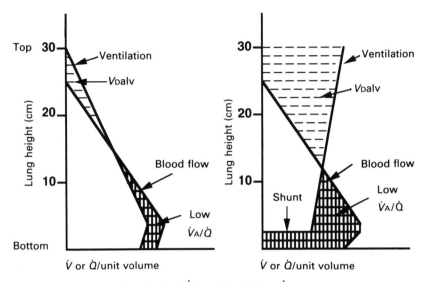

Fig 5.4 Distribution of ventilation ($\dot{V}$) and blood flow ($\dot{Q}$) plotted against lung height during spontaneous respiration (left) and during anaesthesia with controlled ventilation (right). Note that the small alveolar dead space (V_{Dalv}) associated with zone 1 conditions during spontaneous respiration is increased by the greater ventilation to non-dependent zones during controlled ventilation. In elderly people there is often an area with low ventilation–perfusion ($\dot{V}_A/\dot{Q}$) ratios at the base of the lung associated with airway closure. General anaesthesia usually results in the development of a shunt in dependent lung zones as a result of compression collapse.

During controlled ventilation the distribution of ventilation is determined by the shape of the total respiratory (lung plus chest wall) pressure–volume curve because the inspiratory muscles are no longer active. Furthermore, in the supine position, the hydrostatic pressure produced by the semiliquid abdominal contents exerts an upward pressure on the dependent areas of the diaphragm so that ventilation is preferentially directed into non-dependent zones. As the distribution of blood flow is still gravitationally determined there is gross mismatching of ventilation and perfusion (figs 5.3 and 5.4). The situation is exacerbated if there is a decrease in pulmonary artery pressure resulting from a reduction in blood volume, peripheral pooling of blood, or the administration of oxygen or a pulmonary vasodilator drug, because this will result in an increase in zone 1 with a further increase in alveolar dead space. Similar changes may occur if mean alveolar pressure is increased by mechanical ventilation with positive end expiratory pressure (PEEP), or if the emptying of the lung is delayed in patients with increased airway resistance (auto or intrinsic PEEP). When there is an increase in dead space/tidal volume ratio in the spontaneously breathing patient with normal respiratory control mechanisms, minute ventilation will tend to increase to compensate for the increased dead space so that P_{CO_2} is maintained at normal levels, but if the minute volume is controlled by a ventilator, P_{CO_2} may increase. If the rest of the lung is normal there will be no effects on P_{ao_2} other than those arising from any increase in P_{CO_2}.

In most patients undergoing anaesthesia or intensive care there is some alveolar collapse in dependent lung zones and this creates an intrapulmonary right to left shunt.[10] This is usually quantified by expressing the shunt as a percentage of the cardiac output. The P_{ao_2} resulting from a given shunt depends on the alveolar P_{O_2} (P_{AO_2}) (which in turn depends on the inspired P_{O_2} (P_{IO_2}), the alveolar P_{CO_2} (P_{ACO_2}) and the respiratory exchange ratio) and on the mixed venous P_{O_2} ($P_{\bar{v}O_2}$) (fig 5.5). Normally, it is assumed that an increase or decrease in the percentage shunt means that the volume of collapsed lung has increased or decreased. The percentage shunt may, however, change with no alteration of the volume of collapsed lung if the *proportion* of blood flowing through the oxygenated and collapsed zones is changed by an alteration in the pulmonary vascular pressures. For example, blood flow through a collapsed area of lung is maximal when it is in the dependent position but can be reduced by rotating the patient so that the collapsed area is uppermost, with a resultant decrease in shunt and increase

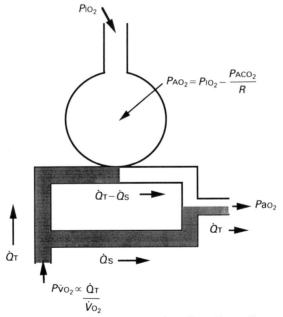

Fig 5.5 Factors governing arterial oxygen tension. P_{IO_2}, P_{AO_2}, P_{ACO_2}, inspired and alveolar gas tensions; R, respiratory exchange ratio (normally 0·8); P_{ao_2}, $P_{\bar{v}O_2}$, arterial and mixed venous oxygen tensions; $\dot{Q}s$ and $\dot{Q}T$, shunt flow and cardiac output; $\dot{V}_{O_2}$, oxygen consumption per minute. Note that the P_{ao_2} depends on both the proportion of blood flowing through the shunt and the $P_{\bar{v}O_2}$. $P_{\bar{v}O_2}$ depends on the relationship between $\dot{Q}T$ and $\dot{V}_{O_2}$.

147

in Pa_{O_2}.[11] (The improvement in oxygenation is not, however, usually sustained because collapse soon develops in the areas of lung now made dependent, whereas the collapse in the non-dependent zones disappears.)

The opposite effect may be seen in patients with dependent zone collapse when pulmonary artery pressure and cardiac output are decreased by vasodilator drugs. Under such circumstances the continued flow through the dependent zone with reduced flow to the ventilated area of lung will cause an apparent increase in the *proportion* of shunt, even though the actual flow through the shunt is unchanged (fig 5.6). The application of a high peak airway pressure or PEEP will also reduce flow through the ventilated non-dependent zones and so will have a similar effect. Another example is the redistribution of flow which may be seen during anaesthesia for thoracic surgery with a double lumen tube. When the upper lung is collapsed the effects of gravity and hypoxic vasoconstriction in the upper lung decrease the upper lung blood flow so that the shunt is only 20–30% instead of the 45–55% predicted from the relative volume of each lung. If the mean airway pressure in the dependent lung is increased, however, by the use of high peak or end expiratory pressures, shunt will increase because the compression of capillaries in the dependent lung increases pulmonary artery pressure and so diverts blood flow into the non-dependent collapsed lung (fig 5.7). The injection of pulmonary vasoconstrictor drugs will have a similar effect.

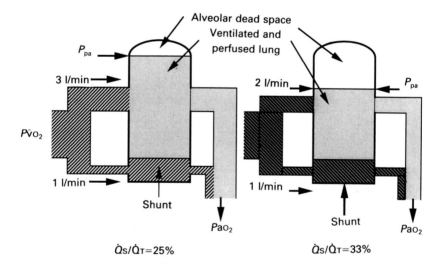

Fig 5.6 The effect of a decrease in pulmonary artery pressure (P_{pa}) resulting from a decrease in cardiac output on percentage shunt in the presence of dependent zone collapse or consolidation. If flow to the ventilated area of lung is decreased from 3 l/min to 2 l/min whilst flow through the shunt remains at 1 l/min the percentage shunt ($\dot{Q}_S/\dot{Q}_T$) will increase from 25% to 33%. Note that the resulting fall in arterial P_{O_2} (Pa_{O_2}) will be accentuated by the decrease in mixed venous P_{O_2} ($P\bar{v}_{O_2}$) resulting from the decrease in output.

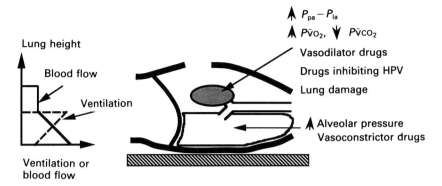

Fig 5.7 Factors that may increase flow through the non-dependent collapsed lung during one lung anaesthesia in the lateral position. The distribution of blood flow and ventilation with lung height is shown on the left of the diagram.

Another factor that affects the Pa_{O_2}, even when the areas of shunt are scattered throughout the lung and are not changed by alterations in lung volume, is the direct relationship between shunt and cardiac output. The increase in shunt with cardiac output occurs when the output is changed by altering blood volume or the administration of inotropic drugs and the cause is not properly understood. It is possible that the increase in flow increases pulmonary artery pressure and so opposes hypoxic vasoconstriction. However, an increase in output will usually increase $P\bar{v}_{O_2}$ and this may also reduce the magnitude of the vasoconstrictor response (see below). Although the increase in $P\bar{v}_{O_2}$ may increase the proportion of shunt it will also increase the oxygen saturation of the blood flowing through the shunt and so tend to offset the effects of the increased percentage shunt on Pa_{O_2}. Obviously, these interactions may lead to very variable effects on Pa_{O_2}.

Hypoxic pulmonary vasoconstriction

The pulmonary circulation differs from other vascular beds in that it constricts in response to hypoxia. The response is characterised by three important features:

- First, the response is present in an isolated perfused lung preparation and so must be controlled by some local mechanism.
- Second, the magnitude of pulmonary vasoconstriction is related to the PA_{O_2}, the response curve of blood flow against P_{O_2} being sigmoid in shape with the maximum decrease in flow occurring between P_{O_2} values of 8 and 4 kPa, and a reduction in PA_{O_2} to mixed venous levels resulting in a decrease in flow of about 50%. The apparent anomaly of a reduction in alveolar oxygen tension causing constriction of precapillary vessels (the pulmonary arteries <500 μm in diameter) has now been explained by the

149

demonstration that these small vessels are completely surrounded by alveoli so that alveolar gases can easily diffuse to the vessel wall.

- The third feature which characterises the response is that it can also be activated by a reduction in $P\bar{v}o_2$, although a decrease in $P\bar{v}o_2$ has about one third of the effect of a similar decrease in Pao_2. This suggests that the sensor site is situated within the smooth muscle of the arterial wall, but closer to the surrounding alveoli than to the lumen of the vessel.

The exact nature of the constrictor mechanism is still not understood although it now appears that the hypoxia acts directly on some aspect of metabolism in the smooth muscle cell.[12]

Hypoxic vasoconstriction results in a diversion of blood flow away from the hypoxic area of lung, so improving gas exchange.[13] It also produces an increase in pulmonary artery pressure. The magnitude of these effects depends on the volume of lung made hypoxic. If the hypoxic area is large there will be less normal lung to accommodate the diverted flow, so that there will be a greater increase in pressure. As the increase in smooth muscle tone is opposed by the intravascular pressure, there will be less diversion of flow when the rise in pulmonary artery pressure is increased.[14] Thus hypoxic pulmonary vasoconstriction is least effective when the volume of hypoxic lung is large or when pulmonary vascular pressures are increased by disease, fluid overload, or left heart failure.[15] The magnitude of the response to hypoxia is greatest in the newborn, varies between species and between individuals in any given species, and is reduced by hypothermia, sepsis,[16] trauma to the lung, liver cirrhosis,[17] and the action of many drugs.

An increase in Pco_2 has a more variable effect on pulmonary vascular tone, although it usually augments hypoxic pulmonary vasoconstricton and so increases the response to hypoventilation. A reduction in pH has a similar effect. As collapsed lung equilibrates with mixed venous blood gas tensions, the higher Pco_2 augments the diversion of blood flow away from a collapsed area of lung.[18] It now appears that the reduction in blood flow in collapsed lung is almost entirely the result of hypoxic vasoconstriction, and that the mechanical effect produced by narrowing of the extra-alveolar vessels is of only minor importance.

$Paco_2$ has a major effect on airway muscle tone, an increase causing bronchodilatation and a decrease bronchoconstriction. Thus alveolar gas concentrations act on both the airways and the pulmonary circulation in a manner that tends to minimise ventilation–perfusion inequalities.

Nitric oxide and vasomotor tone

In recent years it has become clear that the endothelium plays a major role in controlling vascular tone.[19] Both pulmonary and systemic vessels have been shown to release a labile endothelium derived relaxing factor (EDRF) which modifies the vasopressor response to various pharmacological agents

---

General factors decreasing hypoxic pulmonary vasoconstriction

Chronic hypoxia
Increased mixed venous P_{O_2} ($P\bar{v}_{O_2}$)
Increased pH
Decreased arterial or mixed venous P_{CO_2} (Pa_{CO_2} or $P\bar{v}_{CO_2}$)
Increased vascular pressures
Increased volume of hypoxic lung
Increased transpulmonary pressures
Hypothermia
Handling or trauma to lung
Endotoxin
Pneumonia
Cirrhosis

---

and to acute hypoxia. It is now clear that EDRF is nitric oxide (NO). The NO is synthesised from L-arginine by nitric oxide synthase. It then diffuses within the cell, or to another cell, where it stimulates soluble guanylyl cyclase or other haem containing proteins. This results in an increase in cyclic guanosine monophosphate (GMP) which produces the physiological effect. For example, in smooth muscle cells cyclic GMP decreases cell calcium which leads to relaxation of the muscle cell and vasodilatation. As nitric oxide has a high affinity for haemoglobin with the formation of methaemoglobin, it has a half life measured in seconds. It is also rapidly oxidised to nitrite and nitrate by superoxide radical in the blood vessel wall or by oxygen in free solution.

Vascular tone is controlled by opposing factors which cause constriction or dilatation. Dilatation is induced by acetylcholine, bradykinin, angiotensin converting enzyme inhibitors, and adenine nucleotides, all of which stimulate NO production. It seems likely that pulsatile flow and local shear stress may play an important role in the control of NO release in vivo. There is, however, now evidence that NO may also influence blood pressure by regulating sympathetic nerve activity. Nitric oxide decreases hypoxic vaso-constriction in the lung, and there is evidence that there is either decreased production or increased destruction of NO in systemic and pulmonary hypertension and in ischaemic heart disease. Excessive production of NO may be the cause of the profound vasodilatation in septic shock. Nitric oxide also inhibits platelet aggregation. It modulates glomerular tubular feedback in the kidney, inhibits insulin release, controls the relaxation of sphincters along the gastrointestinal tract, and may also function as a neuro-transmitter.[20]

151

The NO synthase which subserves intercellular communication is Ca^{2+} and cadmodulin dependent, but there is another inducible, Ca^{2+} independent synthase which releases larger quantities of NO over longer periods from activated macrophages, thus causing NO to act as a cytotoxic agent. More recently other NO synthases have been discovered in tissues other than the reticuloendothelial system, so raising the possibility that NO may be implicated in the causation of other types of cell damage.

The rapid inactivation of NO by haemoglobin and the ability to administer the gas by inhalation has enabled NO to be used as a selective pulmonary vasodilator (see page 168).

Methods of studying the effects of drugs on the pulmonary circulation

Drugs may alter the distribution of pulmonary blood flow by altering the total flow or pulmonary vascular pressures, or by modifying pulmonary vascular tone in the oxygenated or hypoxic areas of lung. Secondary effects may be produced by drugs which affect airway tone and so alter total or regional lung volume.

Most studies of drugs use measurements of pulmonary vascular resistance or changes in the distribution of flow as an index of vascular tone. As a result of the complexity of the pulmonary circulation all the results obtained from these methods must be interpreted with caution. The most commonly used methods are summarised in table 5.1.

Methods using the concept of pulmonary vascular resistance

Conceptual problems

This measurement is made by dividing the pressure difference across the lung by the flow:

Table 5.1 Control of variables during studies on the pulmonary circulation

Preparation	Variables not controlled	Abnormalities
Isolated perfused lung (constant flow or pressure)	Perfusate P_{O_2}	No neural control or lymph drainage No other organs in circuit
Lobar perfusion (constant flow or pressure)	Left atrial pressure $P\bar{v}_{O_2}$	No neural control or lymph drainage of lobe
Ventilated or collapsed lobe (flowmeters)	Cardiac output, vascular pressures, $P\bar{v}_{O_2}$	No neural control or lymph drainage of lobe
Unilateral hypoxia (radioisotopes, $\dot{V}_{O_2}$, SF_6)	Cardiac output, vascular pressures, $P\bar{v}_{O_2}$	P_{CO_2} decreases with blood flow
Generalised ventilation hypoxia	Cardiac output, vascular pressures, $P\bar{v}_{O_2}$	Arterial hypoxaemia

$P\bar{v}_{O_2}$, mixed venous P_{O_2}; $\dot{V}_{O_2}$, oxygen consumption.

152

$$PVR = \frac{P_{\overline{pa}} - P_{\overline{la}}}{\dot{Q}}$$

where PVR is pulmonary vascular resistance, $P_{\overline{pa}}$ and $P_{\overline{la}}$ are mean pulmonary artery and left atrial pressures, and $\dot{Q}$ is the cardiac output. The normal value is approximately 1.5 mm Hg/l per min or 0.1 mm Hg/ml per s. To express the result in CGS units it is necessary to multiply the second figure by 1332, so that the normal value is approximately 100 dyn/s per cm⁵. This measurement is useful in that it has conceptual similarities to Poiseuille's law for laminar flow through a parallel sided tube:

$$\text{Resistance} = \frac{\text{Pressure difference}}{\text{Flow}} = \frac{8\eta l}{\pi r^4}$$

This relationship tells us that the resistance increases with increased viscosity (η) of the perfusing fluid, with increasing length (l) of the tube, and is inversely related to the fourth power of the radius (r). Blood is, however, a non-newtonian fluid (with a viscosity that changes with flow), blood flow is pulsatile, and the pulmonary vasculature consists of a branching network of distensible tubes, the cross sectional area of which is augmented by recruitment of extra vessels when flow or pulmonary artery pressure increases. Furthermore, the radius and length of the vessels are affected by changes in transpulmonary pressure and lung volume. It is, therefore, obvious that Poiseuille's equation cannot be applied to the pulmonary circulation and that attempts to do so must frequently yield conflicting results. Nevertheless, the general concept of resistance is of value and the measurement can be used as an index of vascular tone if appropriate precautions are taken to control the variables.

Perfusion preparations

The most reliable measurements are obtained by using one of the various forms of perfused lung preparation in which changes in resistance can be detected by making simultaneous measurements of flow and the pressure difference between pulmonary artery and left atrium. Most commonly the lungs or a lobe is perfused at constant flow, so that resistance changes can be detected by changes in pressure across the lung. Equally valid results can, however, be obtained by perfusing the lungs at a constant input and output pressure, when changes in resistance result in changes in flow. Ideally, a number of measurements are made at each stage of the experiment so that pressure–flow curves can be plotted before and after the intervention (fig 5.8). A shift of the curve then provides strong evidence of a change in vascular tone provided the other variables have been kept constant. The optimal control of variables is obtained in the isolated perfused lung preparation in which the lungs are either retained in the chest or suspended in a box. The lungs are ventilated at constant tidal volume with 5% carbon dioxide in an oxygen–nitrogen mixture. End expiratory pressure is kept

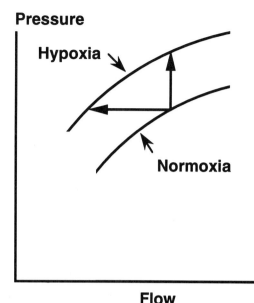

Flow

Fig 5.8 Pressure–flow curves obtained when vasomotor tone is normal or increased by hypoxia. The vertical arrow shows the increase in pressure which would be recorded in response to hypoxia during a constant flow perfusion, whereas the horizontal arrow shows the decrease in flow in response to hypoxia with a constant pressure perfusion.

constant and airway pressure is monitored to ensure that there are no changes in lung mechanics. Alveolar hypoxia can then be induced by reducing the oxygen concentration to 3–5%. In the constant flow type of perfusion, blood from a warmed reservoir is pumped by an occlusive pump through a cannula tied into the pulmonary artery. It is then drained through a cannula in the left atrium, which is connected to an overflow system to ensure that left atrial pressure is maintained constant, and both pulmonary artery and left atrial pressures are measured. Flow can be derived from a previous calibration of the pump, or measured by an electromagnetic flowmeter, or by a timed diversion of flow from the atrial cannula into a parallel calibrated reservoir (fig 5.9).

In the alternative technique a constant pressure perfusion is effected by pumping the blood up to a reservoir in which the surface is maintained at a constant level by means of an overflow, and flow is again measured by collecting the outflow from the lungs over a measured period, or by using an electromagnetic flowmeter. Both types of preparation are effectively denervated, thus eliminating possible reflex responses, and all the other variables are rigidly controlled. Such preparations are ideally suited to the investigation of agents which are administered by inhalation, or of drugs that are

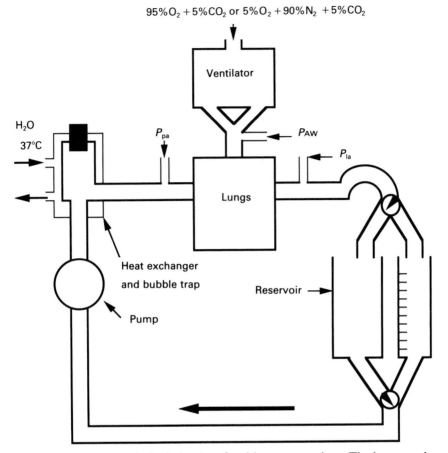

$95\%O_2 + 5\%CO_2$ or $5\%O_2 + 90\%N_2 + 5\%CO_2$

Fig 5.9 Perfusion circuit for isolated perfused lung preparations. The lungs can be ventilated at constant volume with a normoxic or hypoxic gas mixture and the airway (P_{AW}), pulmonary artery (P_{pa}), and left atrial (P_{la}) pressures recorded. Blood flow can be measured by diverting the venous outflow into the measuring cylinder for a known time.

metabolised by the lung. However, there is no bronchial circulation and the normal routes of drug elimination are not included in the circuit. In addition, the ligature round the pulmonary artery occludes the lymphatic drainage so that the preparation tends to become oedematous after several hours of perfusion.

To overcome these problems, many workers use the *in situ* perfused lobe technique. The left lower lobe is usually chosen because it has a long bronchus which can be cannulated easily so that the lobe can be ventilated separately from the rest of the lung. Perfusion of the lobe is achieved by using a constant flow device to pump blood from the right side of the heart into a

155

cannula tied into the left lower lobe artery. The blood drains into the left atrium and then circulates normally. The disadvantage of this technique is that left atrial pressure and $P\bar{v}_{O_2}$ cannot be controlled (although they can be monitored). The whole body is, however, perfused normally so that normal detoxication mechanisms are not interfered with. Innervation and lymphatic drainage are destroyed if the cannula is tied in place with a ligature around the pulmonary artery, but these problems can be overcome in larger animals by floating a catheter with a terminal balloon into the appropriate branch of the artery and by ventilating the lobe with a cuffed endobronchial tube.

In vivo studies: errors in the measurement of pulmonary vascular resistance

Most human studies on the effects of drugs have used the concept of pulmonary vascular resistance. As already pointed out there are many disadvantages to this approach. The first is that the measurements are likely to be very inaccurate. It is difficult to measure any vascular pressure with an error less than 1–2 mm Hg and there are many additional sources of error when left atrial pressure is derived from a pulmonary wedge pressure

---

Factors affecting measurements of pulmonary vascular resistance (PVR)

"Passive" factors	*Change in PVR*
Pulmonary artery pressure increase	Decrease
Left atrial pressure increase	Decrease
Transpulmonary pressure, increase or decrease from functional residual capacity	Increase
Interstitial pressure increase	Increase
Blood viscosity increase	Increase

"Active" factors	
Blood gases	
P_{O_2} decrease	Increase
P_{CO_2} increase	Increase (doubtful in humans)
pH decrease	Increase
Autonomic activity	(Probably negligible in humans)
Endogenous substances	
Catecholamines, angiotensin, histamine	Increase
Acetylcholine, bradykinin, prostacyclin	Decrease

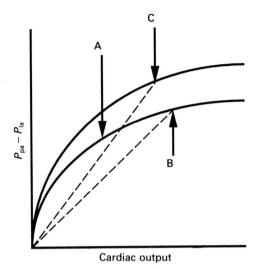

Fig 5.10 Pressure–flow curves are approximately linear over a limited range of flow in the supine subject. When the normoxic curve has been defined by measurements of pulmonary artery pressure minus left atrial pressure $(P_{pa} - P_{la})$ and cardiac output before and after exercise (A, B), a single measurement (C) may suffice to indicate hypoxic vasoconstriction.

measurement. The accuracy of cardiac output measurement is rarely better than ±10% so that the total error in the measurement of resistance may well exceed the change as a result of the experimental intervention. The second disadvantage is that the measured changes may be caused by "passive" or "active" changes in the pulmonary circulation which are not directly related to the action of the drug under test. The major factors that may affect the measurement are shown in the box. From these it may be concluded that a change in pulmonary vascular resistance can only be considered valid if:

1 $(P_{\overline{pa}} - P_{\overline{la}})$ increases or decreases whereas flow and $P_{\overline{la}}$ are unchanged
2 $(P_{\overline{pa}} - P_{\overline{la}})$ decreases when $P_{\overline{la}}$ decreases or is unchanged and flow decreases or is unchanged
3 $(P_{\overline{pa}} - P_{\overline{la}})$ increases when flow is increased or unchanged and $P_{\overline{la}}$ is increased or unchanged.

One other approach is to construct a pressure–flow curve for each individual by exercising the subject in the supine position (when most of the lung vessels are fully distended). Under these circumstances the curve appears to be linear and so can be defined by two points (fig 5.10). If it is assumed that exercise does not in itself alter vasomotor tone, a shift in the curve may be used as an index of vasomotor activity.

Methods using the distribution of flow as an index of pulmonary vascular tone

In human studies it is often possible to reduce the number of variables by studying the regional distribution of blood flow rather than pulmonary vascular resistance. One method of studying the hypoxic response is to measure the redistribution of blood flow in response to unilateral hypoxia induced by the administration of 8–10% oxygen through one limb of a double lumen tube. In the earlier studies the distribution of flow was determined by measuring the oxygen consumption of each lung, because this is directly proportional to blood flow. Attempts were also made to use carbon dioxide output in a similar manner, but this technique proved inaccurate because the carbon dioxide output was also affected by the ventilation to each lung.[21] A much simpler way of measuring the distribution of blood flow is to infuse a solution of a relatively insoluble gas into the pulmonary artery and to measure the concentration evolved into the alveoli on each side. One method is based on the infusion of sulphur hexafluoride and measurement of its concentration in expired gas with infrared analysis.[21] Other methods use a radiolabelled isotope of a relatively insoluble gas such as xenon or krypton.[22] This is dissolved in saline and injected into the right side of the circulation. Most of the radio labelled isotope is evolved into the alveoli during the first passage of the blood through the lungs so that the count rate is directly related to the blood flow. The radioactivity can either be measured in expired gas or detected by scintillation detectors or a gamma camera placed over the chest. The use of the gamma camera has not only enabled blood flow to be measured in areas of collapsed lung, but has also permitted regional variations in perfusion to be studied. The distribution of flow has also been studied by measuring regional radioactivity after the injection of microspheres or macroaggregates labelled with radioactive isotopes. By using radioisotopes with different energies up to six sequential injections may be made at different stages of the experiment. As the counting may be delayed for several hours the method has proved to be of great value when studying the distribution of blood flow in stressful environments such as during zero or exaggerated gravity.

Another method of studying the redistribution of blood flow after the administration of a vasoactive drug is to measure the effects on gas exchange. This can be done by the standard method of calculating percentage shunt and dead space/tidal volume ratio from the oxygen and carbon dioxide tensions in arterial and mixed venous blood, and mixed expired gas. Greater precision is, however, obtained by the Wagner inert gas technique in which a solution of six inert gases of different solubilities is infused into the pulmonary circulation at a constant rate, and the retention/excretion ratios are measured from an arterial and mixed expired gas sample. By using a computer to fit the data to a 50 compartment model of the lung, it is possible to derive values for

158

shunt, dead space, and compartments with intermediate ventilation–perfusion ratios.[23] As with other in vivo measurements it is important to remember that any alterations in the distribution of blood flow which occur may be caused by changes in lung volume or haemodynamics, as well as by changes in vasomotor tone.

It is obvious that the conditions outlined above severely limit the number of useful observations that can be made. Furthermore, as the normal pulmonary vascular bed has very little tone, the action of pulmonary vasodilator drugs can only be studied after constriction has been induced by some other agent (such as hypoxia). Obviously, vasodilator drugs must also be studied in the patients in whom they are likely to be used, but such studies often produce variable results owing to differences in the aetiology of the pulmonary hypertension in each patient. For these reasons we will first consider the actions of drugs on the normal pulmonary circulation and on hypoxic pulmonary vasoconstriction. In the last section we shall consider the problem of pulmonary hypertension and the effects of vasodilator drugs.

Effect of drugs on the normal pulmonary circulation

It has already been pointed out that the distribution of pulmonary blood flow is primarily controlled by the interrelationship of the pulmonary vascular pressures, the transpulmonary pressure difference, and the effects of gravity, and it has been shown how changes in these variables may affect distribution and gas exchange in the normal and abnormal lung. Many drugs given during anaesthesia have profound haemodynamic effects which will produce major effects on flow distribution. The changes in cardiac output may also affect $P\bar{v}o_2$ which will, in turn, affect the partitioning of blood flow between normoxic and hypoxic areas of lung. A number of these drugs may affect pulmonary vasomotor tone and so further modify the distribution of blood flow. Their effect depends on the pre-existing level of vascular tone. In normoxic areas of lung pulmonary vascular tone is low so that pulmonary vasodilators have little effect whereas constrictors produce major changes. In areas with hypoxic pulmonary vasoconstriction the reverse is the case. When analysing the effects of drugs on the pulmonary circulation, one must, therefore, consider not only the changes in pulmonary haemodynamics and $P\bar{v}o_2$, but also their effects on vasomotor tone in the normoxic and hypoxic areas of lung (see box).

Anaesthetic drugs

Experimental studies

Although Buckley and colleagues[24] had reported that nitrous oxide increased the pressor response to alveolar hypoxia in dogs, whereas 0·5% halothane decreased it, reversible depression of the hypoxic vasoconstrictor

---

Drugs affecting hypoxic pulmonary vasoconstriction

Decrease
Inhalational anaesthetic agents
β Agonists
Pulmonary vasodilators
   α Blockers
   Sodium nitroprusside
   Calcium channel blockers
   Nitric oxide

Increase
Cyclo-oxygenase inhibitors
Propranolol
Almitrine
Lignocaine (lidocaine)

---

response by inhalational agents such as trichloroethylene, halothane, and ether was not demonstrated in an isolated perfused lung preparation until 1972.[25] Subsequent studies using the isolated perfused lung preparation have demonstrated that halothane decreases vasomotor tone in the normoxic lung and that diethyl ether, halothane, methoxyflurane, enflurane, and isoflurane produce a dose dependent depression of vasoconstriction in the hypoxic lung. Intravenous anaesthetic agents such as thiopentone, pentobarbitone, pentazocine, fentanyl, droperidol, ketamine, and diazepam appear to have no effect on hypoxic vasoconstriction.[26 27]

In another series of experiments the left lower lobe was ventilated independently of the rest of the lung and electromagnetic flowmeters used to measure the partition of flow between the lobe and the rest of the lung. Ventilation of the lobe with nitrogen reduced the blood flow by 53% and this reduction in flow was approximately halved when isoflurane or fluroxene were added to the nitrogen in a concentration of 2 MAC; 0·3 MAC nitrous oxide produced slight but significant inhibition of the response although halothane and enflurane had little effect (MAC = minimum alveolar concentration). Similar effects were produced when the agent was added to the whole lung while the lobe was hypoxic.[27]

The inhalational agents have also been studied in the intact animal. The hypoxic stimulus was provided by unilateral ventilation hypoxia and the distribution of blood flow between the two lungs measured by radioisotope methods. In these experiments anaesthetic concentrations of trichlorethylene, ether, and nitrous oxide reduced the magnitude of hypoxic vasoconstriction, whereas 0·5–1·5% halothane had little effect. In intact dogs submitted to whole lung ventilation hypoxia, isoflurane inhibited the pressor response whereas halothane and enflurane had no effect.

The difference in results between the isolated perfused lung experiments and those using in vivo preparations are probably caused by the haemodynamic changes associated with the administration of the anaesthetic agent. Agents such as halothane produce a marked decrease in cardiac output, which may be exaggerated when the animal is made hypoxic. If this causes the intravascular pressure to decrease when vascular tone is decreased by inhibition of hypoxic vasoconstriction, there may be little change in flow through the hypoxic segment. There may also be changes in the hypoxic stimulus as a result of changes in $P\bar{v}_{O_2}$.

Human studies

Studies in the human are subject to many variables and must be interpreted with great caution. The first report of the action of anaesthetic drugs on human pulmonary haemodynamics was published by Johnson in 1951.[28] The first evidence that clinically used concentrations of inhalational anaesthetic agents could inhibit hypoxic vasoconstriction was, however, obtained by Bjertnaes in 1978.[29] He used unilateral hypoxia as the stimulus and administered the agent to the hypoxic lung, the blood flow diversion being measured by the injection of radiolabelled macroaggregates. Subsequently, Rodgers and Benumof[30] measured Pa_{O_2} before and after the administration of halothane or isoflurane, during one lung anaesthesia that was induced and maintained with either ketamine or methohexitone, and concluded that approximately 1 MAC concentrations of halothane or isoflurane do not produce significant depression of hypoxic vasoconstriction in humans. These findings were confirmed by Carlsson and colleagues who measured the diversion of flow in response to unilateral ventilation hypoxia with a continuous infusion of sulphur hexafluoride (a relatively insoluble inert gas). They found that inhaled concentrations of 2% enflurane and 1·0–1·5% isoflurane had no effect on the diversion of flow.[31 32] Subsequent studies[33] suggested that, during a more prolonged period of administration, halothane may indeed cause some depression of hypoxic vasoconstriction. It would seem reasonable to conclude that, although there is a large variation in the effect of inhalational agents on hypoxic vasoconstriction, there is no contraindication to the use of the inhalational agents in most patients undergoing one lung anaesthesia.

Other drugs

It was Halmagyi and Cotes[34] who first reported the occurrence of arterial hypoxaemia after the administration of bronchodilator drugs such as adrenaline and aminophylline to patients with asthma. During the next decade similar changes were reported with isoprenaline, salbutamol, and orciprenaline, but it was not clear whether the hypoxaemia resulted from impaired distribution of gas caused by preferential deposition of the aerosol in relatively well ventilated areas of lung, from maldistribution of blood flow secondary to haemodynamic changes, or from impaired hypoxic pulmonary vasoconstriction. Subsequent studies in animals subjected to unilateral ventilation hypoxia showed that bronchodilator drugs such as salbutamol and orciprenaline could inhibit hypoxic vasoconstriction.[35 36] Isoprenaline is known to dilate vessels in both normoxic and hypoxic areas of lung, but the other agents have little effect in normoxia and appear to have a specific action on hypoxic vasoconstriction. These effects have been confirmed by studies using the multiple inert gas elimination method in patients with asthma which have shown that blood flow to low ventilation–perfusion areas was doubled after the administration of nebulised isoprenaline, and that these changes could have accounted for the observed fall in P_{O_2}.[37]

Two other β agonists, dopamine and dobutamine, are of particular interest because, although both increase blood flow to low ventilation–perfusion areas and decrease Pa_{O_2},[38] they appear to produce their effects by different mechanisms, dobutamine inhibiting the hypoxic vasoconstrictor response whereas dopamine vasoconstricts the vessels in the oxygenated lung and so decreases the flow diversion from the hypoxic area by increasing the pulmonary artery pressure.[39] Protamine also produces pulmonary vasoconstriction and produces hypoxaemia by a similar mechanism.[40]

The vasodilator drugs nitroglycerin (predominantly a venodilator) and sodium nitroprusside (acting mainly on the arterial system) have been shown to produce arterial hypoxaemia in humans, and to depress the diversion of blood flow in response to unilateral hypoxia in the dog.[41] They probably act by releasing nitric oxide. In patients with the adult respiratory distress syndrome (ARDS) sodium nitroprusside produced a decrease in pulmonary artery pressure and Pa_{O_2} with an increase in the shunt component measured by the multiple inert gas method.[42] In another study both nitroglycerin and prostaglandin E_1 were found to have similar effects, although PGE_1 administration was accompanied by an increase in cardiac output which increased oxygen delivery.[43] As there was no increase in cardiac output or $P\bar{v}_{O_2}$ with both nitroprusside and nitroglycerin, it seems logical to conclude that the increase in shunt was the result of inhibition of the hypoxic vasoconstrictor mechanism.

The calcium channel blockers also inhibit hypoxic vasoconstriction, although the effects of these drugs in normal humans are somewhat variable.[44] Nifedipine inhibits hypoxic vasoconstriction in experimental preparations[45] and in normal humans.[44] It also reduces pulmonary vascular resistance in patients with primary pulmonary hypertension, or with pulmonary hypertension secondary to chronic obstructive lung disease.[46] Diltiazem has also been shown to decrease Pa_{O_2} and to increase shunt in patients with ARDS.[47]

Drugs that augment hypoxic vasoconstriction

It is apparent that many drugs interfere with the hypoxic vasoconstrictor mechanism and so impair gas exchange. This raises the question as to whether any advantage would be gained by the administration of agents which would augment hypoxic vasoconstriction.

162

The cyclo-oxygenase inhibitors such as aspirin and indomethacin have been shown to augment hypoxic vasoconstriction, both in the experimental situation and in patients.[48] Other agents that appear to have similar actions are alcohol, lignocaine, propranolol, and almitrine.[26] Almitrine seems to have a biphasic action, low doses augmenting the response and high doses obtunding it.[49 50] Although augmentation of the response should improve gas exchange, it also increases pulmonary artery pressure, and this may impair right ventricular function and reduce the efficiency of the hypoxic vasoconstrictor mechanism. There appears therefore to be little clinical indication for the use of such agents at the present time.

Pulmonary hypertension

Pulmonary hypertension is defined as a chronic increase in pulmonary artery systolic pressure above 30 mm Hg or a mean pressure greater than 20–25 mm Hg. From a consideration of Poiseuille's equation (page 153) it is apparent that pulmonary hypertension may be expected to occur in the following circumstances:

1 When there is a reduction in the number of vessels perfused.
2 When there is a narrowing of the vessels as a result of intimal thickening, muscle hypertrophy, vascular spasm, or a decrease in the transmural pressure holding them open.
3 When there is an increase in the pulmonary venous pressure.
4 When there is an increase in blood viscosity (for example, as a result of polycythaemia).

The clinical conditions that may cause pulmonary hypertension are listed in the box. For convenience these are grouped under five main headings:

- those predominantly associated with a reduction in the size of the vascular bed
- those associated with a narrowing of the vessels
- those associated with an increase in pulmonary venous pressure
- primary or idiopathic (cause unknown)[51]
- diverse aetiology.

It will, however, become apparent that such a categorisation is somewhat artificial for there are often a number of factors contributing to the hypertension in each patient.

Reduction in perfused vascular bed

One obvious cause of a reduction in the pulmonary vascular bed is surgical resection. Even if a pneumonectomy is performed, however, the increase in

---

Clinical causes of pulmonary hypertension

1 Reduction of vascular bed:
   Extensive surgical resection
   Pulmonary embolism
   Emphysema
   Pulmonary fibrosis

2 Narrowing of vessels:
   Chronic increases in blood flow
   Increased vascular tone
      Endogenous vasoconstrictors
      Hypoxia and hypercapnia
   Decreased transmural pressure
      Pulmonary oedema
      Increased alveolar pressure

3 Pulmonary venous hypertension

4 Primary (idiopathic)

5 Other: drugs, toxins, parasites HIV, portal hypertension

---

pulmonary artery pressure is only 5–8 mm Hg provided that the remaining lung is normal. Much greater increases in pressure are seen if the remaining lung is affected by disease. A reduction in the area of perfused vascular bed is also produced by pulmonary embolism. This may result from thromboemboli, amniotic fluid, tumour, fat, or gas bubbles. As the normal pulmonary circulation has a low resistance, thromboembolism leads to little increase in pressure until at least 60% of the pulmonary vessels have been occluded. If, however, pulmonary hypertension is already present (for example, from previous embolisation), right heart failure may be induced by a relatively small embolus. It has been suggested that the release of serotonin (5-hydroxytryptamine) or another endogenous substance may accentuate the hypertension resulting from the obstruction, but there is little evidence that this occurs in humans. Pulmonary embolism results in perfusion defects on the lung scan and ventilation of these areas of lung increases the alveolar component of dead space. Arterial hypoxaemia is almost invariably present and is caused mainly by an increase in right to left shunt. This could be the result of right to left shunting through a patent foraman ovale, to redistribution of blood flow to collapsed areas of lung, or to the presence of a high pressure pulmonary oedema.

Amniotic fluid embolism typically occurs during or shortly after labour and is commonly fatal. It is believed that the lethal effects of amniotic fluid emboli result mainly from the thromboses that they induce and from the subsequent development of disseminated intravascular coagulation.

Destruction of the pulmonary vascular bed appears to be the major cause of hypertension in patients with emphysema. There is, however, a poor correlation between the magnitude of the pathological changes and the degree of pulmonary hypertension. It is possible that this is caused by differences in the site of the lesions. For example, right ventricular hypertrophy may occur when as little as 14% of the lung is affected by bronchiolar emphysema, but it rarely develops in patients with panacinar emphysema until 40–70% of the lung is affected.[52]

Large areas of fibrosis occur in the lungs of patients with the pneumoconioses, sarcoidosis, fibrosing alveolitis, and collagen disease such as scleroderma, systemic lupus erythematosus, and rheumatoid arthritis, and these lead to the development of pulmonary hypertension. Pulmonary hypertension has also been reported in patients with advanced tuberculosis and bronchiectasis.

Narrowing of the pulmonary vessels

The presence of pulmonary hypertension in patients with the ARDS was first documented in 1977.[53] In the acute phase narrowing of the pulmonary vessels may be caused by endogenous substances, such as thromboxane A_2 or B_2 and prostaglandin E_2, by an increase in interstitial pressure secondary to pulmonary oedema, and by alveolar hypoxia and hypercapnia secondary to respiratory failure. In the later phases of the disease fibrosis and destruction of the pulmonary vascular bed become important.

Hypoxia and hypercapnia are important causes of pulmonary hypertension in patients with chronic obstructive lung disease and there is now firm evidence that prolonged oxygen therapy has beneficial effects on survival.[54 55] Pulmonary hypertension in patients with chronic bronchitis is increased during acute exacerbations. The administration of oxygen during an acute exacerbation usually results in some reduction in pulmonary artery pressure and an increase in physiological dead space. Although it was originally believed that the increase in $P\text{co}_2$ associated with the administration of oxygen resulted from a decrease in the hypoxic drive to respiration, it now seems probable that the increase is mainly due to the inability of the patients to increase their minute volume to compensate for the increase in dead space induced by the redistribution of blood flow. Alveolar hypoxia is an important cause of pulmonary hypertension in the neonatal respiratory distress syndrome or ARDS, and probably accounts for the prevalence of pulmonary hypertension in patients with kyphoscoliosis. Patients with the primary hypoventilation syndrome and those with obstructive sleep apnoea may also develop pulmonary hypertension during sleep. This responds to nocturnal oxygen therapy.

Alveolar hypoxia also appears to be the main cause of pulmonary hypertension in individuals living at high altitude.[56] There is, however, a wide variation in the response between individuals, whether they are normally domiciled at high altitude or are normally domiciled at sea level and then taken to high altitude. In those living constantly at high altitude there is hypertrophy of the media of the muscular pulmonary arteries. When such people are moved to sea level there is an immediate decrease in pulmonary artery pressure, which is probably caused by the release of hypoxic pulmonary vasoconstriction, followed by a more gradual fall, which is probably related to the involution of the muscle fibres.

Sustained high blood flows, such as those resulting from intracardiac shunts, ultimately produce narrowing of the pulmonary vessels and pulmonary hypertension. Initially there is medial hypertrophy in the small pulmonary arterioles, and this is later combined with intimal proliferation, and plexiform and other dilatational lesions. In the more severe cases pulmonary haemosiderosis and fibrinoid necrosis are seen. The hypertension decreases when oxygen is inhaled and the pathological lesions regress if the heart defect is corrected in the earlier stages of the disease, but, if dilatational lesions and plexogenic arteriopathy have developed, the changes are generally irreversible. The time of onset of these changes depends, to a large extent, on the location of the shunt. In patients with pre-tricuspid shunts (for example, atrial septal defects) the changes tend to develop in young adults or in middle life, whereas patients with post-tricuspid shunts (for example, ventricular septal defects) tend to retain the fetal pattern of pulmonary circulation and so have pulmonary hypertension from birth.

Pulmonary blood vessels may also be narrowed by a decrease in transmural pressure caused by a reduction in lung volume or an increase in interstitial pressure resulting from pulmonary oedema. A more common cause of narrowing is an increase in alveolar pressure as a result of an increase in airway resistance. This appears to be an important cause of pulmonary hypertension in patients with asthma and chronic bronchitis.

Pulmonary venous hypertension

Pulmonary venous hypertension may be caused by mediastinal lesions which compress the pulmonary veins, a myxoma or ball-valve thrombus in the left atrium, mitral or aortic valve disease, or left ventricular failure. It may also result from pulmonary veno-occlusive disease.

An acute increase in pressure in the pulmonary venous system results in pulmonary congestion and a corresponding increase in pulmonary artery pressure. If the congestion is severe pulmonary oedema may result. Chronic increases in venous pressure may lead to pathological changes in the lung but, in contrast to those produced by increases in precapillary pressure, they affect the whole of the pulmonary vasculature. The pulmonary veins and venules show medial hypertrophy, arterialisation, dilatation, and eccentric intimal fibrosis. The microcirculation is characterised by capillary congestion, oedema, dilatation of interstitial and pleural lymphatics, and alveolar haemosiderosis. Pulmonary arterioles are often muscularised and both muscular and elastic arteries may be dilated.[57]

Other causes

There are a number of other clinical conditions in which the cause of the pulmonary hypertension is even more obscure. For example, there was a Swiss epidemic of pulmonary hypertension which appeared to be related to the use of the slimming drug aminorex, and there was another epidemic in Spain associated with the use of contaminated cooking oil. There is an association between portal and pulmonary hypertension, and pulmonary hypertension may occur in patients with schistosomiasis when their ova impact in the lung. Patients with HIV infection may develop pulmonary hypertension, and there is also a condition known as primary or idiopathic pulmonary hypertension in which the aetiology is still far from clear.[51]

Significance of pulmonary hypertension

The most obvious effect of pulmonary hypertension is that it increases the right ventricular pressure, workload, and oxygen consumption, and so may lead to right ventricular failure. As the blood flow to the right ventricle occurs during both systole and diastole it is important to maintain a high systemic pressure to minimise myocardial ischaemia. A second problem resulting from a high pulmonary artery pressure is that it may cause high pressure pulmonary oedema by increasing the pressure in the precapillary vessels. Pulmonary venous hypertension also causes oedema and in both situations severe arterial hypoxaemia may result. Pulmonary embolism and other conditions causing chronic hypertension may cause a maldistribution of blood flow as a result of changes in arteriolar resistance. Localised reductions in flow result in non-perfused alveoli and an increase in alveolar dead space, but the concomitant increases in pressure may also oppose the effects of hypoxic vasoconstriction, which redistributes flow away from underventilated areas of lung, and so may also increase arterial hypoxaemia.

It will be apparent that there are many causes of pulmonary hypertension, and that a number may be present in any one patient. For example, in chronic obstructive airway disease the hypertension may be caused by alveolar hypoxia and hypercapnia, destruction of the vascular bed, polycythaemia (which increases blood viscosity), gas trapping, and water retention (which increases the static pressure throughout the circulation). Although little can be done to alter the size of the vascular bed, all the other causes are amenable to treatment. The effects of treatment will, however, depend on the magnitude and reversibility of the factors involved in each patient. Similarly in ARDS it seems probable that in the early stages pulmonary hypertension is predominantly caused by vasoconstriction from hypoxia and endogenous mediators, augmented by a reduction in the vascular bed as a result of alveolar collapse, and obstruction of small vessels by leucocytes, although in the later stages medial hypertrophy, thrombosis, and interstitial fibrosis dominate the scene. Again, the relative importance of each factor in the individual patient is difficult to determine. Many of the putative mediators are very short lived and difficult to measure, and there is no good animal model of ARDS. As a number of therapeutic strategies currently employed are designed to reduce pulmonary vasomotor tone, it is necessary to consider some of the implications of this type of therapy.

Pulmonary vasodilator drugs

Conventional vasodilator drugs have three main disadvantages in patients with pulmonary hypertension:

1 Most pulmonary vasodilators also dilate the systemic vascular bed and so decrease aortic pressure. This results in a decrease in coronary perfusion which may lead to myocardial ischaemia when right ventricular stroke work and oxygen consumption are increased by an excessive afterload.
2 The decrease in pulmonary artery pressure may decrease the perfusion of non-dependent zones and so increase alveolar dead space.
3 Inhibition of the hypoxic vasoconstrictor mechanism may increase flow to poorly ventilated areas of lung and so increase arterial hypoxaemia.

These disadvantages, and the failure to document improved survival in adult patients treated with conventional pulmonary vasodilator drugs, suggest that there is little indication for their use in adult practice at the present time. (This is not the case in the neonate where pulmonary vasodilators may play an important role in maintaining pulmonary blood flow in patients with persistent pulmonary hypertension.)

The situation has been radically changed by the recent discovery of the role of nitric oxide as a physiological vasodilator.[58] Nitric oxide is also a bronchodilator.[59] It has now been shown that nitric oxide can vasodilate the pulmonary vascular bed when inhaled in concentrations of 10–80 p.p.m. (parts per million). The advantage of the inhalational route of administration is that the nitric oxide only dilates the pulmonary vessels supplying ventilated alveoli, and has no effect on systemic vessels because it is immediately deactivated by combination with haemoglobin.[60] It has now been shown that the inhalation of 18 p.p.m. of nitric oxide decreases pulmonary artery pressure and shunt in patients with ARDS, and that it can be inhaled for many days without apparent toxicity.[61] An even more recent study has demonstrated a significant improvement in oxygenation without any reduction in pulmonary artery pressure when inhaled in concentrations of 60–230 parts per *billion*.[62] Interestingly, this concentration is similar to that produced by endogenous NO production in the nasal mucosa,[63] which is denied the ARDS patient by the use of a tracheal tube! Nitric oxide inhalation has also been used with success in neonates with persistent pulmonary hypertension,[64] and in patients with chronic pulmonary disease. There may also be interactions with anaesthetic agents.[65]

It seems strange that an agent that was once a feared contaminant of nitrous oxide should now be hailed as a therapeutic agent of great promise. However, NO is rapidly oxidised to nitrogen dioxide (NO_2) and requires specially designed apparatus for its administration, together with careful monitoring. As NO is the mediator in so many biological systems, there are many potential side effects of long term administration. This is an exciting new form of treatment which can undoubtedly decrease pulmonary artery pressure and improve arterial oxygenation, but whether it will ultimately affect mortality remains to be seen.

Conclusions

The low resistance of the pulmonary circulation results in relatively poor control of the distribution of blood flow. Distribution is primarily dependent on the interrelationship of transpulmonary and vascular pressures, but is modified at alveolar level by the influence of alveolar and mixed venous gas tensions. Drugs may modify the distribution of flow by changing cardiac output and pulmonary vascular pressures, but a number of drugs may alter distribution by altering pulmonary vascular tone in normoxic or hypoxic areas of lung. Drugs that decrease the effectiveness of hypoxic pulmonary vasoconstriction may increase blood flow to underventilated lung regions and so cause arterial hypoxaemia. Selective vasodilatation of ventilated lung regions by nitric oxide may, however, reduce shunt and pulmonary artery pressure. Although the complexity of the system makes it difficult to predict the effects of drugs on gas exchange, a knowledge of the potential mechanisms will enable the clinician to understand many of the phenomena observed in routine clinical practice, and should thus improve the standard of patient care.

1 Harvey W. *An anatomical dissertation concerning the movement of the heart and blood in living creatures*. Translated by G Whitteridge. Oxford: Blackwell Scientific, 1977.
2 Malpighi M. *Duae epistolae de pulmonibus*. Florence, 1661.
3 Bradford JR, Dean HP. The pulmonary circulation. *J Physiol* 1894; **16**: 34–96.
4 Euler US von, Liljestrand G. Observations on the pulmonary arterial blood pressure in the cat. *Acta Physiol Scand* 1946; **12**: 301–20.
5 Nisell O. Effects of oxygen and carbon dioxide on the circulation of isolated and perfused lungs of the cat. *Acta Physiol Scand* 1948; **16**: 121–7.

169

6 Cournand A, Ranges HA. Catheterization of right auricle in man. *Proc Soc Exp Biol Med* 1941; **46**: 462–6.
7 Bakhle YS. Pharmacokinetic and metabolic properties of lung. *Br J Anaesth* 1990; **65**: 79–93.
8 West JB. Blood flow. In West JB, Ed. *Regional differences in the lung*. London: Academic Press, 1977: 85–165.
9 Chen L, Williams JJ, Alexander CM, Ray RJ, Marshall C, Marshall BE. The effect of pleural pressure on the hypoxic pulmonary vasoconstrictor response in closed chest dogs. *Anesth Analg* 1988; **67**: 763–9.
10 Hedenstierna G. Gas exchange during anaesthesia. *Br J Anaesth* 1990; **64**: 507–14.
11 Gattinoni L, Pelosi P, Vitale G, Pesenti A, D'Andrea L, Mascheroni D. Body position changes redistribute lung computed-tomographic density in patients with acute respiratory failure. *Anesthesiology* 1991; **74**: 15–23.
12 Cutaia M, Rounds S. Review: Hypoxic pulmonary vasoconstriction. Physiological significance, mechanism, and clinical relevance. *Chest* 1990; **97**: 706–18.
13 Marshall BE, Hanson CW, Frasch F, Marshall C. Role of HPV in pulmonary gas exchange and blood flow distribution. *Intensive Care Med* 1994; **20**: 291–7; 379–89.
14 Marshall BE, Marshall C, Benumof J, Saidman LJ. Hypoxic pulmonary vasoconstriction in dogs: effects of lung segment size and oxygen tension. *J Appl Physiol* 1981; **51**: 1543–51.
15 Benumof JL, Wahrenbrock EA. Blunted hypoxic pulmonary vasoconstriction by increased lung vascular pressures. *J Appl Physiol* 1975; **38**: 846–50.
16 Graham LM, Vasil A, Vasil ML, Voelkel NF, Stenmark KR. Decreased pulmonary vasoreactivity in an animal model of chronic *Pseudomonas* pneumonia. *Am Rev Respir Dis* 1990; **142**: 221–9.
17 Rodriguez-Roisin R, Roca J, Agnsti AG, Mastai R, Wagner PD, Bosch J. Gas exchange and pulmonary vascular reactivity in patients with liver cirrhosis. *Am Rev Respir Dis* 1987; **135**: 1085–92.
18 McFarlane PA, Gardaz J-P, Sykes MK. CO_2 and mechanical factors reduce blood flow in a collapsed lung lobe. *J Appl Physiol* 1984; **57**: 739–43.
19 Davies MG. The vascular endothelium: a new horizon. *Ann Surg* 1993; **218**: 593–609.
20 Star RA. Southwestern internal medicine conference: nitric oxide. *Am J Med Sci* 1993; **306**: 348–58.
21 Carlsson AJ, Hedenstierna G, Blomqvist H, Strandberg A. Separate lung blood flow in anesthetized dogs: a comparative study between electromagnetometry and SF_6 and CO_2 elimination. *Anesthesiology* 1987; **67**: 240–6.
22 Sykes MK, Hill AEG, Loh L, Tait AR. Evaluation of a new method for continuous measurement of the distribution of blood flow between the two lungs. *Br J Anaesth* 1977; **49**: 285–92.
23 Kaufman RD, Patterson RW, Lee A StJ. Derivation of V_A/Q distribution from blood-gas tensions. *Br J Anaesth* 1987; **59**: 1599–609.
24 Buckley MJ, McLauchlin JS, Fort L, Saigusa M, Morrow DH. Effects of anesthetic agents on pulmonary vascular resistance during hypoxia. *Surg Forum* 1964; **15**: 183–4.
25 Sykes MK, Loh L, Seed RF, Kafer ER, Chakrabarti MK. The effect of inhalational anaesthetics on hypoxic pulmonary vasoconstriction and pulmonary vascular resistance in the perfused lungs of the dog and the cat. *Br J Anaesth* 1972; **44**: 776–87.
26 Sykes MK. Anesthetics and the pulmonary circulation. In Altura BM, Halevy S, Eds. *Cardiovascular actions of anesthetics and drugs used during anesthesia*. Vol 2. *Regional blood flow and clinical considerations*. Basel: Karger, 1986: 92–125.
27 Eisenkraft JB. Effects of anaesthetics on the pulmonary circulation. *Br J Anaesth* 1990; **65**: 63–78.
28 Johnson SR. Effect of some anaesthetic agents on circulation in man—with special reference to the significance of pulmonary blood volume for the circulatory regulation. *Acta Chir Scand* 1951; **158** (suppl): 1–143.
29 Bjertnaes LJ. Hypoxia-induced pulmonary vasoconstriction in man: inhibition due to diethyl ether and halothane anesthesia. *Acta Anesthesiol Scand* 1978; **22**: 570–88.
30 Rogers SN, Benumof JL. Halothane and isoflurane do not decrease PaO_2 during one-lung ventilation in intravenously anesthetized patients. *Anesth Analg* 1985; **64**: 946–54.
31 Carlsson AJ, Bindslev L, Hedenstierna G. Hypoxia-induced pulmonary vasoconstriction in the human lung; the effect of isoflurane anaesthesia. *Anesthesiology* 1987; **66**: 312–16.

32 Carlsson AJ, Hedenstierna G, Bindslev L. Hypoxia-induced pulmonary vasoconstriction in human lung exposed to enflurane anaesthesia. *Acta Anaesthesiol Scand* 1987; **31**: 57–62.
33 Benumof JL, Augustine SD, Gibbons JA. Halothane and isoflurane only slightly impair oxygenation during one-lung ventilation in patients undergoing thoracotomy. *Anesthesiology* 1987; **67**: 910–15.
34 Halmagyi DF, Cotes JE. Reduction in systemic blood oxygen as a result of procedures affecting the pulmonary circulation in patients with chronic pulmonary disease. *Clin Sci* 1959; **18**: 475–89.
35 Reyes A, Sykes MK, Chakrabarti MK, Tait A, Petrie A. The effect of salbutamol on hypoxic pulmonary vasoconstriction in dogs. *Bull Eur Physiopathol Respir* 1978; **14**: 741–53.
36 Reyes A, Sykes MK, Chakrabarti MK, Carruthers B, Petrie A. Effect of orciprenaline on hypoxic pulmonary vasoconstriction in dogs. *Respiration* 1979; **38**: 185–93.
37 Wagner PD, Dantzker DR, Iacovoni VE, Tomlin WC, West JB. Ventilation–perfusion inequality in asymptomatic asthma. *Am Rev Respir Dis* 1978; **118**: 511–24.
38 Rennotte MT, Reynaert M, Clerbaux Th, *et al*. Effects of two inotropic drugs, dopamine and dobutamine, on pulmonary gas exchange in artificially ventilated patients. *Intensive Care Med* 1989; **15**: 160–5.
39 Gardaz JP, McFarlane PA, Sykes MK. Mechanisms by which dopamine alters blood flow distribution during lobar collapse in dogs. *J Appl Physiol* 1986; **60**: 959–64.
40 Kim YD, Michalik R, Lees DE, Jones M, Hanowell S, Macnamara TE. Protamine induced arterial hypoxaemia: the relationship to hypoxic pulmonary vasoconstriction. *Can Anaesth Soc J* 1985; **32**: 5–11.
41 D'Oliveira M, Sykes MK, Chakrabarti MK, Orchard C, Keslin J. Depression of hypoxic pulmonary vasoconstriction by sodium nitroprusside and nitroglycerine. *Br J Anaesth* 1981; **53**: 11–17.
42 Radermacher P, Huet Y, Pluskwa F, *et al*. Comparison of ketanserin and sodium nitroprusside in patients with severe ARDS. *Anesthesiology* 1988; **68**: 152–7.
43 Radermacher P, Santak B, Becker H, Falke KJ. Prostaglandin E₁ and nitroglycerin reduce pulmonary capillary pressure but worsen ventilation–perfusion distributions in patients with adult respiratory distress syndrome. *Anesthesiology* 1989; **70**: 601–6.
44 Naeije R, Mélot C, Mols P, Hallemans R. Effect of vasodilators on hypoxic pulmonary vasoconstriction in normal man. *Chest* 1982; **82**: 404–10.
45 Kennedy T, Summer W. Inhibition of hypoxic pulmonary vasoconstriction by nifedipine. *Am J Cardiol* 1982; **50**: 864–8.
46 Mélot C, Hallemans R, Naeije R, Mols P, Lejeune P. Deleterious effect of nifedipine on pulmonary gas exchange in chronic obstructive pulmonary disease. *Am Rev Respir Dis* 1984; **130**: 612–6.
47 Mélot C, Naeije R, Mols P, Hallemans R, Lejeune P, Jaspar N. Pulmonary vascular tone improves pulmonary gas exchange in the adult respiratory distress syndrome. *Am Rev Respir Dis* 1987; **136**: 1232–6.
48 Adnot S, Defouilloy C, Brun-Buisson C, Piquet J, de Cremoux H, Lemaire F. Effects of indomethacin on pulmonary hemodynamics and gas exchange in patients with pulmonary artery hypertension, interference with hydralazine. *Am Rev Respir Dis* 1987; **136**: 1243–9.
49 Reyes A, Roca J, Rodriguez-Roisin R, Torres A, Ussetti P, Wagner PD. Effect of almitrine on ventilation-perfusion distribution in adult respiratory distress syndrome. *Am Rev Respir Dis* 1988; **137**: 1062–7.
50 Mélot C, Dechamps P, Hallemans R, Decroly P, Mols P. Enhancement of hypoxic pulmonary vasoconstriction by low dose almitrine bismesylate in normal humans. *Am Rev Respir Dis* 1989; **139**: 111–19.
51 Accp consensus statement: primary pulmonary hypertension. *Chest* 1993; **104**: 236–50.
52 Harris P, Heath D. *The human pulmonary circulation*, 3rd edn. Edinburgh: Churchill Livingstone, 1986: 511.
53 Zapol WM, Snider MT. Pulmonary hypertension in severe acute respiratory failure. *N Engl J Med* 1977; **296**: 476–80.
54 Stuart-Harris C, Bishop JM, Clark TJH, *et al*. Long term domiciliary oxygen therapy in chronic hypoxic cor pulmonale complicating chronic bronchitis and emphysema. *Lancet* 1981; **i**: 681–6.
55 Nocturnal oxygen therapy trial group 1980. Continuous or nocturnal oxygen therapy in

hypoxic obstructive airways disease. *Ann Intern Med* 1980; **93**: 391–8.
56 Rotta A, Cánepa A, Hurtado A, Velásquez T, Chávez R. Pulmonary circulation at sea level and high altitude. *J Appl Physiol* 1956; **9**: 328–36.
57 Edwards WD. Pathology of pulmonary hypertension. *Cardiovasc Clin* 1988; **18**: 321–59.
58 Barnes PJ, Belrisi MG. Nitric oxide and lung disease. *Thorax* 1993; **48**: 1034–43.
59 Dupuy PM, Shore SA, Drazen JM, Frostell C, Hill WA, Zapol WM. Bronchodilator action of inhaled nitric oxide in guinea pigs. *J Clin Invest* 1992; **90**: 421–8.
60 Frostell C, Fratacci M-D, Wain JC, Jones R, Zapol WM. Inhaled nitric oxide. A selective pulmonary vasodilator reversing hypoxic pulmonary vasoconstriction. *Circulation* 1991; **83**: 2038–47.
61 Rossaint R, Falke KJ, López F, Slama K, Pison U, Zapol WM. Inhaled nitric oxide for the adult respiratory distress syndrome. *N Engl J Med* 1993; **328**: 399–405.
62 Gerlach H, Pappert D, Lewandowski K, Rossaint R, Falke KJ. Long-term inhalation with evaluated low doses of nitric oxide for selective improvement of oxygenation in patients with adult respiratory distress syndrome. *Intensive Care Med* 1993; **19**: 443–9.
63 Gerlach H, Rossaint R, Pappert D, Knorr M, Falke KJ. Autoinhalation of nitric oxide after endogenous synthesis in nasopharynx. *Lancet* 1994; **343**: 518–19.
64 Pearl RG. Inhaled nitric oxide. The past, the present, and the future. *Anesthesiology* 1993; **78**: 413–16.
65 Nakamura K, Mori K. Nitric oxide and anesthesia. *Anesth Analg* 1993; **77**: 877–9.

6: Cardiovascular control mechanisms

CHRISTOPHER P HARKIN,
DAVID C WARLTIER

Introduction

Regulation of the cardiovascular system has two major goals: to maintain a relatively constant arterial pressure and to provide sufficient perfusion to tissues to meet regional metabolic demands. When the requirements of an entire organism for blood flow are altered, the compensatory cardiovascular response involves changing the arterial perfusion pressure. On the other hand, when the perfusion to a particular organ system is altered, cardiovascular compensation occurs by adjusting the calibre of specific blood vessels. The most important variable that is controlled in the regulation of the circulation is arterial blood pressure. Arterial pressure has often been related to Ohm's law in physics. This implies that blood pressure (analogous to voltage) is directly proportional to the product of cardiac output (current) and peripheral vascular resistance (resistance). Neutral control and humoral control of arterial pressure are mediated through alterations of both cardiac output and/or peripheral resistance.

Acute mechanisms for regulation of arterial pressure are coordinated in the cardiovascular control centres of the brain stem. These centres regulate both cardiac output and peripheral resistance and, therefore, are able to exert powerful control of arterial pressure. The cardiovascular centres of the brain stem are in turn influenced by impulses from other neural centres, as well as numerous sensors within and external to the circulation.

Further regulation of the circulation is mediated by endogenous chemical substances which are released into the circulation and have a direct effect on the heart and/or blood vessels in both physiological and pathophysiological states. Many tissues have the ability to regulate blood flow by local mechanisms, preferentially altering regional perfusion without changes in cardiac output and systemic vascular resistance. Finally, the kidneys are the long term regulators of the entire circulation by manipulating the overall fluid status of an organism. This chapter will address these different mechanisms individually, but ultimately all are closely integrated and function in unison to regulate the circulation.

Neural control of the heart and vasculature

Central nervous system cardiovascular centres

The critical central nervous system (CNS) cardiovascular control centres are located in the medulla oblongata and lower pons.[1] The centres for circulatory control are in close proximity to those regulating respiration, and together comprise the CNS areas crucial for survival of the organism.

The centres for circulatory control have two major divisions—the vasomotor and the cardiac regions—which supply nervous innervation to the peripheral vasculature and heart respectively.[2 3] The two divisions are neither anatomically nor functionally distinct, because significant overlap in both of these properties exists. Further subdivisions with more specialised functions have also been demonstrated in animal experiments using precise microelectrode stimulation, electrical ablation, and surgical trans-section techniques. These subdivisions function in a highly integrated and coordinated manner to control arterial pressure.

The vasomotor centre is located bilaterally in the reticular substance of the medulla and lower third of the pons.[3] Although the exact organisation of the vasomotor centre has not been fully defined, experiments have identified certain areas which have specific functions. The vasoconstrictor area, also termed C-1, is located in the anterolateral portions of the upper medulla and contains a high concentration of neurons that secrete noradrenaline. The C-1 area has been proposed as one of the sites of action of α_2-adrenoceptor agonists such as clonidine and dexmedetomidine. C-1 neurons descend in the spinal cord and synapse with cells in the intermediolateral cell column. The neurons of the intermediolateral cell column are preganglionic neurons which synapse further with adrenergic neurons. Adrenergic neurons send vasoconstrictor fibres to the periphery via the sympathetic nervous system (SNS).

A vasodilator region, referred to as area A-1, is positioned bilaterally but more medially in the lower half of the medulla.[3] Neurons from this area project rostrally to and inhibit activity of the vasoconstrictor area (C-1), causing vasodilatation. Finally, a sensory area, designated A-2, is located bilaterally in the tractus solitarius in the posterolateral portions of the medulla and lower pons. This region receives sensory neural input predominantly from the glossopharyngeal (cranial nerve IX) and vagus (cranial nerve X) nerves. Neurons arising from A-2 project to the vasoconstrictor and vasodilator areas modulating outputs from these regions. Thus, sensory area A-2 integrates reflex control for multiple circulatory functions. The baroreceptor reflex is a typical example.

The cardiac control centre can also be subdivided.[4] The cardioinhibitory area is well characterised and positioned in the nucleus ambiguus and the dorsal nucleus of the vagus nerve. Parasympathetic vagal efferents arising from this area send impulses to decrease heart rate and, to a lesser extent,

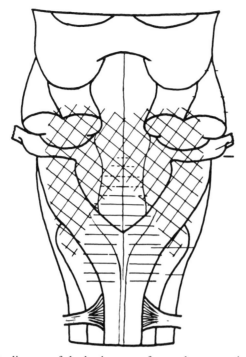

Fig 6.1 Schematic diagram of the brain stem of a cat demonstrating locations of the depressor (horizontal lines) and pressor (cross hatched) areas. (Reprinted with permission from Alexander.[2])

reduce atrial contractility. Few parasympathetic fibres, however, innervate ventricular myocardium. The exact location of the cardiostimulatory area is less well defined, but appears to be present in the lateral medulla. Stimulation of this more diffuse region increases heart rate and myocardial contractility via activation of the SNS.

Both cardiostimulatory and cardioinhibitory areas, as well as the vaso-constrictor area, are tonically active, and these regions continuously emit low levels of efferent impulses at a rate of 0·5–2 impulses/second.[5] Activity of the vasoconstrictor area is responsible for a state of partial arteriolar contraction referred to as vasomotor tone. As the areas that control vasoconstriction and cardiac stimulation lie together in a lateral and superior position in the cardiovascular control centre, these sites constitute the pressor area (fig 6.1).[2] Those areas that cause vasodilatation and cardiac inhibition lie more medially, and form the depressor area (fig 6.1). Microelectrode stimulation of the pressor area increases heart rate, myocardial contractility, and peripheral vascular resistance in experimental animals. Conversely, stimulation of the depressor area reduces rate and arterial pressure.

The cardiovascular control centres receive neural input from other regions

Table 6.1 Nerve fibre classification

Fibre type	Diameter (μm)	Myelin	Conduction velocity (m/s)
Type A			
α	12–20	+	120
β	5–12	+	120
γ	3–6	+	5–40
δ	2–5	+	5–40
ε	2	+	5
Type B	<3	+	3–15
Type C	0·3–1·2	−	0·5–2

+ , Myelinated.
− , Unmyelinated.

within the brain.[6] The reticular substance of the pons, mesencephalon, and diencephalon sends both excitatory and inhibitory impulses into the cardiovascular centres. The hypothalamus also has significant excitatory or inhibitory control, especially of the vasoconstrictor region. Finally, numerous areas of the cerebral cortex (for example, motor cortex, anterior temporal lobe, frontal cortex, anterior cingulate gyrus, amygdala, septum, and hippocampus) also project into the cardiovascular centres and elicit cardiovascular alterations associated with emotions.

Autonomic nervous system

The cardiovascular control centres of the brain stem ultimately activate/deactivate the autonomic nervous system (ANS) which provides innervation of cardiac and vascular smooth muscle. The ANS represents the efferent or motor component of cardiovascular control and consists of two complementary divisions—the sympathetic and parasympathetic nervous systems (SNS and PNS, respectively). The SNS and PNS are commonly considered physiologically antagonistic, producing opposite effects on innervated tissues.

The SNS and PNS are bipolar, each consisting of two interconnected neurons.[7] The first, proximal neuron originates within the CNS, but does not make direct contact with the effector organ. This neuron is referred to as the preganglionic neuron and relays impulses from the CNS to the autonomic ganglion. Autonomic ganglia contain the cell bodies of the second, distal neuron (the postganglionic neuron), which innervates the effector organ. Both sympathetic and parasympathetic divisions have preganglionic neurons which are myelinated, slow conducting, type B fibres with diameters of less than 3 μm (table 6.1). Impulses are conducted in these fibres at 3–15 m/s. Postganglionic neurons of both divisions are unmyelinated type C fibres with diameters of less than 2 μm and conduct impulses at 0·5–2 m/s (table 6.1).

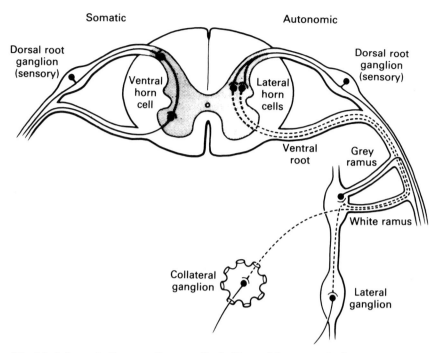

Fig 6.2 Schematic diagram of preganglionic fibres of the sympathetic nervous system. Preganglionic fibres exiting white rami can make synaptic connections in one of three fashions: (1) synapse can occur in paravertebral ganglia at the level of exit; (2) preganglionic fibres can travel up or down the paravertebral sympathetic chain and synapse at other levels; and (3) fibres can exit the paravertebral chain without synapsing and travel to peripheral collateral ganglia. (– – –) Preganglionic fibres; (——) postganglionic fibres. (Reprinted with permission from Lawson.[8])

Sympathetic nervous system

Preganglionic neurons of the SNS arise from the thoracic and first two lumbar (T1–L2) segments of the spinal cord.[8] The cell bodies of the preganglionic neurons are located in the intermediolateral grey column of the 14 spinal cord segments and have fibres that leave the spinal cord in the ventral (anterior) motor nerve roots (fig 6.2). These fibres pass via white (myelinated) communicating rami into one of 22 pairs of ganglia which make up the paravertebral sympathetic chain. Once in the ganglia of the paravertebral sympathetic chain, the preganglionic fibre may follow any one of three courses:

1 The fibre may synapse with the cell bodies of the postganglionic neuron in the ganglion at the level of exit.
2 The fibre may course upwards or downwards in the paravertebral sympathetic chain and synapse with postganglionic neurons at other levels.

3 Preganglionic fibres may travel for variable distances through the paravertebral chain and exit without synapsing to more peripheral, unpaired collateral sympathetic ganglia where synapse with postganglionic neurons occurs (fig 6.2).[8]

Thus, the cell bodies of postganglionic neurons are located either in the ganglia of the paired paravertebral sympathetic chains or in the more peripheral unpaired collateral ganglia. In contrast to the PNS, the SNS ganglia are almost always positioned closer to the spinal cord than the effector organs innervated. The coeliac and inferior mesenteric ganglia represent examples of unpaired peripheral collateral ganglia which are formed by the convergence of preganglionic neurons with numerous postganglionic cell bodies. Many fibres from postganglionic neurons pass back into spinal nerves via grey (unmyelinated) communicating rami. These neurons subsequently travel with the spinal nerves to innervate vascular smooth muscle.

The distribution of the SNS neurons to each organ is determined in part by the embryonic position from which the organ originates.[9] This is significant because the first five thoracic preganglionic neurons ascend into the neck to form three unique paired ganglia. These ganglia are the superior cervical, middle cervical, and stellate ganglia, the stellate ganglia being formed by fusion of the inferior cervical and first thoracic SNS ganglia. These three pairs of ganglia provide sympathetic innervation to the head, neck, upper extremities, heart, and lungs.

Parasympathetic nervous system

The cell bodies of the preganglionic neurons of the PNS are located in the brain stem and the sacral segments of the spinal cord. Cranial nerves III (oculomotor), VII (facial), IX (glossopharyngeal), and X (vagus) all contain preganglionic PNS neurons.[8] The preganglionic cell bodies of the second, third, and fourth sacral nerves are located in the intermediolateral grey column of the spinal cord. The paired vagus nerves contain about 75% of all fibres of the PNS and have the most extensive distribution of any of the parasympathetic nerves, including innervation of the heart.

Preganglionic neurons of the PNS are quite different from the analogous preganglionic nerves in the SNS. PNS preganglionic fibres are longer and pass uninterrupted to ganglia near or in the innervated organ which are generally not visible. As a consequence, the postganglionic neurons of the PNS are short because of the location of the corresponding ganglion. Proximity of the PNS ganglia to the effector organs limits the distribution of the postganglionic neurons in contrast to postganglionic SNS fibres which are more widespread.

- In the ANS, all preganglionic neurons of either division release the neurotransmitter acetylcholine and are classified as cholinergic.

- In the PNS, the neurotransmitter released from postganglionic neurons is acetylcholine.
- In the SNS, the neurotransmitter between postganglionic adrenergic neurons and effector organs is noradrenaline.

ANS effects on the circulation

The heart and peripheral vasculature are innervated by both the SNS and PNS. Alterations in heart rate (chronotropism), the strength of contraction (inotropism), and coronary blood flow are produced by both divisions of the ANS (table 6.2). Cardiac vagal fibres are primarily distributed to the sinoatrial and atrioventricular nodes and the atria, but are only minimally distributed to ventricular myocardium. PNS stimulation leads to decreases in the rate of sinoatrial node discharge and reduces atrioventricular node excitability, causing slowing of impulse conduction to the ventricles via muscarinic receptors. Strong vagal discharge may cause complete sinoatrial node arrest or interrupt impulse conduction from the atria to the ventricles. The PNS has little effect on myocardial contractility because of the lack of vagal efferent distribution to the ventricles. Any decrease in contractile force following PNS stimulation is probably secondary to declines in heart rate. The human heart is tonically stimulated by both the PNS and SNS but vagal tone predominates, the degree of vagal tone being greatest in young individuals. Total pharmacological ANS blockade or cardiac denervation (for example, heart transplantation) results in higher heart rates by inhibition of this dominant vagal tone.

The SNS has the same supraventricular distribution as the PNS but also provides greater innervation of ventricular myocardium.[10] Postganglionic fibres of the SNS arise in the paired stellate ganglia. The right stellate ganglion sends fibres primarily to the anterior epicardial surface and interventricular septum of the heart. Stimulation of these fibres leads to

Table 6.2 Effects of adrenergic and cholinergic stimulation on the cardiovascular system

	Adrenergic response	Cholinergic response
Heart		
Sinoatrial node	Tachycardia	Bradycardia
Atrioventricular node	Increased conduction	Decreased conduction
His Purkinje system	Increased automaticity and conduction velocity	Minimal
Myocardium	Increased contractility	Minimal
Vasculature		
Skin and mucosa	Constriction	Dilatation
Skeletal muscle	Constriction $(\alpha_1)>$ dilatation (β_2)	Dilatation
Coronary	Constriction (α_1) and dilatation (β_2)	Dilatation (EDRF) and constriction
Pulmonary	Constriction	Dilatation (?)

increases in heart rate via activation of β_1-adrenergic receptors. The left stellate ganglion distributes fibres to the lateral and posterior surfaces of both ventricles. Left stellate ganglion stimulation increases ventricular contractility while causing only minimal increases in heart rate. Experimental investigations have revealed that normal basal sympathetic tone maintains cardiac contractility at approximately 20% greater levels than the denervated heart.

SNS activation causes coronary arteriolar vasodilatation through increases in myocardial oxygen consumption and coupling of myocardial metabolic requirements to blood flow.[11] Simultaneous α-adrenergic activation causes large epicardial coronary artery vasoconstriction, however, limiting metabolically driven coronary vasodilatation by about 30%. Parasympathetic activation causes coronary vasodilatation in experimental animal models because of an acetylcholine mediated release of endothelium derived relaxing factor (EDRF). The direct stimulation of human coronary vascular smooth muscle by PNS in the absence of a normally functioning vascular endothelium may produce constriction leading to coronary spasm.

The peripheral vasculature is innervated by both divisions of the ANS, but the SNS has far greater importance in the regulation of vascular tone.[12] The distribution of parasympathetic nerves is relatively limited and PNS stimulation dilates vessels partially via endothelial mechanisms; the SNS causes vasoconstriction by stimulation of α-adrenergic receptors. Vasculature of the skin, kidneys, spleen, and mesentery has extensive sympathetic innervation, although vascular beds of the brain, heart, and muscle have significantly less innervation.

Vascular tone is the sum of the muscular forces intrinsic to the blood vessel wall opposing an increase in vessel diameter.[5] The degree of tone is influenced by ANS activity, humoral and local metabolic substances, and autacoids with dilator or constrictor actions. Basal vasomotor tone results partially from low level, continuous impulses (0·5–2 impulses/second) from the lateral portion of the vasomotor centre in the medulla oblongata which pass via the SNS to maintain partial arteriolar and venular constriction. Circulating adrenaline from the adrenal medulla may add to regional constriction dependent on the relative concentration of α-constrictor versus β_2-vasodilator receptors.

Basal vasomotor tone is normally maintained at about half maximum constriction, enabling the arteriole to constrict or dilate further. Without basal vasomotor tone, the arteriole could only constrict during SNS stimulation. Thus, vasodilatation can be produced by a reduction in the tonic sympathetic nerve activity without elicitation of "opposing" PNS. Basal vasomotor tone produces little resistance to flow in the venule as compared with the arteriole. However, the importance of the degree of SNS stimulation on the venous circulation is to increase or reduce venous capacitance. A small change in venous capacitance can produce large alterations in venous return and cardiac preload because up to 80% of the total blood volume can be stored in the veins.

Humoral control of the circulation

Catecholamines

The adrenal medulla is unique in that this gland is innervated by preganglionic SNS fibres which pass directly to it from the spinal cord.[8][13] Embryologically, cells of the adrenal medulla are derived from neural tissue and are analogous to postganglionic neurons. The adrenal medulla secretes primarily adrenaline (80%) and also noradrenaline in response to SNS stimulation. As adrenaline and noradrenaline are released into the blood and exert functions at distal sites, these catecholamines function as hormones.

The release of catecholamines by the adrenal medulla occurs after acetylcholine is secreted by preganglionic SNS fibres. The cardiovascular response to the secreted adrenaline and noradrenaline is similar to direct stimulation by the SNS. The effects of these hormones are, however, significantly prolonged (10–30 seconds) compared with the duration of action of noradrenaline as a neurotransmitter. Adrenal medullary secretion may be considered as additive to that of SNS stimulation in that some poorly innervated vessels are also constricted by circulating catecholamines.

Renin–angiotensin system

The renin–angiotensin system is another important humoral regulator of the cardiovascular system, particularly under conditions of stress.[14][15] The enzyme renin is synthesised in and released from juxtaglomerular cells of the renal cortex. Juxtaglomerular cells are modified vascular smooth muscle cells located in the tunica media of the afferent arteriole immediately proximal to the glomerulus. Renin is secreted into the blood in response to a decrease in renal artery pressure, reduced sodium delivery to the distal tubule (sensed by osmoreceptors of the macula densa region), and SNS stimulation via activation of β_1-adrenergic receptors. Renin cleaves the hepatically synthesised α_2-globulin, angiotensinogen, to form the decapeptide, angiotensin I. Angiotensin I is physiologically inactive but is rapidly hydrolysed to form the octapeptide angiotensin II by angiotensin converting enzyme which is found in high concentration in the vascular endothelium of the lungs.

Angiotensin II produces vasoconstriction of arterioles in most vascular beds. It also stimulates SNS ganglion cells and facilitates impulse transmission in the SNS. Activation of presynaptic angiotensin receptors increases noradrenaline release. Angiotensin II directly stimulates the adrenal cortex to synthesise and secrete aldosterone, which causes salt and water retention leading to expansion of plasma volume; this increases arterial pressure even more. Angiotensin II is metabolised by aminopeptidases to a series of inactive metabolic products and the heptapeptide angiotensin III. Angiotensin III is a less potent vasoconstrictor but has equal or greater potency as a stimulator of aldosterone secretion.

Decreases in blood pressure or declines in sodium delivery to the macula densa (for example, haemorrhage, dehydration) therefore lead to formation of angiotensin II and III. Angiotensin II and III increase arterial pressure by elevating peripheral vascular resistance and by causing aldosterone secretion with subsequent salt and water retention. The renin–angiotensin system does not play a major role in the maintenance of arterial pressure in the normal, sodium replete individual. This system is, however, of major importance in maintaining blood pressure during periods of hypovolaemia, sodium deprivation, or inadequate cardiac output.

Vasopressin

Vasopressin or antidiuretic hormone is a peptide synthesised in the supraoptic and paraventricular nuclei of the brain stem, which is transported to and released from the posterior pituitary gland.[16] Vasopressin secretion from the pituitary occurs in response to multiple physiological stimuli including the following:

- an increase in plasma osmolality sensed by osmoreceptors located in the hypothalamus
- a decrease in plasma volume detected by cardiopulmonary receptors, particularly in the left atrium
- increased plasma concentrations of angiotensin II.

Vasopressin binds to specific receptors which cause the collecting ducts of the kidney to increase free water reabsorption (inhibit diuresis). An increase in plasma volume occurs which has a negative feedback on further vasopressin release.

The vasoconstriction produced by vasopressin is generalised, affecting most regional circulations. Skin and gastrointestinal tract arteries are markedly constricted, although large epicardial coronary arteries and pulmonary arteries are constricted to a lesser extent. Severe and preferential constriction of small coronary collaterals can result in areas of regional ischaemia. Large quantities of vasopressin are released by the posterior pituitary gland during haemorrhage, and the constrictor action exerts an adjunctive pressor effect to that produced by baroreceptor reflexes.

Endothelium derived relaxing factor

Endothelium derived relaxing factor/nitric oxide (EDRF/NO) is a cell messenger that has important physiological and pathophysiological actions.[17 18] The primary effect of NO on the circulation is to relax vascular smooth muscle. A variety of endogenous mediators and pharmacological agents exert haemodynamic effects by causing release of NO from vascular endothelium. For example, acetylcholine will produce vasodilatation in the presence of an intact endothelium in isolated vascular ring preparations. In contrast, acetylcholine causes vasoconstriction following endothelial denudation.

NO is synthesised by at least two major NO synthase isoforms. One is expressed constitutively in neurons and vasculature, and requires calcium and calmodulin binding for activation. This constitutive enzyme is involved in cell communication and is activated by an increase in intracellular calcium. The enzyme is in a soluble form in neural tissue, but it is membrane bound in vascular endothelium. The other isoenzyme is expressed after induction by cytokines or endotoxin and participates in host defence. This inducible isoform has calmodulin bound as a subunit and produces NO continuously with no requirement for calcium. This isoenzyme may contribute to the pathophysiology associated with syndromes characterised by an overproduction of cytokines, such as septic shock. It is present in macrophages but is not normally found in endothelial cells or vascular smooth muscle unless induced by cytokines.

The NO synthases are mixed function mono-oxygenases which use NADPH (nicotinamide adenine dinucleotide—reduced form). L-Arginine is oxidised in a stepwise manner to form NO and citrulline as primary products. NO synthases can be specifically and competitively inhibited by L-arginine analogues (for example, N_ω-nitro-L-arginine methyl ester (L-NAME) and N_ω-monomethyl-L-arginine (L-NMMA)). The inhibitors have been used to elucidate the physiological and pathophysiological roles of NO. Administration of inhibitors of NO synthesis to experimental animals leads to considerable increases in arterial pressure, substantiating the premise that a basal release of NO normally occurs and defects in NO synthesis may play a role in the aetiology of hypertension. The same inhibitors may also be useful in increasing arterial pressure in septic shock.

The primary biological function of NO appears to be the activation of soluble guanylyl cyclase which subsequently increases the cyclic guanosine monophosphate (cGMP) content of several tissues including vascular smooth muscle. cGMP may cause relaxation of vascular smooth muscle by several mechanisms. These include the activation of cGMP dependent protein kinase, which in turn activates a calcium ATPase, causing extrusion of calcium from the cell or improving calcium uptake into the sarcoplasmic reticulum.

Atrial natriuretic peptide

Atrial natriuretic factor (ANP) is a peptide synthesised and stored in human atrial myocytes; it is secreted in response to distension of the atria (increased vascular volume or increased atrial pressure), adrenaline, vaso-pressin, or morphine.[19] Studies have determined that there is a larger amount of ANP synthesised and stored in the right than in the left atrium. ANP acts directly on the arterial and venous vasculature and kidneys to reduce arterial pressure and intravascular volume. It decreases blood pressure by relaxing vascular smooth muscle and sympathetic tone. ANP inhibits renin release and aldosterone secretion thereby interfering with sodium retention, leading to natriuresis. Further renal effects include dilatation of afferent arterioles and possible constriction of efferent arterioles of the glomerulus, leading to an increased filtration fraction and diuresis. Controversy exists as to whether ANP inhibits sodium uptake in the inner medullary collecting ducts causing further natriuresis. ANP suppresses antidiuretic hormone secretion. No direct inotropic or chronotropic effects caused by this peptide have been observed, but some evidence indicates that at least a portion of the vasodilator action of ANP is mediated by EDRF/NO.

Other humoral substances

There are several other endogenous substances that can be released into the circulation and affect the heart and vasculature. These include adenosine, histamine, the plasma kinins (kallidin and bradykinin), serotonin, and endothelins.

Adenosine is a ubiquitous endogenous nucleotide which stimulates A_1 and A_2 receptors to produce haemodynamic actions.[9] It has inhibitory effects on cardiac impulse conduction through the atrioventricular node (negative dromotropic effect). Adenosine is also a potent vasodilator. The local regulation of flow in the coronary circulation and other regions during an increase in oxygen demand is at least partially related to the release of adenosine.[13]

Histamine is one of several naturally occurring endogenous substances collectively referred to as autacoids.[6] Other autacoids include prostaglandins, angiotensin II, serotonin, and plasma kinins. Histamine is located in mass cells in the lungs, skin, and gastrointestinal tract and in basophils throughout the blood. The predominant circulatory effects of histamine are the result of dilatation of arterioles and capillaries. Histamine causes vasodilatation by binding to H_1 and H_2-receptors directly on blood vessels. Histamine induced vasodilatation leads to flushing, decreased systemic vascular resistance, reduced arterial pressure, and increased capillary permeability. This autacoid also has positive inotropic properties by directly stimulating cardiac H_2-receptors and indirectly by causing adrenaline release from the adrenal medulla. Stimulation of cardiac H_2-receptors also causes positive chronotropic effects. Finally, coronary arteries have been shown to be vasoconstricted as a result of H_1-receptor stimulation and vasodilated after H_2-receptor stimulation.[20]

Plasma kinins are among the most potent endogenous vasodilators known.[21] Two examples of plasma kinins are kallidin and bradykinin, which are polypeptides formed by cleavage of α_2-globulin kininogens by kallikrein enzymes. Plasma kinins are about 10 times more potent as vasodilators than histamine. Kinins also cause increased capillary permeability and tissue oedema. Vasodilatation leads to a marked reduction in arterial pressure. In contrast, plasma kinins have been shown to constrict large veins which subsequently elevates venous return. This increase in venous return increases stroke volume and cardiac output. Bradykinin is inactivated by a converting enzyme, the same enzyme responsible for activation of the potent vasoconstrictor, angiotensin II. Many of the actions of bradykinin are mediated by release of NO from vascular endothelium.

Serotonin is also an endogenous vasoactive autacoid synthesised from tryptophan.[22] About 90% of endogenous serotonin exists in enterochromaffin cells of the gastrointestinal tract and the remainder in the CNS and platelets. The circulatory actions of serotonin are dependent on the specific vascular bed. It produces vasodilatation in blood vessels in skeletal muscles and skin, while causing vasoconstriction particularly in splanchnic and renal vessels, and to a lesser degree in cerebral and pulmonary vessels. It is also a potent venoconstrictor, although the resulting effects of increased venous return on cardiac output may be obscured by reflex mediated baroreceptor responses.

Vascular endothelium is also responsible for the production of a group of potent vasoconstricting agents called endothelins. Endothelins are polypeptides that have an undetermined physiological role but they cause intense and prolonged vasoconstriction when administered intravenously.

Reflex control of the circulation

Intrinsic reflexes

Cardiovascular reflexes represent rapidly acting mechanisms to control the circulation using the central and autonomic nervous systems.[23] Reflex control of the circulation can be initiated either from within the cardiovascular system (intrinsic reflexes) or from other organs or systems (extrinsic reflexes). Intrinsic reflexes are the most important short term regulators of arterial pressure, and are produced by changes in arterial pressure or special chemical stimuli. Alterations in blood pressure are sensed by stretch receptors, pressoreceptors, baroreceptors, or mechanoreceptors. Chemoreceptors are sensitive to chemical stimuli, regulate respiration, and, secondarily, also influence the circulation.

Arterial baroreceptor reflexes

Arterial baroreceptors are specialised pressure sensitive nerve endings in walls of the aortic arch and internal carotid arteries just above the carotid bifurcation (carotid sinus) (fig 6.3). Afferent fibres from the baroreceptors travel in the aortic and carotid sinus nerves, which join the vagus and glossopharyngeal nerves, respectively, and connect with the cardiovascular centres in the medulla, commonly in the nucleus tractus solitarius. Cells from the nucleus tractus solitarius project to the C-1 area and inhibit this region by secretion of γ-aminobutyric acid (GABA). There is a small tonic discharge from baroreceptor afferents at a normal arterial pressure. When the baroreceptor endings are stretched, action potentials are generated and propagated at a frequency that is roughly proportional to the pressure change in the artery. Hence, increased arterial pressure sensed by the baroreceptors will increase the frequency of impulses travelling to the CNS. Afferent input produces greater activity in the medullary depressor area and inhibits the pressor and cardiac areas, causing decreases in myocardial contractility and heart rate, and reducing vasoconstrictor tone of both arterioles and veins. Therefore, increased blood pressure leads to reflex activity aimed at reducing the pressure back to a normal set point (the depressor reflux). The opposite

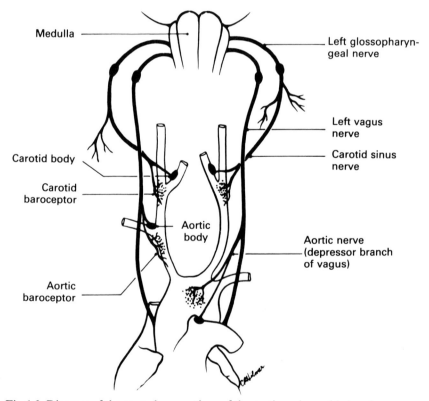

Fig 6.3 Diagram of the central connections of the aortic and carotid sinus baroreceptors. (Reprinted with permission from Smith and Kampine.[6])

effect for declines in blood pressure is also true (the pressor reflex). The arterial baroreceptor reflex provides a negative feedback mechanism for homoeostasis of arterial pressure.[23]

The baroreceptor reflex plays an important role in rapid control of arterial pressure, for example, when rising from a recumbent position. The baroreceptor response can be elicited experimentally during sudden decreases or increases in arterial pressure produced by intravenous administration of sodium nitroprusside or phenylephrine, respectively (Smyth's procedure) (fig 6.4). The slope of the plot of heart rate (or R–R interval) versus systolic pressure during rapid changes in pressure obtained by this technique is a measure of the "sensitivity" of the baroreflex.[24] It has been proposed that such sensitivity may be reduced in patients at risk of sudden death. Clamping of the common carotid artery or damage to the carotid sinus nerve during carotid endarterectomy surgery may elicit dramatic haemodynamic changes through alterations in the arterial baroreflex.

Arterial baroreceptors respond most effectively to the rate of change of arterial pressure. The response is greatest to changes of arterial pressure in the physiological range (80–150 mm Hg). Arterial baroreceptors respond more actively to declines in arterial pressure than increases. Evidence suggests that the carotid baroreceptors are more sensitive to pressure changes than the aortic baroreceptors and operate at lower ranges of arterial pressure. Experimental investigations have determined that arterial baroreceptors primarily influence reflex control of cardiac rate and contractility. Control of systemic vascular resistance is of secondary importance. The vessels most influenced by arterial baroreceptors are splanchnic arterioles and venules; the venules are important in increasing venous return to the heart during the

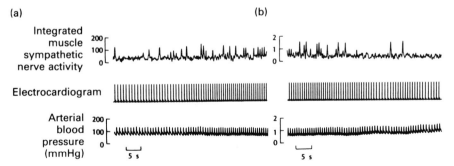

Fig 6.4 Baroreceptor reflex in a human subject. Panel (a) is a recording of the baroreceptor response following intravenous infusion of sodium nitroprusside. Note the increase in heart rate and sympathetic nerve activity in response to the decline in blood pressure. Panel (b) shows the baroreceptor mediated decrease in heart rate and sympathetic nerve activity following an intravenous infusion of phenylephrine. (Reprinted with permission from Ebert.[24])

187

pressor reflex. Evidence also suggests that the arterial baroreceptors participate in stimulating the renin–angiotensin system via an increase in sympathetic tone.[5] Decreased baroreceptor responsiveness occurs with advancing age,
hypertension, and coronary artery disease.

An important property of arterial baroreceptors is the ability to adapt to
prolonged changes in arterial pressure. Arterial baroreceptors continue to
function in hypertensive individuals or even during acute hypertensive
episodes or exercise, but reset at a higher blood pressure range.[25] The higher
pressure ultimately forms a new baseline range, which can be reversed if the
increase in presence is relieved. This resetting of the baroreceptor range
demonstrates that these reflexes probably have no role in long term blood
pressure regulation but, instead, only respond to acute changes in arterial
pressure. In fact, resetting can be demonstrated within minutes to hours.
The efferent portion of the baroreceptor reflex arc is blocked by many drugs
used for the treatment of hypertension, and as a result, orthostatic hypotension commonly occurs and, if severe, may lead to syncope. This condition
may also be present secondary to pathological processes such as diabetes.
Such "autonomic insufficiency" can lead to a lack of haemodynamic
compensation especially during anaesthesia.

Atrial and vena caval low pressure baroreceptors

The right and left atria and inferior and superior vena cava near the
junction with the right atrium also contain specialised low pressure mechanoreceptors which respond to increases in central venous pressure.[6] These
baroreceptors respond to pressure change but in a much lower range than
arterial baroreceptors. The low pressure baroreceptors send impulses via
large myelinated fibres in the vagus nerves to the CNS when the atria or vena
cava are distended. The efferent portion of the reflex consists of SNS fibres to
the sinoatrial node and subsequently causes tachycardia. This increase in
heart rate caused by atrial stretch is known as the Bainbridge reflex and is
abolished by vagotomy. Although the Bainbridge reflex has been observed in
numerous species, the heart rate response to atrial filling in humans is
complicated by numerous other factors, including the dominant arterial
baroreflex, so this reflex probably plays only a secondary role.

Other baroreceptors have been isolated that are also stimulated by filling
and distension of the atria, but send impulses via unmyelinated vagal fibres to
the CNS.[9] The reflex heart rate response is the opposite of that which occurs
in the Bainbridge reflex, and the overall response is analogous to that of the
arterial baroreceptors. An increase in venous return increases and positive
pressure ventilation reduces discharge from the receptors. Arterial distension
results in decreases in SNS activity causing a decline in vasoconstriction of
skeletal muscle, renal, and mesenteric arterioles, an increase in splanchnic
venous capacitance, and a reduction in heart rate. The decrease in SNS
activity is accompanied by a decline in renin secretion. Reduced circulating

angiotensin and aldosterone also decrease arteriolar vasoconstriction and lead to a decrease in plasma volume.

In a similar manner to arterial baroreceptors, atrial baroreceptors adapt to a continuous increase in pressure by resetting.[6] This has been demonstrated in experimental animals where congestive heart failure leads to prolonged atrial distension, increased atrial pressure, and attenuation of this reflex. This adaptation is reversed if the heart failure is relieved. It is also important to note that these atrial baroreceptors are not only stimulated by stretch, but also by atrial muscle contraction. Hence, it is believed that the diuresis observed in certain clinical and experimental pathological conditions, such as paroxysmal atrial tachycardia and atrial fibrillation, may be the result of the unusual contractile activity in the atrial wall. The low pressure baroreceptors play an important role in control of extracellular fluid volume. When volume is reduced, these receptors cause a reflex release of vasopressin and enhanced sympathetic tone which activates the renin–angiotensin–aldosterone axis. In addition, SNS reflex constriction of the afferent arterioles occurs to conserve intravascular volume.[12] These actions increase volume and homoeostasis occurs.

Ventricular reflexes

The ventricles contain receptors which are also stimulated by stretch or by strong ventricular contraction.[6] These receptors provide afferent input to the medulla via unmyelinated vagal fibres. The medulla responds by decreasing sympathetic tone and causing bradycardia and vasodilatation. A very similar reflex response (that is, bradycardia and vasodilatation accompanied by apnoea) can be elicited by injecting the drug veratridine into the heart or coronary circulation (especially the left circumflex perfusion territory in canine experiments). The unusual coronary chemoreceptor response is referred to as the Bezold–Jarisch reflex (fig 6.5). Investigation suggests that this reflex may also be triggered by intracoronary injections of other pharmacological agents, including serotonin, capsaicin, nicotine, bradykinin, histamine, and digitalis. A similar reflex has been noted following injection of contrast media during coronary angiography and in certain pathological conditions when specific metabolites accumulate in the coronary circulation, for example, in myocardial necrosis. It has been proposed that the coronary chemoreceptor reflex may be elicited during inferior wall myocardial infarction.

Arterial chemoreceptors

There are also arterial chemoreceptors located in the carotid and aortic bodies, small masses of tissue lying in close proximity to the carotid sinus and the aortic arch receptors (see fig 6.3), which have prominent effects on respiration and the circulation. The carotid body is the major chemoreceptor. The special nerve endings respond to decreases in the arterial partial pressure

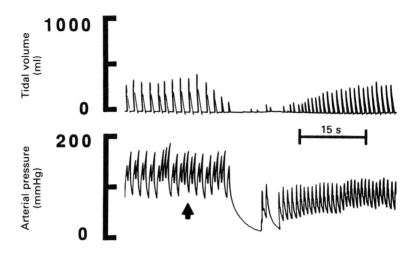

Fig 6.5 Bezold–Jarisch reflex following intravenous injection of veratridine (4 μg/kg) in a conscious dog. Note the apnoea, decreased arterial pressure, and bradycardia caused by this agent. (Courtesy of Dr P. Clifford, Department of Anesthesiology, Medical College of Wisconsin.)

of oxygen, increases in the arterial partial pressure of carbon dioxide, and increases in the arterial hydrogen ion concentration. The afferent pathway is located in the same nerves as the adjacent baroreceptors. Arterial chemoreceptors serve primarily to cause an increase in respiratory minute volume, but their secondary effect is to produce sympathetic vasoconstriction during hypotension. This response is additive to that produced by arterial baroreceptors. The "secondary" circulatory reflex actions improve oxygen delivery to heart and brain through generalised peripheral vasoconstriction and increased arterial pressure. Increased arterial pressure occurs during hypotension secondary to severe depletion of intravascular volume and subsequent reduction in blood flow and ischaemia of the carotid and aortic bodies. The chemoreceptor response also contributes to formation of Mayer waves. Decreases in perfusion of the chemoreceptors during hypotension causes activation of the reflex and results in increases in arterial pressure. Increases in flow then deactivate the chemoreceptors and decreases in arterial pressure occur. The repetitive cyclisation leads to large swings in pressure (Mayer waves) at a frequency of 2–3 cycles/min.

Extrinsic reflexes

Receptors of the afferent limbs of extrinsic reflexes are external to the circulatory system. These reflexes are less consistent than intrinsic reflexes and, in normal circumstances, play only a minor role in circulatory control.

On the other hand, extrinsic reflexes are important and protective during certain types of environmental stresses and pathophysiological circulatory states. Afferent impulses enter the CNS via somatic nerves, although the central processing of these reflexes is still uncertain. Examples of extrinsic reflexes include pain and cold, oculocardiac, CNS ischaemic, and Cushing's reflexes.

Pain reflex

Pain, depending on severity, produces variable haemodynamic responses. Mild to moderate pain results in tachycardia and increases in arterial pressure mediated by the somatosympathetic reflex. Severe pain, such as that experienced from deep bone trauma or stretching of abdominal or perineal viscera, may elicit bradycardia, hypotension, and at times circulatory collapse and syncope.

Cold reflex

Cutaneous thermosensitive nerve endings respond to cold temperature and send impulses through somatic afferent fibres to the hypothalamus. This results in cutaneous vasoconstriction and piloerection. An example of this reflex is the cold pressor test in which application of intense local cold, such as immersion of a hand in ice water, leads to stimulation of both pain and cold receptors with a subsequent increase in arterial pressure. In certain patients with coronary artery disease, the cold pressor test can produce angina either by reflex coronary vasoconstriction or abruptly increased left ventricular afterload.

Oculocardiac reflex

Receptors stimulated by pressure or stretch in the extraocular muscles, conjunctiva, and globe send impulses through the ophthalmic division of the trigeminal nerve (cranial nerve V) to the CNS.[26] This leads to bradycardia and hypertension and possibly more severe cardiac arrhythmias including asystole. With repeated stimulation, this reflex does have a tendency to fatigue, probably at the level of the cardioinhibitory centre.

Central nervous system ischaemic reflex

The CNS ischaemic response occurs when severe hypotension such as that occurring in circulatory shock reduces perfusion and causes hypoxia of the medullary vasomotor centre.[27] Chemoreceptors in the vasomotor centre sense local increases in P_{CO_2} and decreases in pH. As a result, there is an intense increase in SNS activity leading to a profound and generalised vasoconstriction. Simultaneously, an increase in PNS activity reduces heart rate. This reflex does not become active until mean arterial pressure decreases below 50 mm Hg and is maximal at mean pressures of 15–20 mm Hg. The CNS ischaemic response does not participate in regulation of normal arterial pressure but is an emergency control system for restoring cerebral blood flow when it is dangerously reduced.

191

Cushing's reflex

This is another reflex that has an origin directly in the CNS. When intracranial pressure is acutely raised, cerebral vessels are compressed. The decrease in cerebral perfusion pressure causes a reduction in arterial blood flow, and the CNS ischaemic response occurs. The decrease in blood flow to the vasomotor area results in an increase in SNS activity. This leads to progressive elevations in arterial pressure in an effort to exceed intracranial pressure and maintain adequate cerebral perfusion. Simultaneous decreases in heart rate are observed which are mediated by the baroreceptor reflex.

Spinal shock and autonomic hyperreflexia

When the spinal cord is acutely trans-sected, all cord functions, including reflexes mediated through the CNS, are interrupted below the level of injury.[26] Vasoconstrictor tone regulated by the ANS is disrupted below the cord lesion, and if the spinal cord injury occurs at a high level (that is, C6–C7), spinal shock may result. Spinal shock is characterised by a fall in blood pressure as a result of lack of arteriolar and venular constriction, as well as a loss of skeletal muscle pump action. The efferent limb of cardiovascular reflexes cannot compensate for the reduction in arterial pressure. This condition is analogous to the loss of control of blood pressure during spinal anaesthesia. Spinal shock typically lasts from one to three weeks.

After this period, local reflexes in the spinal cord below the level of disruption gradually return and a chronic stage, characterised by SNS overactivity or autonomic hyperreflexia, begins. Hyperreflexia occurs in response to cutaneous or visceral stimulation below the level of that cord lesion in 85% of patients with spinal cord injury at or above the T6 level. The stimulus sends afferent impulses into the spinal cord causing local activation of preganglionic sympathetic nerves and subsequent vasoconstriction. This reflex is normally modulated by inhibitory impulses from higher centres, but because of the trans-section, such impulses are blocked. The vasoconstriction causes hypertension and elicits the baroreceptor depressor reflex. The reflex mediated decline in SNS activity and increase in PNS activity occurs only above the level of the cord trans-section, whereas vasoconstriction continues below this level. With high levels of trans-section, circulatory reflexes are insufficient to offset the effects of vasoconstriction, leading to persistent and sometimes severe hypertension.

Local regulation of the circulation

Pressure autoregulation

Flow is locally controlled in certain vascular beds by a process termed 'autoregulation' (fig 6.6).[28] By definition, autoregulation is the ability of an organ to maintain a relatively constant blood flow in the presence of changes in arterial perfusion pressure. The kidneys, brain, and heart are organs that exhibit autoregulation, whereas the skin and lungs are organs with a minimal ability for autoregulation.

A schematic diagram of the changes in blood flow to an organ over a wide range of perfusion pressures in the presence or absence of autoregulation is shown in fig 6.6. In the absence of autoregulation, pressure–flow relationships are linear, and increases in driving pressure lead to direct increases in perfusion. An autoregulatory curve is characterised by a large range of pressures during which flow remains relatively constant. Vasodilatation is achieved at lower perfusion pressures by relaxation of smooth muscle, and vascular smooth muscle constriction occurs at higher perfusion pressures to maintain constant flow. The ability to autoregulate assumes that a set point of basal vasomotor tone allows this dilatation or constriction to occur. Flow varies directly with pressure when the limits of autoregulation are exceeded. In regional beds that are maximally vasodilated, for example, by a drug such as dipyridamole, the process of autoregulation is eliminated and flow is directly dependent on driving pressure (fig 6.6).[29] Autoregulation of blood flow is affected to only a small extent by neural and humoral influences. Experimental investigations have demonstrated that the ability to autoregulate flow is largely an intrinsic property and even occurs in denervated tissues. As a result of this, autoregulation is considered a local phenomenon affected primarily by the active tone of arterioles.

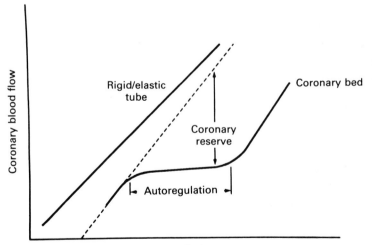

Fig 6.6 Pressure autoregulation in the normal coronary circulation. Note that during maximum vasodilatation, autoregulation is abolished (dashed line) and pressure–flow relationships resemble that of a rigid/elastic tube. (Reprinted with permission from Goldberg and Warltier.[29])

Two major theories have been advanced to explain the mechanism of autoregulation.[28] The first of these is the myogenic theory suggesting that elevations in perfusion pressure lead to stretch and increases in tension of vascular smooth muscle cells. The distension of the smooth muscle directly causes vasoconstriction to maintain flow constant in spite of an increased driving pressure. Conversely, at low perfusion pressures, there is less muscle tension, vascular smooth muscle cells relax, and blood flow is maintained in spite of the decrease in pressure. Therefore, the degree of tension that smooth muscle is exposed to is the stimulus for regulation, and subsequent constriction/dilatation serves as the mediator of this mechanism. Autoregulation is advantageous to vital organs such as the brain, heart, and kidneys because blood flow is optimised even during periods of hypotension and hypertension. It has also been proposed that the myogenic mechanism protects capillaries from excessively high blood pressures which could cause these fragile vessels to rupture.

The metabolic theory of autoregulation is based on the state of oxygenation in the surrounding tissues. A reduction in perfusion pressure leads to a decrease in blood flow and tissue P_{O_2} with concomitant increases in tissue P_{CO_2} and other metabolites related to normal cellular activity (for example, lactic acid, adenosine, potassium, and hydrogen ions). The reduced P_{O_2}, increased P_{CO_2}, and vasodilator substances directly cause arteriolar relaxation, and blood flow increases. High perfusion pressures supply ample oxygen, remove carbon dioxide, and wash out vasodilators, leading to vasoconstriction and decreases in tissue blood flow. Regardless of the validity of either the myogenic or the metabolic theory, both are based on the premise that autoregulation of tissue flow is a negative feedback mechanism, maintaining constancy of arterial flow during large changes in perfusion pressure.

Matching of flow and metabolism

When tissues have greater metabolic activity, such as skeletal muscle during exercise or myocardium during increases in heart rate, arterioles in the tissue dilate and flow increases independent of changes in perfusion pressure. This process is referred to as active or functional hyperaemia.[25] The mechanism of functional hyperaemia is very similar to the metabolic theory of autoregulation. As the tissue requirement for oxygen increases, there is a concomitant accumulation of metabolic byproducts. For example, as more ATP is consumed during periods of increased metabolic activity, adenosine is released into the interstitium. The accumulation of this and other vasodilator substances leads to smooth muscle relaxation in arterioles with increases in tissue perfusion. This represents a powerful regulator of flow in which perfusion is closely coupled with metabolic demands. Investigations have

194

demonstrated that during intense exercise, active hyperaemia can increase skeletal muscle blood flow as much as 20-fold.

Reactive hyperaemia

When blood flow is interrupted by an arterial occlusion for a brief period and then suddenly restored, the resulting flow greatly exceeds previous levels for a short time before returning to the usual resting levels (fig 6.7). The increase in flow during early reperfusion is termed "reactive hyperaemia". Reactive hyperaemia is probably related to the metabolic theory of tissue perfusion; lack of perfusion causes a deprivation of oxygen and an accumulation of vasodilating metabolites. The resulting degree and duration of the excess blood flow during the reactive hyperaemic response are proportional to the length of the blood flow interruption and severity of oxygen debt (fig 6.7).[30] This response emphasises a close connection between delivery of nutrients to tissues and the regulation of tissue perfusion. Reactive hyperaemia will occur after ischaemia (partial or total occlusion of arterial supply) or hypoxia (decreased arterial partial pressure of oxygen). The heart and brain have large, skeletal muscle has intermediate, and liver, lung, and skin have relatively small reactive hyperaemia responses.

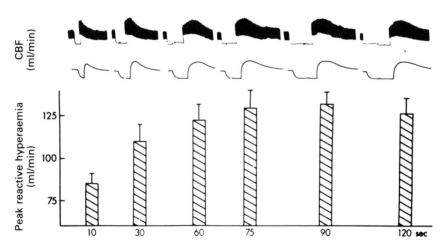

Fig 6.7 Average values (lower histogram) and chart recordings (top panel) of canine coronary blood flow (CBF) reactive hyperaemic responses after 10, 30, 60, 75, 90, and 120 seconds of total coronary occlusion. Note that with increasing time of occlusion there is an increasing hyperaemic response. (Reprinted with permission from Warltier et al.[30])

195

Long term regulation of circulation

Whereas circulatory reflexes provide acute and rapid control of the circulation, the concept of long term regulation is based on the balance of blood volume and urinary output.[13] The kidneys provide the major long term control of the circulation. Reflex changes in haemodynamics as mediated by baroreceptors play no important role in long term adjustments because the receptors rapidly adapt to continued increases or decreases in pressure. Long term regulation follows a simple renal body fluid mechanism: increases in arterial pressure produce increases in salt and water output through the kidneys, hence reducing extracellular fluid volume, blood volume, and venous return. Reduced venous return decreases cardiac output and arterial pressure. After several weeks, cardiac output returns to previous levels whereas reductions in systemic vascular resistance develop to maintain the lower arterial pressure. Conversely, a decline in blood pressure stimulates the kidneys to retain fluid which ultimately results in elevation of arterial pressure. Renal perfusion pressure and urinary output are directly related. This process occurs independent of any hormonal actions but is significantly amplified by the renin–angiotensin system.

The renal body fluid mechanism is continuous, overriding, and undergoes no adaptation. It requires that small alterations in fluid volume lead to substantial changes in arterial pressure. It is also unique because it has the ability to return the blood pressure completely back to normal values. This is in contrast to short term regulating mechanisms which cannot entirely re-establish normal arterial pressure. Overall, the renal body fluid mechanism develops over hours to days and regulates the circulation over an infinite time span.

Conclusion

Several mechanisms involving the CNS, ANS, humoral and chemical substances, and circulatory reflexes act together to provide homoeostasis of the circulation. By functioning together to regulate cardiac output, peripheral vascular resistance, and venous capacitance, relatively constant arterial pressure and adequate tissue perfusion are maintained. The cardiovascular control mechanisms act in unison to provide important adaptive responses to stresses such as haemorrhage or exercise. Without such reflexes, even the simple act of assuming an upright position would be met with abrupt and large declines in cardiac output and arterial pressure threatening the status of the organism.

This work was supported by Anesthesiology Research Training Grant GM 08377.

1 Dampney RA, Goodchild AK, Tan E. Identification of cardiovascular cell groups in the brain stem. *Clin Exp Hypertens [A]* 1984; **6**: 205–20.

2 Alexander RS. Tonic and reflex functions of medullary sympathetic cardiovascular centers. *J Neurophysiol* 1946; **9**: 205.
3 Hilton SM, Spyer KM. Central nervous regulation of vascular resistance. *Annu Rev Physiol* 1980; **42**: 399–411.
4 Levy MN, Martin PJ, Stuesse SL. Neural regulation of the heart beat. *Annu Rev Physiol* 1981; **43**: 443–54.
5 Calaresu FR, Yardley CP. Medullary basal sympathetic tone. *Annu Rev Physiol* 1988; **50**: 511–24.
6 Smith JJ, Kampine JP. *Circulatory physiology: the essentials*. Baltimore: Williams & Wilkins, 1990.
7 Janig W. Pre- and postganglionic vasoconstrictor neurons: Differentiation, types and discharge properties. *Annu Rev Physiol* 1988; **50**: 525–40.
8 Lawson NW. Autonomic nervous system physiology and pharmacology. In Barash PG, Cullen BF, Stoelting RK, eds, *Clinical anesthesia*. Philadelphia: JB Lippincott, 1992: 319–84.
9 Katz AM. *Physiology of the heart*. New York: Raven Press, 1992.
10 Hoffman BB, Lefkowitz RJ. Adrenergic receptors in the heart. *Annu Rev Physiol* 1982; **44**: 475–84.
11 Feigl EO. Coronary physiology. *Physiol Rev* 1983; **63**: 1–205.
12 Donald DE, Shepherd JT. Autonomic regulation of the peripheral circulation. *Annu Rev Physiol* 1980; **42**: 429–39.
13 Vatner SF, Cox DA. Circulatory function and control. In Kelley WN, ed, *Textbook of internal medicine*. Philadelphia: JB Lippincott, 1992.
14 Mirenda JV, Grissom TE. Anesthetic implications of the renin-angiotensin system and angiotensin-converting enzyme inhibitors. *Anesth Analg* 1991; **72**: 667–83.
15 Reid IA, Morris BJ, Ganong WF. The renin angiotensin system. *Annu Rev Physiol* 1978; **40**: 377–410.
16 Hays RM. Agents affecting the renal conservation of water. In Gilman AG, Goodman CS, Rall TW, Murad R, eds, *Pharmacological basis of therapeutics*. New York: Macmillan, 1985: 908–19.
17 Johns RA. Endothelium, anesthetics, and vascular control. *Anesthesiology* 1993; **79**: 1381–91.
18 Rich GF, Johns RA. Nitric oxide and the pulmonary circulation. *Adv Anesth* 1994; **11**: 1–25.
19 Cogan MG. Renal effects of atrial natriuretic factor. *Annu Rev Physiol* 1990; **52**: 699.
20 Ginsberg R, Bristow MR, Stinson EB, Harrison DC. Histamine receptors in the human heart. *Life Sci* 1980; **26**: 2245.
21 Regoli D. Neurohumoral regulation of precapillary vessels: The kallikrein–kinin system. *J Cardiovasc Pharmacol* 1984; **6**: S401–12.
22 Marwood JF, Stokes GS. Serotonin (5HT) and its antagonists: Involvement in the cardiovascular system. *Clin Exp Pharmacol Physiol* 1984; **11**: 439.
23 Shepherd JT, Mancia G. Reflex control of the human cardiovascular system. *Rev Physiol Biochem Pharmacol* 1986; **105**: 1–99.
24 Ebert TJ. Autonomic balance and cardiac function. *Curr Opin Anaesth* 1992; **5**: 3–10.
25 Ludbrook J. Reflex control of blood pressure during exercise. *Annu Rev Physiol* 1983; **45**: 155–68.
26 Stoelting RK, Dierdorf SF. *Anesthesia and co-existing disease*. New York: Churchill Livingstone, 1993.
27 Guyton AC. Acute hypertension in dogs with cerebral ischemia. *Am J Physiol* 1948; **154**: 45–54.
28 Olsson RA. Local factors regulating cardiac and skeletal muscle blood flow. *Annu Rev Physiol* 1981; **43**: 385–95.
29 Goldberg AH, Warltier DC. The coronary circulation: Importance for anesthesiologists. *Semin Anesth* 1990; **9**: 232.
30 Warltier DC, Gross GJ, Brooks HL. Pharmacologic vs. ischemia-induced coronary artery vasodilation. *Am J Physiol* 1981; **240**: H767–74.

7: Cerebral circulation

DAVID K MENON

The brain receives 15% of the resting cardiac output (700 ml/min in the adult) and accounts for 20% of basal oxygen consumption. Mean resting cerebral blood flow (CBF) in young adults is about 50 ml/100 g brain per min. This mean value represents two very different categories of flow: 70 and 20 ml/100 g per min for grey and white matter respectively. Regional CBF (rCBF) and glucose consumption decline with age, along with marked reductions in brain neurotransmitter content, and less consistent decreases in neurotransmitter binding.[1]

Functional anatomy of the cerebral circulation

Arterial supply

Blood supply to the brain is provided by the two internal carotid arteries and the basilar artery, which divides into the two posterior cerebral arteries. The anastomoses between these two sets of vessels gives rise to the circle of Willis (fig 7.1). Functionally significant hypoplasia of the anterior and posterior communicating arteries is, however, common, and a classic "normal" polygonal anastomotic ring is found in less than 50% of brains.[2]

In spite of the anatomical variations described, certain patterns of regional blood supply from individual arteries are generally recognised. Cerebral ischaemia associated with systemic hypotension classically produces maximal lesions in areas where the zones of blood supply from two vessels meet, resulting in "watershed" infarctions. The presence of anatomical variants may, however, substantially modify patterns of infarction following large vessel occlusion. For example, in some individuals, the proximal part of one anterior cerebral artery is hypoplastic, and flow to the ipsilateral frontal lobe is largely provided by the contralateral anterior cerebral, via the anterior communicating artery. Occlusion of the single dominant anterior cerebral artery in such a patient may result in massive infarction of both frontal lobes—the unpaired anterior cerebral artery syndrome.

Microcirculation

The cerebral circulation is protected from systemic blood pressure surges by a specially designed branching system and two resistance elements: the

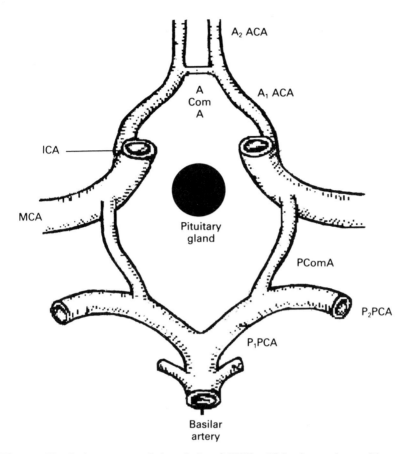

Fig 7.1 Classical anatomy of the circle of Willis. ICA = internal carotid artery; AComA = anterior communicating artery; ACA = anterior cerebral artery (A_1 = precommunicating segment of ACA; A_2 = postcommunicating segment of ACA); MCA = middle cerebral artery; PComA = posterior communicating artery; PCA = posterior cerebral artery (P_1 = precommunicating segment of PCA; P_2 = postcommunicating segment of PCA).

first of these lies in the large cerebral arteries and the second in vessels of diameter less than 100 μm. The architecture of the cerebral microvasculature is highly organised and follows the columnar arrangement seen with neuronal groups and physiologically functional units.[3] Pial vessels on the surface of the brain give rise to arterioles that penetrate the brain at right angles to the surface and give rise to capillaries at all laminar levels. Each of these arterioles supplies a hexagonal column of cortical tissue, with intervening boundary zones, an arrangement that is responsible for columnar patterns of local blood flow, redox state,[4] and glucose metabolism seen in the cortex during hypoxia or ischaemia.[5] Capillary density in the cortex is one third of adult levels at birth, doubles in the first year, and reaches adult levels at four years. In the adult animal capillary density is related to the number of synapses, rather than number of neurons or mass of cell bodies in a given region,[6] and can be closely correlated with the regional level of oxidative metabolism.[7 8] Conventionally, functional activation of the brain is thought to result in "capillary recruitment," implying that some parts of the capillary network are non-functional during rest. Recent evidence suggests, however, that all capillaries may be persistently open,[8] and "recruitment" involves changes in capillary flow rates with homogenisation of the perfusion rate in a network.[9]

Venous drainage

The brain is drained by a system of intra- and extracerebral venous sinuses, which are endothelialised channels in folds of dura mater. These sinuses drain into the internal jugular veins, which, at their origin, receive minimal contributions from extracerebral tissues. Measurement of oxygen saturation in the jugular bulb (SjO_2) thus provides a useful measure of cerebral oxygenation. It has been suggested that the supratentorial compartment is preferentially drained by the right internal jugular vein, whereas the infratentorial compartment is preferentially drained by the left internal jugular vein; this statement is probably incorrect. Available evidence suggests that about 70% of the flow to each internal jugular vein is from ipsilateral tissues, about 3% is from extracranial veins, whereas the remainder arises from the contralateral cerebral hemisphere.

Cerebral blood volume: physiology and potential for therapeutic intervention

Most of the intracranial blood volume of about 200 ml is contained in these venous sinuses and pial veins, which constitute the capacitance vessels of the cerebral circulation; reduction in this volume can buffer rises in the volume of other intracranial contents (the brain and CSF). Conversely, when compensatory mechanisms to control intracranial pressure (ICP) have been exhausted, even small increases in cerebral blood volume (CBV) can result in steep rises in ICP (fig 7.2). The position of the system on this curve can be expressed in terms of the pressure–volume index (PVI), which is defined as the change in intracranial volume that produces a tenfold increase in ICP. This is normally about 26 ml,[10] but may be markedly lower in patients with intracranial hypertension, who are on the steep part of the intracranial pressure–volume curve (see effects of PCO_2 on CBV).

With the exception of mannitol induced oedema reduction, the only intracranial constituent whose volume can be readily modified by the

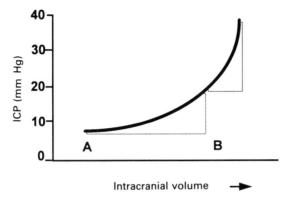

Fig 7.2 Intracranial pressure–volume curve: the pressure–volume index (PVI), defined as the change in intracranial volume required to cause a tenfold increase in ICP, increases non-linearly, from approximately 25 ml in normals (point A on the curve) to as little as 5 ml in patients with raised ICP (point B on the curve).

anaesthetist through physiological or pharmacological interventions is the CBV. Although the CBV forms only a small part of the intracranial volume, and such interventions only produce small absolute changes (typically about 10 ml or less), they may result in marked reductions in ICP in the presence of intracranial hypertension. Conversely, inappropriate anaesthetic management may cause the CBV to increase. Again, although the absolute magnitude of such increase may be small, it may result in steep rises in ICP in the presence of intracranial hypertension.

Determinants of cerebral perfusion

The inflow pressure to the brain is equal to the mean arterial pressure (MAP) measured at the level of the brain. The outflow pressure from the intracranial cavity depends on the ICP, because collapse of intracerebral veins is prevented by the maintenance of an intraluminal pressure 2–5 mm Hg above ICP. The difference between the MAP and the ICP thus provides an estimate of the effective cerebral perfusion pressure (CPP):

$$CPP = MAP - ICP$$

Microcirculatory transport and the blood–brain barrier

Endothelial cells in cerebral capillaries contain few pinocytic vesicles, and are sealed with tight junctions, with no anatomical gap. Consequently, unlike other capillary beds, the endothelial barrier of cerebral capillaries presents a high electrical resistance and is remarkably non-leaky, even to small molecules such as mannitol (molecular weight or M_r of 180 daltons). This

201

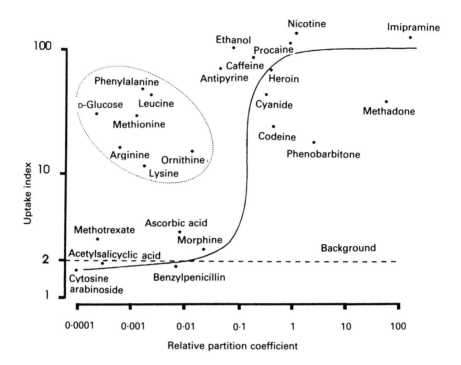

Fig 7.3 Correlation between brain uptake index and oil/water partition coefficients for different substrates. Although blood–brain barrier permeability, in general, increases with lipid solubility, note that several substances including glucose and amino acids show high penetration as a result of active transport or facilitated diffusion. (After Oldendorf.[12])

property of the cerebral vasculature, termed the "blood–brain barrier," is a function of the cerebral microenvironment rather than an intrinsic property of the vessels themselves, and leaky capillaries from other vascular beds develop a blood–brain barrier if they are transplanted to the brain or exposed to astrocytes in culture.[11] Passage through the blood–brain barrier is not simply a function of molecular weight; lipophilic substances traverse the barrier relatively easily, and several hydrophilic molecules (including glucose) cross the blood–brain barrier via active transport systems to enter the brain interstitial space[12] (fig 7.3). In addition, the blood–brain barrier maintains a tight control of relative ionic distribution in the brain extracellular fluid. These activities are energy requiring and explain the fact that the mitochondrial density is exceptionally high in these endothelial cells, accounting for 10% of cytoplasmic volume.[13] Although the blood–brain barrier is disrupted by ischaemia, this process takes hours or days rather than minutes, and much of the cerebral oedema seen in the initial period after ischaemic insults is cytotoxic rather than vasogenic. Consequently, "membrane stabilising agents" such as corticosteroids are ineffective in this phase of the process, and mannitol retains its ability to reduce cerebral oedema in the early phases of acute brain injury.

Measurement of rCBF

All clinical and many laboratory methods of measuring CBF or rCBF are indirect and may not produce directly comparable measurements. It is also important to treat results from any one method with caution, and attribute any observed phenomena to physiological effects only when demonstrated by two or more independent techniques. Methods of measuring CBF may be regional or global, and applicable either to humans or primarily to experimental animals. All of these methods have advantages and disadvantages (table 7.1). All methods that provide absolute estimates of rCBF use one of two principles: they either measure the distribution of a tracer or estimate rCBF from the wash-in or wash-out curve of an indicator. Other techniques do not directly estimate rCBF, but can be used either to measure a related flow variable (such as arterial flow velocity) or to infer changes in flow from changes in metabolic parameters. Some techniques that have been used for the measurement of CBF are described briefly.

The Kety–Schmidt technique[14]

The Kety–Schmidt technique involves the insertion of catheters into a peripheral artery and the jugular bulb. A diffusible tracer such as 10–15% inhaled nitrous oxide (N_2O) is administered, and paired arterial and jugular venous samples of blood are obtained at rapid intervals for measurement of N_2O levels. The resultant plot of concentration versus time produces an arterial and a venous curve (fig 7.4). The jugular venous level of N_2O rises more slowly than the arterial levels, because N_2O is being taken up by the brain as it is delivered. The rate of equilibration of the two curves measures the rate at which N_2O is being delivered to the brain, and thus provide a means of measuring global CBF.

Xenon-133 wash-out

An array of collimated scintillation counters is positioned over the head to plot the regional decay in radioactivity after the intracarotid[15] or intra-aortic injection of ^{133}Xe. The wash-out curve for radioactivity is biexponential, and may be resolved into two monoexponential components, which represent a fast wash-out and a slow wash-out component. Although these are often referred to as grey matter and white matter components, it must be

Table 7.1 Methods of measuring CBF

Technique	Global/regional	Comments
Human and laboratory methods		
Kety–Schmidt[14]	Global	Uses rate of uptake of N_2O to measure global CBF. Requires jugular bulb and arterial catheters. Repeated measures possible
[133]Xe wash-out[15 16]	Regional	Classic method uses wash-out curve of radioactive xenon after intracarotid injection to estimate CBF. Summated curves show fast and slow wash-out components (? grey and white matter). Primarily looks at cortex, poor resolution. Modifications include intravenous/inhalational/intra-aortic administration of xenon. Repeated measures possible
Dynamic CT	Regional	Looks at wash-out of stable xenon[16a]/intravenous contrast[16b] after inhalation. Repeated measures possible, but not at rapid intervals
PET ($H_2^{15}O$)[17]	Regional	Uses distribution of radiolabelled marker to estimate rCBF. Repeated measures possible. Expensive equipment. Good resolution
SPECT[18]	Regional	Uses distribution of radiolabelled tracer to estimate rCBF. Cheaper than PET, but resolution poorer, repeated measurements difficult
NIROS (+ O_2 wash-in)[19]	?Regional	Detects rate of change of cerebral oxygenation state after step change in F_{IO_2}. Poorly defined volume and resolution. ? Accurate
Laboratory methods H_2 clearance[20]	Regional	Measures wash-out of H_2 after inhalational administration. Very localised measurement (1–2 mm^3) with hydrogen electrode
		Requires craniotomy. Repeated measures possible
Autoradiography[21]	Regional	Uses distribution of radiolabelled tracer ([14C]iodoantipyrine) to estimate rCBF. Excellent resolution. Single measurement only
Radiolabelled[22] microspheres	Regional	Uses distribution of radiolabelled microspheres (15 μm diameter) to estimate rCBF resolution not as good as autoradiography. Repeated measurements with different radiolabels possible. Radiolabel injection in left atrium or aorta
Indirect or non-quantitative measures MRI[23]	Regional	Uses change in regional oxygenation during functional activation to show changes in rCBF. Superb resolution, absolute measures not possible. Excellent resolution, repeated measures easy. Modification with external label may permit quantitation, but repeated measures more restricted
Doppler ultrasonography[24]	(Regional)	Measures flow velocity in middle cerebral artery using Doppler ultrasonography. Indirect measure of CBF
NIROS[25]	(Regional)	Measures regional Hb oxygenation and cytochrome redox state in restricted and poorly defined volume
MRS[23]	Regional	Provides information regarding intracellular pH and tissue levels of ATP and lactate. Poor resolution, repeatable

PET, positron emission tomography; SPECT, single photon emission tomography; NIROS, near infrared optical spectroscopy; MRI, magnetic resonance imaging; MRS, magnetic resonance spectroscopy.

emphasised that there is no basis to support such an anatomical distinction, because the two curves represent pharmacokinetic compartments, rather than specific neuroanatomical structures. The technique does provide two dimensional information regarding rCBF, but is invasive and primarily looks at superficial cortical blood flow. Further, intracarotid injection only permits the assessment of a single cerebral hemisphere at a time. One modification involves the inhalational[16] or intravenous administration of ^{133}Xe; although this makes the technique less invasive, problems arise because of recircula-

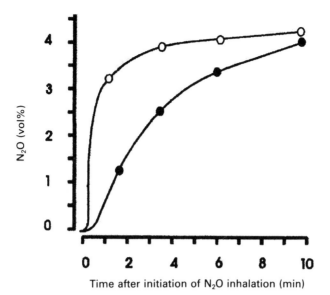

Fig 7.4 The Kety–Schmidt method of measuring global cerebral blood flow. The rate of increase in arterial (–○–) and jugular venous (–●–) N$_2$O concentrations of a diffusible tracer gas (N$_2$O in this instance) are compared. A rapid equilibration implies high CBF, whereas a slow equilibration is evidence of low CBF.

tion and contamination by extracranial tissues. The simultaneous presence of activity in both cerebral hemispheres also leads to the "look-through" phenomenon, where rCBF reductions on one side may be missed because of activity sensed in deeper or contralateral tissues.

Tomographic rCBF measurement: dynamic CT, SPECT, PET, and fMRI

Tomographic information regarding rCBF may be obtained by quantifying the wash-out of a radiodense contrast agent, using rapid sequential X-ray computed tomography (dynamic CT). In the past, inhaled stable xenon has been used most often as the contrast agent. More recent studies have been performed using standard radioiodinated intravenous contrast agents (fig 7.5).

Single photon emission tomography (SPECT) and positron emission tomography (PET) use γ emitting and positron emitting isotopes, respectively, to produce tomographic images of rCBF. Functional magnetic resonance imaging (fMRI) produces tomographic images of rCBF in one of two ways. One technique uses an intravenous MR contrast agent (for example, gadopentate dimeglumine, Magnevist) in much the same way as techniques mentioned previously use other agents. MRI can also produce, without the use of external contrast agents, tomographic images of *changes* in rCBF following functional activation, through the imaging of increases in MR signal intensity produced by the decreases in regional deoxyhaemoglobin levels which occur during flow metabolism coupling (see page 209).

Detailed discussion of these techniques is beyond the scope of this chapter, and the interested reader is referred to the references in table 7.1 for details.

Continuous clinical monitoring of the adequacy of cerebral perfusion, in general, tends to use techniques other than those outlined in table 7.1[27] (fig 7.6). The parameter most commonly monitored in head injured patients is the cerebral perfusion pressure, although many centres are increasingly using fibreoptic jugular venous oximetry[28] and transcranial Doppler measurement of middle cerebral artery flow velocity.[29] Monitoring of the processed EEG[30] or evoked potentials[31] provides information about the consequences of reduced CBF, and this technique has been used in the context of cardiopulmonary bypass and carotid endarterectomy. Near infrared optical spectro-

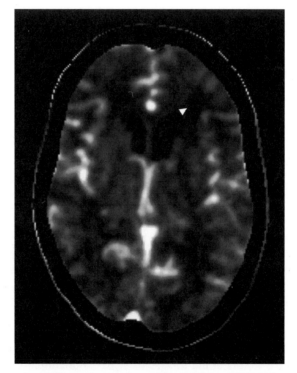

Fig 7.5 Grey scale rCBF map in a patient with a left frontal infarct (arrow) secondary to vasospasm following aneurysmal subarachnoid haemorrhage. The image was obtained with a dynamic CT scan of the brain after intravenous injection of radioiodinated contrast agent. Note the hypoperfusion surrounding the infarcted region. (Image courtesy of Mr Hayball and Dr Miles.)

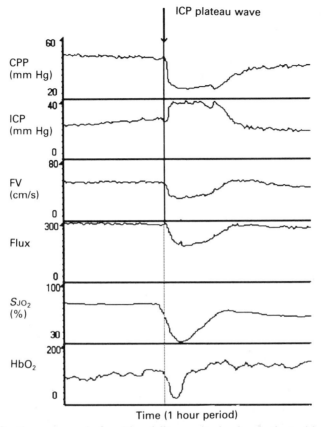

Fig 7.6 Continuous record of multimodality monitoring in a patient with acute head injury during a plateau wave in the ICP. Note the fall in the CPP and reduction in the middle cerebral artery flow velocity (FV) measured using transcranial Doppler and reduction in laser Doppler signal intensity (flux measured in arbitrary units), suggesting reduced capillary flow. The ischaemia associated with the reduction in CPP produces a jugular venous desaturation ($S\text{JO}_2$ catheter) and a fall in oxyhaemoglobin signal (NIROS) measured in arbitrary units. (Recording courtesy of Dr Marek Czosnyka.)

scopy and laser Doppler flowmetry[32] are investigational techniques whose roles have not been clearly defined.

Physiological determinants of regional cerebral blood flow and volume

Flow–metabolism coupling

Increases in local neuronal activity are accompanied by increases in regional cerebral metabolic rate (rCMR). Until recently, the increases in

207

rCBF and oxygen consumption produced during such functional activation were thought to be closely coupled to the cerebral metabolic rate of use of O_2 (CMRo$_2$) and glucose (CMRGlu). However, it has now been clearly shown that increases in rCBF during functional activation tend to track glucose use but may be far in excess of the increase in oxygen consumption.[33] This results in regional *anaerobic* glucose utilisation, and a consequent local decrease in oxygen extraction ratio and increase in local haemoglobin saturation. The resulting local decrease in deoxyhaemoglobin levels is used by functional MRI techniques to image the changes in rCBF produced by functional activation. In spite of this revision of the proportionality between increased rCBF and CMRo$_2$ during functional activation in the brain, the relationship between rCBF and CMRGlu is still accepted as linear. These regulatory changes have a short latency (about 1 s) and may be mediated by either metabolic or neurogenic pathways. The former category includes the increases in perivascular K^+ or adenosine concentrations that follow neuronal depolarisation. The cerebral vessels are richly supplied by nerve fibres, and the mediators thought to play an important part in neurogenic flow metabolism coupling are acetylcholine[34] and nitric oxide,[35] although roles have also been proposed for 5-hydroxytryptamine (serotonin), substance P, and neuropeptide Y.

Autoregulation

Autoregulation refers to the ability of the cerebral circulation to maintain CBF at a relatively constant level in the face of changes in CPP by altering cerebrovascular resistance (CVR) (fig 7.7). Although autoregulation is maintained irrespective of whether changes in CPP arise from alterations in MAP or ICP, autoregulation tends to be preserved at lower levels when falls in CPP result from increases in ICP rather than from decreases in MAP caused by hypovolaemia.[36 37] One possible reason for this may be the cerebral vasoconstrictive effects of the massive levels of catecholamines secreted in haemorrhagic hypotension. For similar reasons, lower MAP levels are tolerated in hypotension if the fall in blood pressure is induced by sympatholytic agents,[38 39] or occurs in the setting of autonomic failure.[40] Autoregulatory changes in CVR probably arise from myogenic reflexes in the resistance vessels, but these may be modulated by activity of the sympathetic system or the presence of chronic systemic hypertension.[41] Thus, sympathetic blockade or cervical sympathectomy shifts the autoregulatory curve to the left, whereas chronic hypertension or sympathetic activation shifts it to the right. These modulatory effects may arise from angiotensin mediated mechanisms.

In reality, the clear cut autoregulatory thresholds seen with varying CPP in fig 7.7 are not observed; the autoregulatory "knees" tend to be more gradual, and there may be wide variations in rCBF at a given value of CPP in

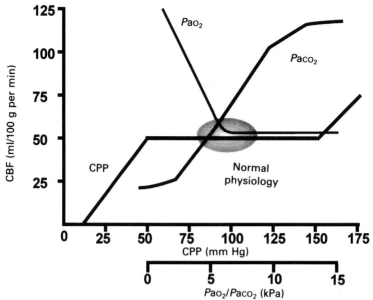

Fig 7.7 Effect of changes in CPP, Paco$_2$, and Pao$_2$ on CBF. The shaded area outlines the normal physiological fluctuations in Paco$_2$ and CPP, but does *not* include the normal range of Pao$_2$. Note the increase in slope of the CBF/Paco$_2$ curve as basal CBF increases from 20 ml/100 g per min (white matter) to 50–70 ml/100 g per min (grey matter).

experimental animals and even in neurologically normal individuals.[42] It has been demonstrated that symptoms of cerebral ischaemia appear when the MAP falls below 60% of an individual's lower autoregulatory threshold.[43] However, generalised extrapolation from such individualised research data to the production of "safe" lower limits of MAP for general clinical practice is hazardous for several reasons:

1 There may be wide individual scatter in rCBF autoregulatory efficiency, even in normal subjects.
2 The coexistence of fixed vascular obstruction (for example, carotid atheroma or vascular spasm) may vary the MAP level at which rCBF reaches critical levels in relevant territories.
3 The autoregulatory curve may be substantially modulated by the mechanisms used to produce hypotension. Earlier discussion made the distinction of reductions in CPP produced by haemorrhagic hypotension, intracranial hypertension, or pharmacological hypotension. The effects on autoregulation may also vary with the pharmacological agent used to produce hypotension. Thus, neuronal function is better preserved at similar levels of hypotension produced by halothane, nitroprusside, or isoflurane in comparison with trimetaphan.[44]

209

4 Autoregulatory responses are not immediate: estimates of the latency for compensatory changes in rCVR range from 10 s to 60 s.[45]

Some recent studies suggest that, especially in patients with impaired autoregulation, the cardiac output and pulsatility of large vessel flow may be more important determinants of rCBF than CPP itself.[46]

Arterial carbon dioxide tension

CBF is proportional to $Paco_2$, subject to a lower limit below which vasoconstriction results in tissue hypoxia and reflex vasodilatation, and an upper limit of maximal vasodilatation (fig 7.7). On average, in the middle of the physiological range, each kilopascal change in $Paco_2$ produces a change of about 15 ml/100 g per min in CBF. The slope of the $Paco_2$/CBF relationship depends, however, on the baseline normocapnic rCBF value, being maximal in areas where it is high (for example, grey matter, cerebrum) and least in areas where it is low (for example, white matter, cerebellum, and spinal cord). Moderate hypocapnia ($Paco_2$ of about 3·5 kPa) has long been used to reduce CBV in intracranial hypertension, but this practice is under review for two reasons:

1 The CO_2 response is directly related to the change in perivascular pH; consequently, the effect of a change in $Paco_2$ tends to be attenuated over time (hours) as brain ECF bicarbonate levels fall to normalise interstitial pH.[47]
2 It has now been shown that "acceptable" levels of hypocapnia in head injured patients can result in dangerously low rCBF levels.[48]

Prostaglandins may mediate the vasodilatation produced by CO_2,[49] more recent work suggesting that nitric oxide may also be involved.[50]

Effects on CBV and ICP

Grubb et al[51] studied the CBF/$Paco_2$ response curve in primates and demonstrated that the CBF changed by about 1·8 ml/100 g per min for each mm Hg change in $Paco_2$. In the same experiment, however, the CBV/$Paco_2$ curve was much flatter (about 0·04 ml/100 g per mm Hg (0·3 ml/100 g per kPa) change in $Paco_2$). It follows from these figures that although a reduction in $Paco_2$ from 5·3 to 4 kPa (40 to 30 mm Hg) would result in about a 40% reduction in CBF (from a baseline of about 50 ml/100 g per min), it would only result in a 0·4% reduction in intracranial volume. This may seem trivial, but in the presence of intracranial hypertension, the resultant 5 ml decrease in intracranial volume in an adult brain could result in a halving of ICP because the system operates on the steep part of the intracranial compliance curve.[52]

Arterial oxygen pressure and content

CBF is unchanged until Pa_{CO_2} levels fall below approximately 7 kPa, but rises sharply with further reductions[53] (see fig 7.7). This is because tissue oxygen delivery governs CBF, and the sigmoid shape of the haemoglobin–O_2 dissociation curve means that the relationship between Ca_{O_2} (arterial O_2 content) and CBF is inversely linear. These vasodilator responses to hypoxaemia appear to show little adaptation with time,[54] but may be substantially modulated by Pa_{CO_2} levels.[55 56] Nitric oxide does not appear to play a role in the vasodilatory response to hypoxia.[50]

Some studies suggest that hyperoxia may produce cerebral vasoconstriction, with a 10–14% reduction in CBF with inhalation of 85–100% O_2, and a 20% reduction in CBF with 100% O_2 at 3·5 atmospheres.[57] There are no human data to suggest that this effect is *clinically* significant.

Haematocrit

As in other organs, optimal O_2 delivery in the brain depends on a compromise between the oxygen carrying capacity and the flow characteristics of blood; previous experimental work suggests that this may be best achieved at a haematocrit of about 40%. Some recent studies in the setting of vasospasm following subarachnoid haemorrhage have suggested that modest haemodilution to a haematocrit of 30–35% may improve neurological outcome by improving rheological characteristics[58] and increasing rCBF. This may result, however, in a reduction in O_2 delivery if maximal vasodilatation is already present, and as clinical results in the setting of acute ischaemia have not been uniformly successful, this approach must be viewed with caution.

Autonomic nervous system

The autonomic nervous system mainly affects the larger cerebral vessels, up to and including the proximal parts of the anterior, middle, and posterior cerebral arteries. β_1-Adrenergic stimulation results in vasodilatation whereas α_2-adrenergic stimulation vasoconstricts these vessels. The effect of systemically administered α or β agonists is less significant. Significant vasoconstriction, however, can be produced by extremely high concentrations of catecholamines (for example, haemorrhage) or centrally acting α_2 agonists (for example, dexmetetomidine).

Pharmacological modulation of CBF

Inhaled anaesthetics

All the potent fluorinated agents have significant effects on CBF and CMR. The initial popularity of halothane as a neurosurgical anaesthetic agent was

211

reversed by the discovery that it was a potent cerebral vasodilator, producing decreases of 20–40% in cerebrovascular resistance in normocapnic individuals at 1·2–1·5 MAC (MAC = minimum alveolar concentration).[59 60] In another study 1% halothane was shown to result in clinically significant elevations in ICP in patients with intracranial space occupying lesions.[61] Preliminary studies with enflurane and isoflurane suggested that these agents might produce smaller increases in cerebrovascular resistance (CVR) at equivalent doses.[62] As enflurane may produce epileptogenic activity[63] its use in the context of neuroanaesthesia decreased. Several studies, however, compared the effects of isoflurane and halothane on CBF, with conflicting results. Although some studies showed that halothane produced larger decreases in CVR, others found no difference. Examination of the patterns of rCBF produced by these two agents provides some clues to the origin of this discrepancy. Halothane selectively increases cortical rCBF while markedly decreasing subcortical rCBF, whereas isoflurane produces a more generalised reduction in rCBF.[64 65] A review of published comparisons of the CBF effects of the two agents suggests that studies that estimated CBF using techniques that preferentially looked at the cortex (for example, ^{133}Xe wash-out) tended to show that halothane was a more potent vasodilator, whereas most studies that have used more global measures of hemispherical CBF (for example, the Kety–Schmidt technique) have found little difference between the two agents at levels of around 1 MAC (fig 7.8).

Both agents tend to reduce global CMR, although the regional pattern of such an effect may vary, with isoflurane producing greater cortical metabolic suppression[64] (reflected by its ability to produce EEG burst suppression at higher doses). Both the rCBF and rCMR effects of the two anaesthetics are markedly modified by baseline physiology and other pharmacological agents. Thus, CBF increases produced by both agents are attenuated by hypocapnia (more so with isoflurane[77 78]), and thiopentone attenuates the increases in cortical rCBF produced by halothane. It is difficult to predict accurately what the effect of either agent would be on CBF in a given clinical situation, but this would be a balance of its suppressant effects on rCMR (with autoregulatory vasoconstriction) and its direct vasodilator effect (which is partially mediated via nitric oxide[35]).

Although initial reports suggested that halothane could "uncouple" flow and metabolism[71] more recent studies clearly show that at concentrations commonly in use for neuroanaesthesia (0·5–1 MAC) neither isoflurane[79] nor halothane[80] completely disrupts flow–metabolism coupling, although their vasodilator effects may alter the slope of this relationship. These vasodilator effects may become more prominent at higher concentrations.

In equivalent MAC doses, nitrous oxide is probably a *more* powerful vasodilator than either halothane[81] or isoflurane;[82] this fact, coupled with its lack of CMR depression,[83] produces a particularly unfavourable pharmacodynamic profile in patients with raised ICP.[84 85] Further, the vasodilatation

212

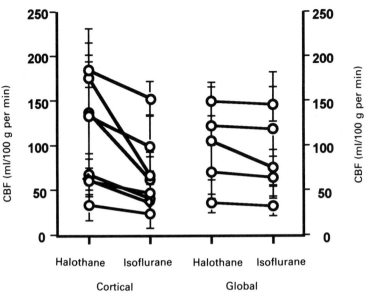

Fig 7.8 Comparison of mean±SD CBF in animals or patients anaesthetised with 0·5–1·5 MAC isoflurane or halothane, either in the same study or in comparable studies from a single research group with identical methodology within a single publication year.[64 66–76] In studies shown on the left, CBF was estimated using techniques likely to be biased towards cortical flow (for example, ^{133}Xe wash-out) and show that halothane produces greater increases in CBF. In studies on the right, CBF was estimated using techniques that measured global CBF (for example, the Kety–Schmidt method); the difference in effects on CBF between the two agents is much less prominent.

produced by nitrous oxide is not decreased by hypocapnia,[86] although the resulting increases in ICP can be attenuated by the administration of other CMR depressants such as the barbiturates.[87]

Desflurane[88] and sevoflurane[89] have effects on the cerebral vasculature that appear very similar to isoflurane, but a few points are worth highlighting. Although high dose desflurane, like isoflurane, can produce EEG burst suppression, this effect may be attenuated over time.[90] It is not known whether this adaptation represents a pharmacokinetic or a pharmacodynamic effect. Initial clinical reports suggest that desflurane may cause a clinically significant rise in ICP in patients with supratentorial lesions,[91] in spite of its documented ability to reduce CMR_{O_2} as documented by EEG burst suppression.[90 92]

Intravenous anaesthetics

Thiopentone,[93] etomidate,[94] and propofol[95 96] all reduce global CMR to a minimum of approximately 50% of baseline, with a coupled reduction in

CBF, although animal studies suggest small differences in the distribution of rCBF changes with individual agents. Decreases in CBV have been demonstrated with barbiturates[97] and probably occur with propofol and etomidate as well. Maximal reductions in CMR are reflected in an isoelectric EEG, although burst suppression is associated with only slightly less CMR depression.[93] Initial doubts that CBF reductions produced by propofol were secondary to falls in MAP have proved to be unfounded.[95 96]

Even high doses of thiopentone or propofol[98] do not appear to affect autoregulation, CO_2 responsiveness, or flow–metabolism coupling.

Opiates

Although high doses of morphine (3 mg/kg) and moderate doses of fentanyl (15 µg/kg) have little effect on CBF and CMR, high doses of fentanyl (50–100 µg/kg)[99] and sufentanil[100] depress CMR and CBF. Results with alfentanil, in doses of 0·32 mg/kg, show no reduction in rCBF.[101] These effects are variable and may only be prominent in the presence of nitrous oxide, where CMR may be reduced by 40% from baseline.[102] Bolus administration of large doses of fentanyl or alfentanil may be associated with increases in ICP in patients with intracranial hypertension,[103] probably as a result of reflex increases in CBF which follow an initial decrease in CBF (caused by reductions in MAP and cardiac output produced by large bolus doses of these agents). These effects are unlikely to be clinically significant if detrimental haemodynamic and blood gas changes can be avoided.

Other drugs

Ketamine can produce increases in global CBF and ICP,[104] with specific increases in rCMR and rCBF in limbic structures.[105] These changes may be partially attenuated by hypocapnia, benzodiazepines, or halothane.[106] Sedative doses of benzodiazepines tend to produce small decreases in CMR and CBF;[107] however, there is a ceiling effect and increasing doses do not produce greater reductions in these variables.[108] Most non-depolarising neuromuscular blockers have little effect on CBF or CMR, although large doses of d-tubocurarine may increase CBV and ICP secondary to histamine release and vasodilatation. In contrast suxamethonium (succinylcholine) can produce increases in ICP, probably secondary to increases in CBF mediated via muscle spindle activation. These effects are, however, transient and mild,[109 110] and can be blocked by prior precurarisation[111] if necessary; they provide no basis for avoiding suxamethonium in patients with raised ICP when its rapid onset of action is desirable for clinical reasons.[29]

214

CBF in disease

Ischaemia

Graded reductions in CBF are associated with specific electrophysiological and metabolic consequences (table 7.2). Some of these thresholds for metabolic events are well recognised, but others, such as the development of acidosis, cessation of protein synthesis and the failure of osmotic regulation, have only recently received attention.[112] Ischaemia is thus a continuum between normal cellular function and cell death; cell death is not, however, merely a function of the severity of ischaemia, but is also dependent on its duration and several other circumstances that modify its effects. Thus, the effects of ischaemia may be ameliorated by the CMR depression produced by hypothermia or drugs, exacerbated by increased metabolic demand associated with excitatory neurotransmitter release, or compounded by other mechanisms of secondary neuronal injury (such as cellular calcium overload or reperfusion injury).

Head injury

Severe head injury is accompanied by both direct and indirect effects on cerebral blood flow and metabolism. CBF may be high, normal, or low soon after the ictus.[113] Thirty per cent of patients undergoing CBF studies within 6–8 hours of a head injury have significant cerebral ischaemia.[114] Global hypoperfusion in these studies was associated with a 100% mortality rate at 48 hours, and regional ischaemia with significant deficits. Blood flow tends to be reduced in the immediate vicinity of intracranial haematomas, and clinically significant vasospasm has been reported in the context of acute head injury.[115] Elevations in intracranial pressure result in reductions in CPP and cerebral ischaemia, which lead to secondary neuronal injury. There is strong evidence that maintenance of a CPP above 60 mm Hg improves outcome in patients with head injury and raised ICP.[116] Traditionally, patients with intracranial hypertension have been nursed head up in an effort to reduce

Table 7.2 Electrophysiological and metabolic consequences of graded reductions in CBF

CBF (ml/100 g per min)	Electrophysiological/metabolic consequence
>50	Normal neuronal function
?	Immediate early gene activation
?	Cessation of protein synthesis
?	Cellular acidosis
20–23	Reduction in electrical activity
12–18	Cessation of electrical activity
8–10	ATP rundown, loss of ionic homoeostasis
<8	Cell death (also depends on other modifiers: duration, CMR, etc)

215

ICP. It is important to realise, however, that such manoeuvres will also reduce the effective MAP at the level of the head and run the risk of reducing CPP. Feldmann et al[117] suggest that a 30° head up elevation may provide the optimal balance by reducing ICP without decreasing CPP.

Hypertensive encephalopathy

Current concepts of the causation of hypertensive encephalopathy are based on the forced vasodilatation hypothesis.[41][118] Severe acute or sustained elevations in mean arterial pressure overcome autoregulatory vasoconstriction in the resistance vessels and result in forced vasodilatation. These vasodilated vessels, exposed to high intraluminal pressures, leak fluid and protein, and result in cerebral oedema, which is multifocal and later diffuse.

Subarachnoid haemorrhage

Cerebral autoregulation and CO_2 responsiveness are grossly distorted after subarachnoid haemorrhage (SAH), more so in patients in worse clinical grades.[119] Such patients may be unable to compensate for reductions in MAP produced by anaesthetic agents and develop clinically significant deficits.[120] Clinically significant vasospasm after SAH occurs in up to 30–40%[121] of patients, typically several days after the initial bleed, and may be the result of one or more of several mechanisms. Nitric oxide (NO) may be taken up by haemoglobin in the extravasated blood or be inactivated to peroxynitrite $(ONOO^-)$ by superoxide radicals $(O^{\pm})$ produced during ischaemia and reperfusion. Alternatively, spasm may be secondary to lipid peroxidation of the vessel wall by various oxidant species including superoxide and peroxynitrite. Other authors have proposed a role for endothelin.[122][123] Vasospasm tends to be worst in patients with the largest amounts of subarachnoid blood,[124] suggesting that the blood in itself contributes to the phenomenon. Vasospasm is associated with parallel reductions in rCBF and CMR_{O_2} in the regions affected.

The clinical impact of late vasospasm has been substantially modified by the routine use of Ca^{2+} channel blockers such as nimodipine,[125] and by the routine use of hypertensive hypervolaemic haemodilution (triple H therapy).[121] Triple H (3H) therapy involves the use of colloid administration (with venesection if needed) to increase filling pressures and reduce haematocrit to 30–35%. If moderate hypertension is not achieved with volume loading, vasopressors and inotropes are used to maintain systolic blood pressures between 150 and 200 mm Hg. The hypertensive element of this therapy protects non-autoregulating portions of the cerebral vasculature from hypoperfusion, whereas the haemodilution element improves rheological characteristics of blood and facilitates flow through vessels whose calibre is reduced by spasm. Such interventions have been shown to produce clinically useful improvements in rCBF in regions of ischaemia.[126]

Mechanisms in rCBF control

Some of the mechanisms involved in cerebrovascular control are shown in fig 7.9. Several of these have been referred to earlier. In addition, the level of free Ca^{2+} is important in determining vascular tone, and arachidonate metabolism can produce prostanoids that are either vasodilators (for example, prostacyclin, PGI_2) or vasoconstrictors (for example, thromboxane TA_2).

Nitric oxide in the regulation of cerebral haemodynamics[50]

Recent interest has focused on the role of nitric oxide (NO) in the control of cerebral haemodynamics. NO is synthesised in the brain from the amino

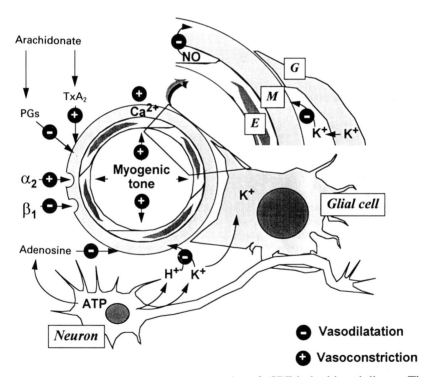

Fig 7.9 Mechanisms involved in the regulation of rCBF in health and disease. The diagram shows a resistance vessel in the brain in the vicinity of a neuron and a glial cell (G). Other abbreviations: E = endothelium; M = muscular layer; PGs = prostaglandins; TxA_2 = thromboxane A_2; NO = nitric oxide. The inset box shows detail of the vessel wall and adjacent glial cell process. See text for details.

acid L-arginine by the constitutive form of the enzyme nitric oxide synthase. This form of the enzyme is calmodulin dependent and requires Ca^{2+} and tetrahydrobiopterin for its activity, and differs from the inducible form of the enzyme which is present in mononuclear blood cells and is activated by cytokines. Under basal conditions endothelial cells synthesise NO which diffuses into the muscular layer and, via a cyclic GMP mediated mechanism, produces relaxation of vessels. There is strong evidence to suggest that NO exerts a tonic dilatory influence on cerebral vessels. It is important to emphasise that data on NO obtained from peripheral vessels cannot always be translated to the cerebral vasculature; for example, some of the endothelium derived relaxing factor activity in cerebral vessels may result from compounds other than NO.[127]

NO plays an important role in cerebrovascular responses to functional activation, excitatory amino acids, hypercapnia, ischaemia, and subarachnoid haemorrhage. Further, NO may play an important part in mediating the vasodilatation produced by volatile anaesthetic agents,[50] although other mechanisms, including a direct effect on the vessel wall, cannot be excluded.

1 Edvinsson L, Mackenzie ET, McCulloch J. The aged brain. In: *Cerebral blood flow and metabolism*. New York: Raven Press, 1993: 647–60.
2 Alpers BJ, Berry RG, Paddison RM. Anatomical studies in the circle of Willis in normal brains. *Arch Neurol Psychiatr* 1959; **81**: 409–18.
3 Collins RC. Intracortical localization of 2-deoxyglucose metabolism on-off metabolic columns. In: Passonneau JV, Hawkins RA, Lust WD, Welsh FA, eds, *Cerebral metabolism and neural function*. Baltimore: Williams & Wilkins, 1980: 338–51.
4 Welsh FA. Regional evalution of ischaemic metabolic alterations. *J Cereb Blood Flow Metab* 1984; **4**: 309–16.
5 Pulsinelli WA, Duffy TE. Local cerebral glucose metabolism during controlled hypoxaemia in rats. *Science* 1979; **204**: 626–9.
6 Dunning HS, Wolff HG. The relative vascularity of various parts of the central and peripheral nervous system in the cat and its relation to function. *J Comp Neurol* 1937; **67**: 433–50.
7 Sokoloff L, Reivich M, Kennedy C, *et al*. The [14C]-deoxyglucose method for measurement of local cerebral glucose utilization: Theory, procedure, and normal values in the conscious and anesthetized albino rat. *J Neurochem* 1977; **28**: 897–916.
8 Göbel U, Theilen H, Kuschinsky W. Congruence of total and perfused capillary network in rat brains. *Circ Res* 1990; **66**: 271–81.
9 Kuschinsky W, Paulson OB. Capillary circulation in the brain [review]. *Cerebrovascular and Brain Metabolism Reviews* 1992; **4**: 261–86.
10 Shapiro K, Marmarou A, Shulman K. Characterization of clinical CSF dynamics and neural axis compliance using the pressure–volume index. I. The normal pressure–volume index. *Ann Neurol* 1980; **7**: 508–13.
11 Janzer RC, Raff MC. Astrocytes induce blood–brain barrier properties in endothelial cells. *Nature* 1987; **325**: 253–57.
12 Oldendorf WH. Lipid solubility and drug penetration of the blood–brain barrier. *Proc Soc Exp Biol Med* 1974; **147**: 813–16.
13 Oldendorf WH, Cornford ME, Brown WJ. The large apparent work capability of the blood brain barrier. A study of the mitochondrial content of capillary endothelial cells in brain and other tissues of the rat. *Ann Neurol* 1977; **1**: 409–17.
14 Kety SS, Schmidt CF. The determination of cerebral blood flow in man by use of nitrous oxide in low concentrations. *Am J Physiol* 1945; **143**: 53–66.

15 Ingvar DH, Lassen NA. Quantitative determination of regional cerebral blood flow in man. *Lancet* 1961; ii: 806–7.

16 Mallett BL, Veall N. Investigation of cerebral blood flow in hypertension, using radioactive xenon inhalation and extracranial recording. *Lancet* 1963; i: 1081–2.

16a Yonas H, Gur D, Latchaw RE, Wolfson SK. Xenon computed tomographic blood flow mapping. In: Wood JH, ed, *Cerebral blood flow. Physiologic and clinical aspects*. New York: McGraw-Hill, 220–42.

16b Miles KA, Hayball M, Dixon AK. Colour perfusion imaging: a new application of computed tomography. *Lancet* 1991; 337: 643–5.

17 Herscovitch MD, Powers WJ. Measurement of regional cerebral blood flow by positron emission tomography. In: Wood JH, ed, *Cerebral blood flow. Physiologic and clinical aspects*. New York: McGraw-Hill, 1987: 257–71.

18 Holman BL, Hill TC. Perfusion imaging with single-photon emission computed tomography. In: Wood JH, ed, *Cerebral blood flow. Physiologic and clinical aspects*. New York: McGraw-Hill, 1987: 243–56.

19 Elwell CE, Owen-Reece H, Cope M, *et al*. Measurement of adult cerebral haemodynamics using near infrared spectroscopy. *Acta Neurochir* 1993; suppl 59: 74–80.

20 Farrar JK. Hydrogen clearance technique. In: Wood JH, ed, *Cerebral blood flow. Physiologic and clinical aspects*. New York: McGraw-Hill, 1987: 275–87.

21 Ginsberg MD. Autoradiographic measurement of local cerebral blood flow. In: Wood JH, ed, *Cerebral blood flow. Physiologic and clinical aspects*. New York: McGraw-Hill, 1987: 299–308.

22 Warner DS, Kassell NF, Boarini DJ. Microsphere cerebral blood flow determination. In: Wood JH, ed, *Cerebral blood flow. Physiologic and clinical aspects*. New York: McGraw-Hill, 1987: 288–98.

23 Prichard JW, Rosen BR. Functional study of the brain by NMR. *J Cereb Blood Flow Metab* 1994; 14: 365–72.

24 Newell DW, Aaslid R, eds. *Transcranial Doppler 1992*. New York: Raven Press.

25 Wyatt JS. Noninvasive assessment of cerebral oxidative metabolism in the human newborn [review]. *J R Coll Physicians Lond* 1994; 28: 126–32.

26 Prough DS, Stump DA, Roy RC, *et al*. Response of cerebral blood flow to changes in carbon dioxide tension during hypothermic cardiopulmonary bypass. *Anesthesiology* 1986; 64: 576–81.

27 Cruz J, Raps EC, Hoffstad OJ, Jaggi JL, Gennarelli TA. Cerebral oxygenation monitoring [review]. *Crit Care Med* 1993; 21: 1242–6.

28 Bodenham A, Webster NR. New practical bedside procedures on the intensive care unit. *Ballière's Clin Anesthesiol* 1992; 6: 425–41.

29 Mayberg TS, Lam AM. Management of central nervous system trauma. *Current Opinion in Anesthesiology* 1993; 6: 764–71.

30 Faught E. Current role of electroencephalography in cerebral ischaemia [review]. *Stroke* 1993; 24: 609–13.

31 Zentner J, Schramm J. Monitoring the central nervous system. *Current Opinion in Anesthesiology* 1993; 6: 784–90.

32 Bolognese P, Miller JI, Heger IM, Milhorat TH. Laser–Doppler flowmetry in neurosurgery [review]. *J Neurosurg Anesthesiol* 1993; 5: 151–8.

33 Fox PT, Raichle ME, Mintun MA, Dence C. Nonoxidative glucose consumption during focal physiologic neural activity. *Science* 1988; 241: 462–4.

34 Edvinsson L, Mackenzie ET, McCulloch J. Perivascular nerve fibres in brain vessels. In: *Cerebral blood flow and metabolism*. New York: Raven Press, 1993: 57–91.

35 Kontos HA. Nitric oxide and nitrosothiols in cerebrovascular and neuronal regulation [review]. *Stroke* 1993; 24: 1155–8.

36 Miller JD, Stanek A, Langfitt TW. Concepts of cerebral perfusion pressure and vascular compression during intracranial hypertension. *Prog Brain Res* 1972; 35: 411–32.

37 Miller JD, Stanek AE, Langfitt TW. Cerebral blood flow regulation during experimental brain compression. *J Neurosurg* 1973; 39: 186–96.

38 Fitch W, MacKenzie ET, Harper AM. Effects of decreasing arterial blood pressure on cerebral blood flow in the baboon: Influence of the sympathetic nervous system. *Circ Res* 1975; 37: 550–7.

39 Heistad DD, Marcus ML, Sandberg S, Abboud FM. Effect of sympathetic nerve stimulation on cerebral blood flow and on large cerebral arteries of dogs. *Circ Res* 1977; **41**: 342–50.

40 Thomas D, Bannister RG. Preservation of autoregulation of cerebral blood flow in autonomic failure. *J Neurol Sci* 1980; **44**: 205–12.

41 Strandgaard S, Olesen J, Skinhoj E, Jassen NA. Autoregulation of brain circulation in severe arterial hypertension. *BMJ* 1973; **i**: 507–10.

42 Bentsen N, Larsen B, Lassen NA. Chronically impaired autoregulation of cerebral blood flow in long-term diabetics. *Stroke* 1975; **6**: 497–502.

43 Strandgaard S. Autoregulation of CBF in hypertensives. The modifying influence of prolonged antihypertensive treatment on the tolerance to acute, drug induced hypotension. *Circulation* 1976; **53**: 720–7.

44 Michenfelder JD, Theye RA. Canine systemic and cerebral effects of hypotension induced by hemorrhage, trimethaphan, halothane, or nitroprusside. *Anesthesiology* 1977; **46**: 188–95.

45 Aaslid R, Lindegaard K-F, Sorteberg W, Nornes H. Cerebral autoregulation dynamics in humans. *Stroke* 1989; **20**: 45–52.

46 Davis DH, Sundt TM Jr. Relationship of cerebral blood flow to cardiac output, mean arterial pressure, blood volume, and alpha and beta blockade in cats. *J Neurosurg* 1980; **52**: 745–54.

47 Koehler RC, Traystman RJ. Bicarbonate ion modulation of cerebral blood flow during hypoxia and hypercapnia. *Am J Physiol* 1982; **243**: H33–40.

48 Stringer WA, Hasso AN, Thompson JR, Hinshaw DB, Jordan KG. Hyperventilation-induced cerebral ischaemia in patients with acute brain lesions: demonstration by Xenon-enhanced CT. *Am J Neuroradiol* 1993; **14**: 465–84.

49 Pickard JD, MacKenzie ET. Inhibition of prostaglandin synthesis and the response of baboon cerebral circulation to carbon dioxide. *Nature (New Biol)* 1973; **245**: 187–8.

50 Maktabi MA. Role of nitric oxide in regulation of cerebral circulation in health and disease. *Current Opinion in Anesthesiology* 1993; **6**: 799–83.

51 Grubb RL Jr, Raichle ME, Eichling JO, Ter-Pogossian MM. The effects of changes in Pa_{CO_2} on cerebral blood volume, blood flow and vascular mean transit time. *Stroke* 1974; **5**: 630–9.

52 Kosteljanetz M. Acute head injury: pressure–volume relations and cerebrospinal fluid dynamics. *Neurosurgery* 1986; **18**: 17–24.

53 McDowall DG. Interrelationships between blood oxygen tension and cerebral blood flow. In: Payne JP, Hill DW, eds, *Oxygen measurements in blood and tissues*. London: Churchill, 1966: 205–14.

54 Krasney JA, Jensen JB, Lassen NA. Cerebral blood flow does not adapt to sustained hypoxia. *J Cereb Blood Flow Metab* 1990; **10**: 759–64.

55 Krasney JA, McDonald B, Matalon S. Regional circulatory responses to 96 hours of hypoxia in conscious sheep. *Respir Physiol* 1984; **57**: 73–88.

56 Krasney JA, Hajduczok G, Miki K, Matalon S. Peripheral circulatory responses to 96 hours of eucapnic hypoxia in conscious sheep. *Respir Physiol* 1985; **59**: 197–211.

57 Purves MJ. *The physiology of the cerebral circulation.* Cambridge: Cambridge University Press, 1972.

58 Adams HP. Prevention of brain ischaemia after aneurysmal subarachnoid haemorrhage. *Neurol Clin* 1992; **10**: 251–68.

59 Christensen MS, Hoedt-Rasmussen K, Lassen NA. Cerebral vasodilation by halothane anaesthesia in man and its potentiation by hypotension and hypercapnia. *Br J Anaesth* 1967; **39**: 927.

60 Wollman H, Alexander SC, Cohen PJ, Chase PE, Melman E, Behar MG. Cerebral circulation of man during halothane anesthesia. Effects of hypocarbia and of *d*-tubocurarine. *Anesthesiology* 1964; **25**: 180–4.

61 Jennett WB, Barker J, Fitch W, McDowall DG. Effects of anaesthesia on intracranial pressure in patients with space-occupying lesions. *Lancet* 1969; **i**: 61–4.

62 Murphy FL, Kennell EM, Johnstone RE. The effects of enflurane, isoflurane, and halothane on cerebral blood flow and metabolism in man. *Abstracts of the meeting of The American Society of Anesthesiologists* 1974: 61–2.

63 Neigh JL, Garman JK, Harp JR. The electroencephalographic pattern during anesthesia with Ethrane: effects of depths of anesthesia, $Paco_2$ and nitrous oxide. *Anesthesiology* 1971; **35**: 482–7.

64 Hansen TD, Warner DS, Todd MM, Vust LJ, Trawick DC. Distribution of cerebral blood flow during halothane versus isoflurane anesthesia in rats. *Anesthesiology* 1988; **69**: 332–7.

65 Hansen TD, Warner DS, Todd MM, Vust LJ. Effects of nitrous oxide and volatile anaesthetics on cerebral blood flow. *Br J Anaesth* 1989; **63**: 290–5.

77 Scheller MS, Todd MM, Drummond JC. Isoflurane, halothane and regional cerebral blood flow at various levels of $Paco_2$ in rabbits. *Anesthesiology* 1986; **64**: 598–604.

78 Drummond JC, Todd MM. The response of the feline cerebral circulation to $Paco_2$ during anesthesia with isoflurane and halothane and during sedation with nitrous oxide. *Anesthesiology* 1985; **62**: 268–73.

79 Maekawa T, Tommasino C, Shapiro HM, Kiefer-Goodman J, Kohlenberger RW. Local cerebral blood flow and glucose utilisation during isoflurane anesthesia in the rat. *Anesthesiology* 1986; **65**: 144–51.

80 Kuramoto T, Oshita S, Takeshita H, Ishikawa T. Modification of the relationship between cerebral metabolism, blood flow, and the EEG by stimulation during anesthesia in the dog. *Anesthesiology* 1979; **51**: 211–17.

81 Sakabe T, Kuramoto T, Kumagae S, Takeshita H. Cerebral responses to the addition of nitrous oxide to halothane in man. *Br J Anaesth* 1976; **48**: 957–62.

82 Lam AM, Mayberg TS, Eng CC, Cooper JO, Bachenberg KL, Mathisen TL. Nitrous oxide–isoflurane anesthesia causes more cerebral vasodilation than an equipotent dose of isoflurane in humans. *Anesth Analg* 1994; **78**: 462–8.

83 Reasoner D, Warner DS, Todd MM, McAllister A. Effects of nitrous oxide on cerebral metabolic rate in rats anaesthetized with isoflurane. *Br J Anaesth* 1990; **65**: 210–15.

84 Henriksen HT, Jorgensen PB. The effect of nitrous oxide on intracranial pressure in patients with intracranial disorders. *Br J Anaesth* 1973; **45**: 486–92.

85 Moss E, McDowall DG. ICP increases with 50% nitrous oxide in oxygen in severe head injuries controlled ventilation. *Br J Anaesth* 1979; **51**: 757–61.

86 Kaieda R, Todd MM, Warner DS. The effects of anesthetics and $Paco_2$ on the cerebrovascular, metabolic, and electroencephalographic responses to nitrous oxide in the rabbit. *Anesth Analg* 1989; **68**: 135–43.

87 Phirman JR, Shapiro HM. Modification of nitrous oxide induced intracranial hypertension by prior induction of anesthesia. *Anesthesiology* 1977; **46**: 150–1.

88 Young WL. Effects of desflurane on the central nervous system. *Anesth Analg* 1992; **75** (suppl 4): 32–7.

89 Scheller MS, Tateishi A, Drummond JC, Zornow MH. The effects of sevoflurane on cerebral blood flow, cerebral metabolic rate for oxygen, intracranial pressure and the electroencephalogram are similar to those of isoflurane in the rabbit. *Anesthesiology* 1988; **68**: 548–51.

90 Lutz LJ, Milde JH, Milde LN. The cerebral functional, metabolic, and hemodynamic effects of desflurane in dogs. *Anesthesiology* 1990; **73**: 125–31.

91 Muzzi DA, Losasso TJ, Dietz NM, Faust RJ, Cucchiara RF, Milde LN. The effect of desflurane and isoflurane on cerebrospinal fluid pressure in humans with supratentorial mass lesions. *Anesthesiology* 1992; **76**: 720–4.

92 Rampil IJ, Lockhart SH, Eger EI, Weiskopf RB. Human EEG dose response to desflurane. *Anesthesiology* 1990; **73**: A1218.

93 Kassel NF, Hitchon PW, Gerk MK, Sokoll MD, Hill TR. Alterations in cerebral blood flow, oxygen metabolism, and electrical activity produced by high dose sodium thiopental. *Neurosurgery* 1980; **7**: 598–603.

94 Milde LN, Milde JH, Michenfelder JD. Cerebral functional, metabolic, and hemodynamic effects of etomidate in dogs. *Anesthesiology* 1985; **63**: 371–7.

95 Ramani R, Todd MM, Warner DS. The cerebrovascular, metabolic and electroencephalographic effects of propofol in the rabbit—a dose response study. *J Neurosurg Anesth* 1992; **4**: 110–19.

96 Van Hemelrijck J, Van Aken H, Plets C, Goffin J, Vermaut G. The effects of propofol on intracranial pressure and cerebral perfusion pressure in patients with brain tumours. *Acta Anaesthesiol Belg* 1989; **40**: 95–100.

97 Weeks J, Todd MM, Warner DS, Katz J. The influence of halothane, isoflurane, and pentobarbital on cerebral plasma volume in hypocapnic and normocapnic rats. *Anesthesiology* 1990; **73**: 461–6.

98 Fox J, Gelb AW, Enns J, Murkin JM, Farrar JK, Manninen PH. The responsiveness of cerebral blood flow to changes in arterial carbon dioxide is maintained during propofol–nitrous oxide anesthesia in humans. *Anesthesiology* 1992; **77**: 453–6.

99 Carlsson C, Smith DS, Keykhah MM, Englebach I, Harp JR. The effects of high dose fentanyl on cerebral circulation and metabolism in rats. *Anesthesiology* 1982; **57**: 375–80.

100 Keykhah MM, Smith DS, Carlsson C, Safo Y, Englebach I, Harp JR. Influence of sufentanil on cerebral metabolism and circulation in the rat. *Anesthesiology* 1985; **63**: 274–80.

101 McPherson RW, Krempasanka E, Eimerl D, Traystman RJ. Effects of alfentanil on cerebral vascular reactivity in dogs. *Br J Anaesth* 1985; **57**: 1232–8.

102 Murkin JM, Ferrar JK, Tweed WA, McKenzie FN, Guiraudon G. Cerebral autoregulation and flow/metabolism coupling during cardiopulmonary bypass: the influence of Pa_{CO_2}. *Anesth Analg* 1987; **66**: 825–32.

103 Sperry RJ, Bailey PL, Reichman MV, Peterson PB, Pace NL. Fentanyl and sufentanil increase intracranial pressure in head trauma patients. *Anesthesiology* 1992; **77**: 416–20.

104 Åkeson J, Björkman S, Messeter K, Rosén I, Helfer M. Cerebral pharmacodynamics of anaesthetic and subanaesthetic doses of ketamine in the normoventilated pig. *Acta Anaesthesiol Scand* 1993; **37**: 211–18.

105 Davis DW, Mans AM, Biebuyck JF, Hawkins RA. The influence of ketamine on regional brain glucose use. *Anesthesiology* 1988; **69**: 199–205.

106 Menon DK, Burdett NG, Carpenter TA, Hall LD. Functional MRI of ketamine-induced changes in rCBF: An effect at the NMDA receptor? (abstract). *Br J Anaesth* 1993; **71**: 767.

107 Forster A, Juge O, Morel D. Effects of midazolam on cerebral blood flow in human volunteers. *Anesthesiology* 1982; **56**: 453–5.

108 Fleischer JE, Milde JH, Moyer TP, Michenfelder JD. Cerebral effects of high-dose midazolam and subsequent reversal with RO 15-1788 in dogs. *Anesthesiology* 1988; **68**: 234–42.

109 Ducey JP, Deppe AS, Foley FT. A comparison of the effects of suxamethonium, atracurium and vecuronium on intracranial haemodynamics in swine. *Anaesth Intensive Care* 1989; **17**: 448–55.

110 Kovarik WD, Lam AM, Slee TA, Mathisen TL. The effect of succinylcholine on intracranial pressure, cerebral blood flow velocity and electroencephalogram in patients with neurologic disorders [abstract]. *Anesthesiology* 1991; **75**: 207.

111 Stirt JA, Grosslight KR, Bedford RF, Vollmer D. "Defasciculation" with metocurine prevents succinylcholine-induced increases intracranial pressure. *Anesthesiology* 1987; **67**: 50–3.

112 Siesjo BK. Pathophysiology and treatment of focal cerebral ischaemia. Part I: Pathophysiology. *J Neurosurg* 1992; **77**: 169–84.

113 Robertson CS, Contant CF, Gokaslan ZL, Narayan RK, Grossman RG. Cerebral blood flow, arteriovenous oxygen difference, and outcome in head injured patients. *J Neurol Neurosurg Psychiatry* 1992; **55**: 594–603.

114 Bouma GJ, Muizelaar JP, Stringer WA, Choi SC, Fatouros P, Young HF. Ultra early evaluation of regional cerebral blood flow in severely head-injured patients using xenon-enhanced computerized tomography. *J Neurosurg* 1992; **77**: 360–9.

115 Martin NA, Doberstein C, Zane C, Caron MJ, Thomas K, Becker DP. Posttraumatic cerebral arterial spasm: transcranial Doppler ultrasound, cerebral blood flow and angiographic findings. *J Neurosurg* 1992; **77**: 575–83.

116 Chan KH, Dearden NM, Miller JD, Andrews PJ, Midgley S. Multimodality monitoring as a guide to treatment of intracranial hypertension after severe brain injury. *Neurosurgery* 1993; **32**: 547–52.

117 Feldman Z, Kanter MJ, Robertson CS, *et al.* Effect of head elevation on intracranial pressure, cerebral perfusion pressure and cerebral blood flow in head injured patients. *J Neurosurg* 1992; **76**: 207–11.

118 Lassen NA, Agnoli A. The upper limit of autoregulation of cerebral blood flow on the pathogenesis of hypertensive encephalopathy. *Scand J Clin Lab Invest* 1973; **30**: 113–16.

119 Voldby B, Enevoldsen EM, Jensen FT. Cerebrovascular reactivity in patients with ruptured intracranial aneurysm. *J Neurosurg* 1985; **62**: 59–67.

120 Pickard JD, Matheson M, Patterson J, Wyper D. Prediction of late ischemic complications after cerebral aneurysm surgery by the intraoperative measurement of cerebral blood flow. *J Neurosurg* 1980; **53**: 305–8.

121 Kassell NF, Peerless SJ, Durward QJ, Beck DW, Drake CG, Adams HP. Treatment of ischaemic deficits from vasospasm with intravascular volume expansion and induced arterial hypertension. *Neurosurgery* 1982; **11**: 337–43.

122 Yamaura I, Tani E, Maeda Y, Minami N, Shindo H. Endothelin-1 of canine basilar artery in vasospasm. *J Neurosurg* 1992; **76**: 99–105.

123 Clozel M. Watanabe H. BQ-123, a peptidic endothelin ET_A receptor antagonist, prevents the early cerebral vasospasm following subarachnoid hemorrhage after intracisternal but not intravenous injection. *Life Sci* 1993; **52**: 825–34.

124 Jakobsen M, Skjødt T, Enevoldsen E. Cerebral blood flow and metabolism following subarachnoid hemorrhage: effect of subarachnoid blood. *Acta Neurol Scand* 1991; **8**: 226–33.

125 Pickard JD, Murray GD, Illingworth R, *et al*. Effect of oral nimodipine on cerebral infarction and outcome after subarachnoid hemorrhage: British aneurysm nimodipine trial. *BMJ* 1989; **298**: 636–42.

126 Darby JM, Yonas H, Marks EC, Durham S, Snyder RW, Nemoto EM. Acute cerebral blood flow response to dopamine-induced hypertension after subarachnoid hemorrhage. *J Neurosurg* 1994; **80**: 857–64.

127 Rosenblum WI. Endothelium-derived relaxing factor in brain blood vessels is not nitric oxide. *Stroke* 1992; **23**: 1527–32.

8: Renal, splanchnic, skin, and muscle circulations

JOHN A REITAN, NGUYEN D KIEN

Renal circulation

The major functions of the kidneys include:

1 Excretion of the end products of systemic metabolism while retaining essential nutrients
2 Regulation of the volume and composition of body fluids
3 Production of endocrine substances including renin, prostaglandins, and kinins which are important for the control of the pressure, volume, and flow of blood.

Anatomy

The kidneys are bilateral, bean shaped organs which lie in a retroperitoneal position on either side of the vertebral column beneath the diaphragm. An adult human kidney weighs between 115 g and 170 g with the upper and lower borders situated between the twelfth thoracic and third lumbar vertebrae. The right kidney is slightly more caudal in position because of the liver. Located on the concave border facing the vertebral column is an indentation called the hilus through which the ureter, blood and lymph vessels, and a nerve plexus pass into the renal sinus. The cut surface of a bisected kidney reveals an outer region called the cortex and an inner region called the medulla. The cortex is divided into the outer cortical layer and the inner juxtamedullary layer. The medulla consists of 4–18 conical pyramids. The base of each pyramid faces the cortex, whereas the apex (called the papilla) extends into the renal sinus and is covered by a funnel shaped calyx. Through these calyces urine is drained from the kidney into the pelvis and the ureter.

The kidney is innervated by the renal plexus of the sympathetic division of the autonomic nervous system. The nerve fibres enter the kidney alongside the arterial vessels. Their branches supply the renal vasculature throughout the cortex and the outer region of the medulla.

The functional unit of the kidney is the nephron. There are approximately

10^6 nephrons in each kidney. Each nephron consists of a glomerulus, a capillary network through which plasma is filtered, and the uriniferous tubule, a long and cylindrical tube where filtered plasma is modified into urine.

Glomerulus

The glomerulus is composed of a capillary network which invaginates into the dilated blind end of the nephron called Bowman's capsule.[1] The glomerulus is the filtration barrier between blood and urine which is responsible for the production of an ultrafiltrate of plasma. The glomerular capillaries are covered by a thin fenestrated endothelium. The endothelial cells form an initial barrier to the passage of blood constituents from the capillary to the Bowman's capsule. Beneath the endothelium is the basement membrane of the glomerulus. This extracellular membrane, consisting of fibrils in a glycoprotein matrix, serves as a retaining wall of large sized proteins. The largest cells of the glomerulus are the visceral epithelial cells which are partially responsible for the synthesis and maintenance of the glomerular basement membrane. The mesangial cells are similar to the visceral epithelial cells. These cells contain filaments and are capable of phagocytosis. They produce prostaglandins and appear to have a role in the counter-regulation of the effect of vasoconstrictors.

Juxtaglomerular apparatus

The juxtaglomerular apparatus is an area of the nephron where the distal tubule comes in contact with the arterioles.[2] It is composed of:

- juxtaglomerular granular cells
- extraglomerular mesangium
- the macula densa.

The juxtaglomerular granular cells are modified smooth muscle cells which produce, store, and release renin. The extraglomerular mesangium is connected with the intraglomerular mesangium, and is composed of cells that are similar to the mesangial cells. The extraglomerular mesangium has been suggested to serve as a functional link of the mesangium, glomerular arterioles, and macula densa.

The juxtaglomerular apparatus is a major structural component of the renin–angiotensin system. It is involved in the autoregulation of renal blood flow and glomerular filtration rate. Changes in sodium or chloride concentration at the macula densa or alterations in the volume and stretch of the afferent arteriole are thought to affect the control of renin release.

Renal tubule

The renal tubule consists of the proximal tubule, the loop of Henle, and the distal tubule. Bowman's capsule opens into the first section of the renal

225

tubule, called the proximal tubule, which lies within the cortex. The proximal tubule contains a large number of lysosomes which are responsible for the normal turnover of intracellular constituents by autophagocytosis. Proteins are absorbed from the tubular lumen by endocytosis or pinocytosis. The proximal tubule is lined with cuboidal epithelium with microvilli that increase the surface area for reabsorption and secretion. The proximal tubule plays a major role in the reabsorption of various ions, water, and organic solutes such as glucose and amino acids. Approximately half of the filtrate is reabsorbed in the proximal tubule.

The transition from the proximal tubule to the loop of Henle occurs abruptly at the outer layer of the medulla. The loop of Henle consists of a straight segment of the proximal tubule, the thin descending limb, and the thick ascending limb. The thin descending limb has permeability properties that are important for maintaining medullary hypertonicity and the delivery of a dilute fluid to the distal tubule.

The distal tubule begins close to the macula densa and extends into the cortex where two or more nephrons combine to form a cortical collecting duct. The distal tubule is involved in the active transport of sodium chloride. Its function is regulated by various hormones including vasopressin, parathyroid hormone, and calcitonin which exert their effects by activating the adenylate cyclase system. The cells of the distal tubule are similar to those of the proximal tubule, except for fewer microvilli. The distal tubule connects to the collecting duct via the connecting tubule which plays an important role in potassium secretion.

The collecting duct extends from the cortical region through the medulla to the tip of the papilla. It collects fluid from several nephrons, travels along the conical pyramid, and terminates at the minor calyx. The collecting duct is also involved in potassium secretion and urine acidification.

There are two types of nephrons separated by their locations in the kidney. About 85% of nephrons are located in the cortex and are called cortical nephrons. The remaining 15% are found close to the medulla and are called the juxtamedullary nephrons. The nephrons filter approximately 180 litres of plasma each day through the glomerular component. Only 1% is excreted as urine, the remaining plasma fluid being reabsorbed into the circulation through the tubules.

Vascular supply

The renal vasculature is characterised by two capillary networks surrounding the glomerulus and the tubule.[3] The renal artery usually divides into the anterior and posterior main branches before entering the renal parenchyma. These main branches further divide into segmental arteries which give rise to the interlobar arteries in the renal sinus. These vessels advance to the junction of the cortex and medulla where they divide and form arcuate arteries. Their divisions tend to lie in a plane parallel to the kidney surface at the corticomedullary junction. As the arcuate arteries advance towards the kidney surface and branch into the interlobular arteries, further divisions occur to form the afferent arterioles. The arterioles eventually divide into several branches which form the capillary network of the glomerulus. The wall structure of the intrarenal arteries and the afferent arterioles resembles that of arterial vessels found in other organs, indicating that these vessels can regulate the glomerular capillary flow through their well developed smooth muscles.[4]

The glomerular capillaries exit Bowman's capsule to form the efferent arterioles. The efferent arterioles are smaller in size than the afferent arterioles. This size reduction is a contributing factor in raising the glomerular pressure. The efferent arterioles supply the renal tubules in the form of a capillary network called the peritubular capillaries. Additionally, they extend into the medulla to form long loops of thin walled vessels called vasa recta. The peritubular capillaries eventually reunite to form interlobular veins which converge into the arcuate and interlobar veins. They run between the pyramids and give rise to several trunks that leave the kidney through a single renal vein at the hilus. Unlike the arterial system, which lacks collateral vessels, the venous network anastomoses at several levels. This allows normal drainage of blood even when a large venous branch is occluded.

Control of the renal circulation

The kidneys receive approximately 20% of the cardiac output. They are capable of increasing flow even further although they constitute less than 0·5% of the total body weight. This marked renal blood flow is well in excess of that required to provide renal tissue with sufficient oxygen and nutrients. Therefore, renal blood flow is regulated to maintain an optimum delivery of filtrate to the nephrons and adequate reabsorption of fluid back into the vascular system. The factors that control renal circulation are divided into intrinsic factors (autoregulation and the renal nerves) and extrinsic factors (hormonal and other endogenous vasoactive agents).

Autoregulation
Regulation of the renal blood flow closely depends on changes of vascular resistance secondary to constriction or relaxation of vascular smooth muscles. Autoregulation is the intrinsic ability of the kidney to maintain a relatively constant blood flow over a range of renal perfusion pressure from 75 to 180 mm Hg. Outside this pressure range, afferent arteriolar resistance is less responsive and flow becomes pressure dependent.[5] As this vascular reaction is demonstrable in isolated kidneys, autoregulation of renal blood flow is generally assumed to be mediated by factors intrinsic to the kidney. The exact mechanisms by which the kidney autoregulates its flow are not, however, clearly understood.

227

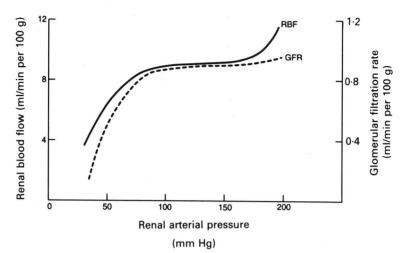

Fig 8.1 An example of autoregulation in the kidney which demonstrates flow and filtration stability between 75 and 180 mm Hg blood pressure. (——) Renal blood flow; (– – –) glomerular filtration rate.

Currently, two theories are proposed to explain the renal autoregulation. One is the myogenic theory first discussed by Bayliss in 1902.[6] It has been shown that a vasoconstrictor is released from renal vessels when the transmural pressure difference increases, supporting a relationship between the endothelium and the vascular smooth muscle which mediates the autoregulation. The second theory postulates a tubuloglomerular feedback mechanism which enables autoregulation of both renal blood flow and glomerular filtration rate. This feedback theory is based on a relationship between the distal tubular Na^+ delivery and the intrarenal release of renin.[7] Changes in distal tubular flow and/or solute can affect renal blood flow and thus modulate glomerular filtration rate. Recent data support a close interaction between tubuloglomerular feedback and the myogenic mechanisms (fig 8.1).

Renal nerves

The renal nerves contain both afferent and efferent nerve fibres which release noradrenaline.[8] Both noradrenaline and adrenaline released from the adrenal medulla activate α_1-adrenoceptors and cause vasoconstriction which decreases both renal blood flow and glomerular filtration rate. Renal nerves also release dopamine which activates specific dopamine receptors existing in abundance in the renal tissues. Activation of the DA_1 receptors causes significant increases in both cortical and medullary blood flows.[9]

Renin–angiotensin system

Renin is a proteolytic enzyme which is synthesised in the epithelial cells of the juxtaglomerular apparatus and secreted into the surrounding interstitium. It cleaves angiotensin I from angiotensinogen. Angiotensin I is converted into angiotensin II which exerts both direct and indirect adrenergic action on renal arterioles. Angiotensin II can also act as a circulating hormone. It is a potent vasoconstrictor; however, its most important action is to stimulate aldosterone production and secretion by the adrenal cortex. Thus, an increase in renin release from the kidney will lead to an increase in Na^+ reabsorption secondary to a higher blood level of aldosterone. The increased reabsorption of Na^+ will facilitate water movement from the interstitial space and increase plasma volume. The renin–angiotensin system shuts off once the volume deficit is corrected.[10] Although angiotensin II is a potent vasoconstrictor of the afferent arterioles, its primary action appears to be on the efferent arterioles. Vasoconstriction of the efferent arterioles can contribute to the maintenance of the glomerular filtration, particularly when renal plasma flow is reduced.

Antidiuretic hormone

This hormone, also called vasopressin, is synthesised in the hypothalamus and released from the posterior pituitary gland. The release of antidiuretic hormone (ADH) can be stimulated by changes in the volume and osmolality of body fluids or by activation of the sympathetic nervous system. This hormone acts on the collecting tubules where it inhibits diuresis and increases water reabsorption leading to increased plasma volume. Although ADH is involved in the maintenance of the volume and osmolality of plasma, the magnitude and direction of such involvement remain controversial. The conflicting results may be caused by different dosages of ADH, varying states of fluid balance, and the influence of other vasoactive agents.

Prostaglandins

PGE_2 and PGI_2 are produced within the kidney during haemorrhagic hypovolaemia. The production of these substances is stimulated by sympathetic nerve activity and angiotensin II. During haemorrhage, prostaglandin synthesis occurs within the kidneys which causes vasodilatation in the afferent and efferent arterioles to prevent severe renal vasoconstriction and ischaemia. Therefore, prostaglandins appear to play a role in modulating the renal vascular effects of other vasoactive agents, including vasoconstrictor hormones and bradykinins. As prostaglandin inhibitors do not significantly alter renal blood flow autoregulation, the contribution of prostaglandins to the control of basal or resting renal blood flow is considered minimal.[11]

Atrial natriuretic peptide

Atrial natriuretic peptide (ANP) is a recently discovered peptide which appears to be involved in the regulation of renal function and Na^+ balance. ANP is released primarily from cardiac atria in response to atrial stretching

229

secondary to volume expansion. This peptide is a rapid acting, potent natriuretic and diuretic substance which can also exert direct vasodilator effects on the systemic vasculature. There are membrane receptors for ANP throughout the renal cortical and medullary vasculature, particularly at the glomerular capillaries. As ANP can inhibit renin secretion and aldosterone release, and increase urinary kallikrein excretion, part of the renal effects of ANP may be indirect. Nevertheless, ANP appears to have an important role in the control of Na^+ balance during conditions of altered plasma volume. The Na^+ excretion may be partially mediated by the vasodilator effect of ANP which increases the glomerular filtration rate.

Adenosine

It has been proposed that adenosine may play a role in the regulation of renal blood flow and glomerular filtration.[12] Administration of adenosine causes significant changes in renal vascular resistance, glomerular filtration rate, and renin release. Responses of renal vascular resistance to intrarenal infusion of adenosine include an initial transient vasoconstriction of the afferent arterioles, possibly by interaction with the renin–angiotensin system, and is followed by a dilatory phase which may be associated with a marked vasodilatation caused by both direct and indirect mechanisms. The vasoconstriction of the afferent arterioles combined with the vasodilatation of the efferent arterioles can result in sustained decreases in glomerular filtration pressure and rate. In addition, adenosine can exert a direct and powerful inhibition of renin release by the juxtaglomerular cells. In general, adenosine appears to be an important mediator in the control of renal blood flow. Further studies are, however, necessary to delineate the effects of adenosine on both the renal and systemic vasculature.

Kinins

Administration of bradykinin released from plasma kallikrein causes marked renal vasodilatation. Infusion of kinin antagonist decreases papillary blood flow by 20% without changing outer cortical blood flow, indicating that kinins exert a vasodilatory influence on the papillary vessels. The role of kinin in regulating medullary haemodynamics is not, however, clear because more than 90% of the renal kallikrein is found in the cortex and a very small fraction in the medulla and papilla.

Nitric oxide

The role of endothelium derived relaxing factor (EDRF) or nitric oxide (NO) is being extensively investigated. Recent data suggest that approximately 30% of renal vascular resistance may be controlled by NO. The collecting duct and vasa recta capillaries seem to be the major sites of NO synthesis.[13] Nitric oxide inhibitor infused into the renal medulla decreases papillary blood flow without changes in cortical blood flow, renal blood flow, or mean arterial pressure.[14] Systemic inhibition of NO, however, significantly decreases renal blood flow without affecting the glomerular filtration rate.[15] The release of NO in response to changes in vessel tension is postulated to be associated with the activation of membrane receptors or to involve a complex enzymatic pathway. Inflammation mediators such as tumour necrosis factor modify the release of NO from either endothelial or non-endothelial cells.[16]

Other vasoactive substances such as serotonin and histamine have been proposed as involved in the control of renal hemodynamics. Current data, however, suggest that their roles in regulating the renal circulation appear to be limited. Future studies should examine the possible role of endothelin in the local control of renal blood flow.

Fig 8.2 demonstrates the main contributors to renal circulatory control.

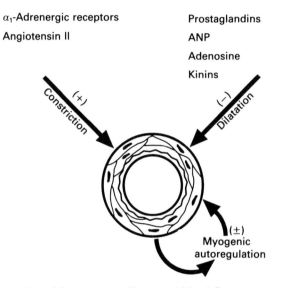

Fig 8.2 An illustration of factors controlling renal blood flow.

Effects of anaesthetic drugs on renal blood flow

Anaesthetic drugs are associated with significant sympathetic and endocrine changes, particularly those with sympathomimetic properties such as pentobarbitone (pentobarbital) and ketamine can stimulate the release of catecholamines. Increased blood level of adrenaline causes significant renal vasoconstriction and triggers renin release from the juxtamedullary nephrons. The formation of angiotensin II from renin leads to profound vasoconstriction of the renal vessels, and associated decreases in both the renal blood flow and glomerular filtration rate. Surgical stress may also induce further releases of catecholamines, ADH, and aldosterone into the circulation. Opiates generally decrease regional vascular resistance by both

231

local and systemically mediated mechanisms, but changes in perfusion pressure are moderated by reflex increases in sympathetic activity. They also appear to have no significant effect on renal blood flow. Low concentration of propofol has no effect on blood pressure, heart rate, and renal nerve activity. At moderate to high doses, renal nerve activity decreased by 22–50%, but the effect of propofol on renal blood flow remains to be elucidated.

In healthy volunteers in the absence of surgical stimuli, as well as patients undergoing surgery, inhalational anaesthetic drugs are associated with dose dependent decreases in renal blood flow, glomerular filtration rate, and urine production. These anaesthetics have both direct and indirect effects on renal blood flow. The direct effects on the renal bed can be intensified in certain clinical conditions including dehydration, pain, and loss of blood volume. They are accompanied by indirect factors such as depressed myocardial performance, altered vascular resistance, or decreased intravascular volume associated with most inhalational anaesthetic agents. Data from laboratory animals clearly demonstrate changes in active ion transport during anaesthesia. It has been suggested that an interaction with adrenaline is involved in the augmented Na^+ transport, whereas the inhibition of Na^+ transport is related to a direct effect of inhalational anaesthetic drugs. At concentrations of 3% or higher, halothane causes significant decreases in renal blood flow and oxygen consumption. The effects of enflurane and isoflurane on renal blood flow are considerably less than that of halothane. All inhalational anaesthetic drugs at high concentrations, however, possess potent vasodilator properties which may lead to loss of autoregulation.

Spinal or epidural anaesthesia may cause significant reductions in glomerular filtration rate and renal plasma flow when arterial blood pressure is markedly reduced. When the reduction of perfusion pressure is corrected, renal haemodynamics are normalised suggesting that perfusion pressure is an important factor in sustaining normal circulation in the kidney. No change in plasma renin levels is observed with either spinal or epidural anaesthesia. Therefore, the decrease in renal blood flow during spinal or epidural anaesthesia is possibly caused by a reduction in venous return and decreased cardiac output.

In summary, anaesthetic drugs are associated with an increase in renal vascular resistance, although whether anaesthetic drugs alter the ability of kidney to autoregulate is still controversial.

Splanchnic circulation

Anatomy

The splanchnic circulation is composed of gastric, small intestinal, colonic, pancreatic, hepatic, and splenic circulations.[17] They are arranged in parallel with one another and fed by three arteries:

1 The coeliac, which perfuses the hepatic artery, the stomach, the spleen, and part of the pancreas
2 The superior mesenteric artery which supplies branches to the pancreas, small intestines, and part of the colon
3 The inferior mesenteric artery which supplies the rest of the colon.

The stomach is composed of three histologically distinct layers: the mucosa, submucosa, and muscularis externa. The mucosa receives approximately three quarters of resting blood flow. Gastric arteries pierce the muscularis layer and form a network of branches into the submucosal area. This submucosal plexus gives rise to smaller branches which form a secondary arcade within the smooth muscles at the base of the mucosa. The venous system is parallel to the arterial vessels.

The mesenteric vasculature to the small and large intestine is composed of several circuits coupled both in series and in parallel. The three parallel circuits serve the muscularis, the submucosa, and the mucosa. Each of these circuits possesses a series coupled component consisting of resistance arterioles, precapillary sphincters, the capillaries themselves, postcapillary sphincters, and the venous capacitance vessels. The resistance arterioles are the primary determinants of vascular resistance and they regulate blood flow both to the splanchnic bed as a whole and through each of the parallel circuits. The mucosa has an enormous surface area for absorption created by villi and microvilli. The mucosa is the metabolically active area in the gut and receives well over half of the total resting organ blood flow. The submucosa and mucosa both have a parallel capillary plexus. Venous drainage from the small intestinal veins join with veins of the colon which subsequently join with splenic veins to form the portal system.[18]

The pancreas receives its blood supply from several branches of the coeliac and superior mesenteric arteries. It drains as well into the portal system.

The splenic circulation is unusual in that the internal red pulp has a complex mesh like structure which filters the blood passing through it. Blood flowing through the spleen may bypass the red pulp and constitutes a fast compartment whereas blood perfusing the red pulp has a considerably increased transit time and may be considered the slow compartment. Splenic blood flow is approximately 250 ml/min. The oxygen content of splenic venous blood is quite high because of the fast compartment and adds significantly to the portal oxygen saturation.

The liver is unique in that it has both an arterial and a venous afferent blood supply. The hepatic artery provides approximately 30–40% of total hepatic blood flow with the rest coming from the portal veins. In the normal resting adult, about 500 ml/min perfuse the liver via the hepatic artery whereas an additional 1300 ml/min flows via the portal system. The portal blood passes through hepatic sinusoids which puts it in close contact with the metabolic cells of the liver parenchyma. Hepatic arterial blood flow also supplies nutrition to connective tissue within the liver itself, especially the walls of the collecting ducts which form the intrahepatic biliary system. The hepatic sinuses are lined with endothelium similar to that found in capillaries, but the permeability of this endothelium is extreme and allows for rapid, easy diffusion of components within the blood into the hepatic parenchyma and back. The sinusoids collect into venules which form the hepatic veins which in turn empty into the inferior vena cava. There is a well organised intrahepatic lymph system as well, which accounts for more than one half of the total body lymph flow.

Overall splanchnic blood flow requires about a quarter of the cardiac output in normal resting adults, whereas the splanchnic capacitance venous system serves as a large reservoir for about a third of the total blood volume of the body.[19]

Control of the splanchnic circulation

The resistance arterioles are the primary determinant of vascular resistance in the splanchnic system and, therefore, regulate blood flow through this bed as a whole and through each parallel circuit. In this sort of control system, the relationship between flow and resistance can be described by the haemodynamic version of Ohm's law:

$$\text{Resistance} = \frac{\text{Pressure}}{\text{Flow}}$$

In the case of the mesenteric circulation, this would be the hydrostatic difference between the arterial and venous pressures divided by flow across the gut.

The control of splanchnic blood flow is by a combination of neuroreflex and hormonal factors.[20] Neural control of the mesenteric circulation is almost exclusively sympathetic in origin. The parasympathetic fibres originating from the vagi have little effect on splanchnic blood flow, although they are most important in the regulation of secretion and motility of the gut. The sympathetic postganglionic fibres act directly on the vascular smooth muscle of the arterioles. In this way increased sympathetic activity decreases blood flow to splanchnic organs. Additionally, sympathetic outflow to the splanchnic bed contracts the venous smooth muscles of the capacitance veins in the splanchnic circulation and may expel a large volume of pooled blood from the splanchnic reservoir into the systemic circulation. Most of these sympathetic ganglia arise from the coeliac plexus with lesser contributions from the superior and inferior mesenteric plexus. Through the sympathetic system, the mechanoreceptor reflexes—particularly the low pressure cardiopulmonary receptor systems—are closely involved in splanchnic arterial and venous vascular tone.[21] Interestingly β_2-adrenoreceptors are also present in the mesenteric circulation and activation of these receptors causes vasodilatation.

Circulating substances that may alter vascular resistance in the splanchnic bed include adrenaline, noradrenaline, angiotensin II, vasopressin, adenosine, and gastrointestinal peptides such as glucagon, VIP (vasoactive intestinal peptide), and cholecystokinin.[22] Most of the gastrointestinal peptides are vasodilators; they rarely reach a concentration high enough to be vasoactive in the systemic circulation as a whole. The catecholamines, including angiotensin and vasopressin, probably achieve a concentration that is centrally vasoactive only under circumstances of significant shock.

In addition to the classic gastrointestinal hormones, various vasoactive substances, including histamine, serotonin, bradykinin, and prostaglandins, which are produced and stored in the splanchnic organs, have been shown to affect organ blood flow in this region.[23] Many of the changes observed with these substances are in patients or study models with compromised splanchnic function.[24] The action of these hormones may be independent or in combination with other regulatory mechanisms.

Autoregulation in the splanchnic circulation is demonstrated by a compensatory dilatation of the resistance arterioles in response to an acute reduction of perfusion pressure which serves to restore the decreased tissue perfusion partially. Splanchnic autoregulation is less pronounced than in the cerebral, cardiac, or renal circulations. The response is evident, however, as a mechanism whereby initial levels of hypoperfusion are rapidly ameliorated by marked arteriolar vasodilatation which partially restores blood flow. This phenomenon is a variation of the postischaemic hyperperfusion mechanism seen in many areas of the body, and is the result of a direct myogenic response to the reduction in perfusion pressure and the accumulation of local ischaemic metabolites in the region, including adenosine, which may be the principal metabolic mediator of autoregulation. Interestingly oxygen consumption in the small intestine is even more rigorously autoregulated than blood flow with the result that oxygen uptake in this organ remains constant when arterial perfusion pressures are varied fourfold.[25] The portal venous system does not autoregulate so that as portal venous pressure and flow are raised, resistance either remains constant or may decrease.

In addition to autoregulation of blood flow within the individual organ as a whole, the splanchnic circulation responds to reduction in perfusion pressures by redistributing blood flow to various degrees within the individual organ. This redistribution is achieved by changes in the relative resistance of the arterioles and precapillary sphincters, gating the parallel vascular circuits in the various layers of the organ. In shock, for example, this response usually favours the mucosa at the expense of the muscularis layers. The gut is protected from ischaemic injury by its unique ability to increase oxygen extraction as much as sixfold, thereby maintaining oxygen consumption at near normal levels over a broad range of flows and avoiding the usual hypoxic sequelae. This protective mechanism is the result not only of the "mass effect" of rapid diffusion of oxygen along a steeper concentration gradient,

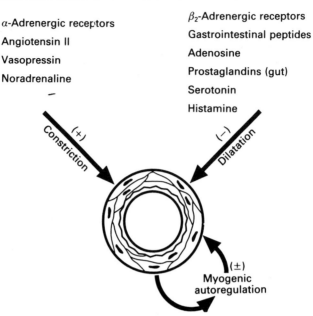

α-Adrenergic receptors
Angiotensin II
Vasopressin
Noradrenaline

β_2-Adrenergic receptors
Gastrointestinal peptides
Adenosine
Prostaglandins (gut)
Serotonin
Histamine

Constriction (+)

Dilatation (−)

(±)
Myogenic
autoregulation

Fig 8.3 Factors influencing blood flow through the splanchnic circulation.

but also of the opening of hypoperfused capillary beds. The net result is an increase in perfused capillary density as flow is reduced within the mucosa of the gut. This provides an important defence mechanism against splanchnic ischaemia.

An illustrated overview of the control mechanisms for splanchnic blood flow is shown in fig 8.3.

The effects of anaesthetic drugs on the splanchnic blood flow

Animal studies have shown that some intravenous anaesthetic drugs, particularly propofol, result in an increase in total liver blood flow with contributions from both the hepatic artery and portal systems. These data mark propofol as a vasodilator in this region. Human studies have, however, indicated an initial fall in hepatic flow followed by return towards normal levels. Barbiturates may also cause a decrease in overall splanchnic blood flow, most pronounced in the portal system because of the relative venoplegia caused by higher doses of these drugs. Midazolam may also reduce splanchnic flow initially, with a rebound increase from the splanchnic reservoir shortly thereafter.

Opiates, in small doses, produce a central sympathetic withdrawal and relative increase in vascular capacitance in this circulation.[26]

The change in splanchnic blood flow following regional anaesthesia of the

236

central neural axis is dictated by the level of block obtained. Spinal and epidural anaesthetic drugs at T10 and below have little effect upon splanchnic flow. Raising the block level to the T4 dermatome reduces total splanchnic blood flow by at least 25% in humans. Inclusion of the sympathetic outflow from the coeliac and mesenteric plexus produces the withdrawal of resting venous tone and the subsequent reduction in transhepatic flow.

With inhalational anaesthetic agents there is most often a reduction in portal blood flow, particularly by halothane. Isoflurane and enflurane apparently increase hepatic arterial blood flow which facilitates an increase in oxygen delivery to the liver with these anaesthetic agents.[27]

Of equal importance in the anaesthetised patient is the physiological consequences of ventilation. During inspiration with controlled ventilation, the diaphragm compresses the liver which causes an increase in hepatic venous pressure and decreased transhepatic conductance. With expiration, there is a reversal of this and splanchnic flow increases dramatically. Positive end expiratory pressure will decrease mesenteric arterial flow, portal blood flow, and total splanchnic blood flow. Interestingly, hypocapnia, which often accompanies controlled ventilation, reduces portal blood flow because of an increase in the resistance in mesenteric and splenic arteries, and portal veins. On the other hand, hepatic arterial resistance is decreased and hepatic arterial blood flow thereby maintained. Increases in circulating carbon dioxide levels most commonly increase portal and total hepatic blood flows, probably mediated through carbon dioxide as a direct vasodilator and the increase in cardiac output resulting from stimulation of the central nervous system. Concurrently there is an initial transient decrease in hepatic arterial flow followed by an increase towards the normocapnic control values. This phenomenon in the hepatic artery is compatible with a typical escape phenomenon of hepatic arterial vasculature from sudden sympathetic stimulation.

Cutaneous circulation

Anatomy

The largest organ in the body is the skin with a surface area of approximately $1\cdot9$ m^2 and a weight of about 2 kg in a 70 kg adult. The blood flow to the skin, including the microcirculation, is approximately 10 times greater than the metabolic needs of the cutaneous system. Under normothermic conditions, the venular plexus in the cutaneous circulation has the potential of being one of the larger reservoirs of blood volume in the body. The gross anatomy of the cutaneous circulation reflects the ability of the skin circulation to dissipate or preserve heat within the body as a whole and the anatomy reflects this functional need.[28]

The cutaneous vascular system is divided into three interconnected levels:

1 The deep subdermal or subcutaneous plexus
2 The middle or cutaneous plexus
3 The superficial or subpapillary plexus.

The subdermal plexus is the major vascular network of the overlying skin. Vessels of this plexus generally run in the subcutaneous fatty or areolar tissue. The arterial blood supply to the skin comes primarily from muscular cutaneous arteries which perforate the subcutaneous tissue from underlying muscle. These arteries and their concomitant veins ascend through the reticular dermis to the papillary dermis. Here the artery forms a superficial arteriolar plexus with terminal arterioles which project into capillary loops through the epidermis. The collecting venous system forms a double layered horizontal network at the subcutaneous dermal junction, and returns into the subcutaneous and muscular area via collecting venules. Total skin flow is made up of the blood perfusing through these vessels as well as bypasses (shunts) at deeper levels—primarily in the hands and feet.[29]

The skin is the primary site of exchange of body heat with the external environment.[30] Hence, changes in cutaneous blood flow in response to various metabolic states and environmental conditions provide the main mechanism by which temperature homoeostasis occurs. Skin blood flow is, under normal circumstances, approximately 5–6% of the resting cardiac output. This can decrease markedly in a cold environment when heat retention is necessary. Alternatively, the skin vessels may dilate to increase flow up to seven times the normal state when heat loss is required by hypermetabolic states. Specialised areas of the skin including the palm, fingers, sole, toes, and the face possess the capability for remarkable vasodilatation and constriction.[31] There may be as much as a 75-fold change in blood flow from cold to hot environments.

Control of the cutaneous circulation

The potential for skin vessels to generate great increases in vascular conductance makes this circulation an important regional flow area during changes in the environment and during anaesthesia.

Cutaneous resistance vessels and the venous plexus in the subcutaneous dermal junction are richly innervated with sympathetic vasoconstrictor nerves which maintain a relatively high degree of neurogenic activity and, hence, vascular tone. This predominant vasoconstrictor tone is mediated by hormonal action of circulating catecholamines at postjunctional α-adrenergic receptors. In addition there is an active dilator system which is activated under thermal, physical, or emotional stress. The mechanism for this active dilatation is not clear and may involve the release of a yet-to-be-determined neurotransmitter on cutaneous blood vessels or, more probably, involves a release of a vasodilator substance from activated sweat glands.[32] The substance most commonly mentioned or identified is bradykinin. Recent studies have shown, however, that calcitonin gene related peptide (CGRP), a vasoactive polypeptide, can increase regional blood flow in the skin under resting conditions at the expense of other organ flow, primarily the splanchnic circulation. From this work it has been proposed that normal, regional, blood flow changes in the skin may be mediated to some extent by CGRP acting as a local vasodilator and produced by neuronal activity.[33]

In the overview of total body circulatory control, investigators have shown that the sympathetic vasomotor fibres in the skin vasculature exert significant influence on overall homoeostasis. Such control is exerted from both the low pressure cardiopulmonary and high pressure arterial baroreceptor areas. These conclusions deviate from the previous literature in which baroreflex sympathetic vasoconstriction in the human skin was proposed to be more or less selectively mediated by cardiopulmonary low pressure receptors.[34]

The afferent control of resistance vessels in the skin is interesting in that arterioles in non-peripheral areas are innervated by two distinct sympathetic nerve types:

1 Adrenergic vasoconstrictor nerves similar to those in all arterioles
2 A specialised sympathetic active vasodilator nerve.

Arterioles in the peripheral skin seem to be innervated solely by sympathetic vasoconstrictor nerves. The remarkable dilatation that occurs in these areas under thermal stress is solely the result of withdrawal of sympathetic support.[35]

Temperature sensors lie predominantly in the preoptic area of the anterior hypothalamus, although they may be situated in the abdominal viscera and spinal cord as well. Increased heat to these areas causes vasodilatation and cold elicits vasoconstriction. Such reflex activity is mediated through the cardiovascular centres in the brain. Increased thermal content in the blood causes inhibition of normal sympathetic vasoconstriction at the preganglionic neuron level which results in opening of arteriovenous anastomoses (shunts) in the extremities, the nose, ears, and mouth. Under normal sympathetic activity, these shunts are closed, and withdrawal of sympathetic activity opens them for thermal regulation. Aortic and carotid chemoreceptor stimulation secondary to acidaemia, hypercapnia, or hypoxaemia may cause a decrease in sympathetic tone to the cutaneous arterioles with subsequent vasodilatation. This effect is the opposite of that seen in the muscle, splanchnic, and renal circulations.[36]

Regional cutaneous blood flow control to non-peripheral areas includes a cholinergic pathway to eccrine sweat glands in the skin. Recent work has shown that some afferent sympathetic preganglionic and postganglionic fibres innervate and activate the glands as well. When the cholinergic and sympathetic pathways to the glands are activated, they trigger the release of bradykinin alone or of other, as yet unknown, local vasodilator substances.

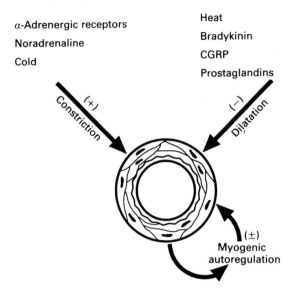

Fig 8.4 An illustration of control mechanisms in the cutaneous circulation.

The only parasympathetic innervation to affect skin blood vessels reaches the sweat glands via the sudomotor nerve. Activation of this system increases the output of the enzyme kallikrein. This substance, in turn, splits the polypeptide bradykinin from globulin in the perivascular interstitial tissues and induces a most potent vasodilatory effect.

Fig 8.4 illustrates the control mechanisms for regulation of cutaneous blood flow.

Effects of anaesthetic drugs on cutaneous blood flow

In humans, propofol administration causes an increase in flow, recorded by laser Doppler, which is probably the result of decreased sympathetic tone caused by the anaesthetic drug plus the direct vasodilating effect of propofol itself. A similar, though smaller, increase in skin blood flow may be observed with thiopentone and other short acting barbiturates as well.

Opiate anaesthesia, in particular morphine anaesthesia, has been shown to increase forearm skin flow and the neurocomponent is thought to be mediated centrally rather than by a local inhibition of adrenergic receptors. Additionally there is a centrally mediated effect upon the venous system, in that a significant venodilatation occurs approximately five minutes after delivery of centrally acting morphine. Most probably, in both cases, sympathetic mediated vasoconstriction is reduced and a resultant vasodilatation occurs.

With local anaesthetic drugs there is vasodilatation of the arterioles and

240

venules at high concentrations; however, small amounts of local anaesthetic drugs have a mild constrictive effect on the precapillary arteriolar vessels. Mepivacaine may also have a postcapillary constrictive effect in small concentrations. Overall, at concentrations used in clinical practice, the direct acting vasodilatory effects of the local anaesthetic drugs predominate.[37]

Most of the potent inhalational anaesthetic agents cause some degree of sympathoplegia from which there is an opening of the arteriovenous anastomoses in the extremities—nose, ears, and mouth. These shunts, normally closed, are opened during anaesthesia and may lead to an accelerated body hypothermia. Indeed, the relative vasodilatation in the cutaneous vessels may be one of the causes of dilated superficial veins whenever these agents are used.

Under regional anaesthesia a relative sympathoplegia occurs and conductance within the skin of the affected limb will increase, whereas blood flow through the cutaneous tissues in non-blocked limbs will decrease by reflex compensatory mechanisms.

In summary the cutaneous circulation is greatly influenced by anaesthesia and, although normally possessing thermoregulatory capacities, it may be sufficiently inhibited by anaesthetic drugs to mimic poikilothermic adaptation.

Muscle circulation

Anatomy

Skeletal muscle comprises approximately 40% of the total body mass. The density of the capillary networks varies greatly between the two basic muscle fibre types that are present in humans.[38] The slow twitch, or red, fibres are numerous in more slowly contracting muscles which help maintain posture and fulfil isometric functions. The fast twitch, or white, fibres are most numerous in the fast contracting muscles such as those used for running and quick movement. Numerous animal studies have demonstrated that resting blood flow and capillary density, as well as oxygen consumption, vary with the type of muscle that is being perfused. In general, the capillary density for slow-twitch fibres is approximately two to three times that seen in fast twitch fibres in the same muscles. Other animal studies have shown that oxidative enzymes, as well as blood flow, are several times higher in the slow contracting muscles compared with the fast twitch muscles which have a much higher activity of glycolytic enzymes and rely more on anaerobic metabolism. Apparently, slow twitch muscles respond better to prolonged activation and long term aerobic function.

In resting muscle, the precapillary arterioles exhibit intermittent asynchronous contractions and relaxations which, in effect, limit the number of capillary beds that are being perfused. This very action allows sudden recruitment and an increase in the number of nutrient capillary beds that perfuse the muscle when muscle activity begins. As a result of this, total blood flow through resting skeletal muscle varies between 2 and 5 ml/min per 100 g. With exercise, this can increase in trained athletes to more than 125 ml/min per 100 g.[39] Dynamic rhythmic exercise has a large, rapid effect on vascular contracture which is not explained by known neural, metabolic, myogenic, or hydrostatic influences.[40] The muscle relaxation between contractions draws blood from the arteries into the veins and effectively reduces arterial driving pressure. During the subsequent contraction venous blood is pumped centrally raising the central venous pressure. The consequent increase in muscle blood flow, coupled with the decrease in arterial pressure and raised central venous pressure, markedly increases the calculated conductance. This rhythmic contraction and relaxation, in effect, pumps blood across the muscle bed.

The anatomical architecture of the muscle and the increase in intramuscular pressure causing hindrance to blood flow itself determine the increase seen in perfusion pressure which attends exercise. In the forearm, the circulation is initially arrested during voluntary isometric contraction of more than 70% maximal. In the calf, tensions of only 20–30% of maximal voluntary contraction are necessary to interrupt blood flow.[38] The increase in vascular resistance during strong muscle contraction occurs chiefly in the larger supply vessels—the branched arteries down into the muscle bed. The manner in which this vascular bed is occluded keeps red cells in the capillary and so provides a continuous, albeit dwindling, supply of nutrient oxygen during contraction.

Overall, the sequence of vascular segments in the muscle beds is similar to those seen in other parts of the bodies—that is, large arteries, small branched arteries, arterioles, precapillary arterioles, capillaries, then postcapillary venules, venules, and collecting veins which return the blood to the central circulation. At the capillary level, only between 20% and 25% of the circuits are open in the resting muscle and these have decreased conductance from sympathetic tone and intramuscular pressure.

Control of the muscle circulation

Blood flow to skeletal muscle depends on the pressure gradient through the vessel complex and the calibre in the resistance vessels. Local modulation of vessel size is dependent on chemical and physical events near or within the environment of the resistance vessels as a result of changes in nervous innervation of the vessels and circulating vasoactive agents.

The resting tone in the resistance arterioles is relatively high in the non-active muscle.[41] There is an intrinsic basal vascular resistance, or contractile property, in these small vessels and those of 50–100 μm in diameter tend to have more myogenic tone than the larger vessels up to 400 μm in diameter. In isolated muscles, the change from continuous to pulsatile perfusion causes a gradual increase in vascular resistance, presumably by the periodic stretch of the arterioles which provides a continuing stimulus to the smooth muscle cells in the vessel walls.[42 43] This phenomenon was a concept initiated by Bayliss early in the century who suggested that distension of the resistance blood vessels by intravascular pressure contributes to the basal vascular resistance through a direct action on the vascular smooth muscle. The phenomenon of autoregulation in the muscle vascular bed relies on this myogenic theory and resides primarily at the precapillary arterioles. Recent observations strongly suggest that myogenic regulatory mechanisms contribute directly or indirectly to circulatory homoeostasis in the following ways: intravascular pressure induces a tonic excitatory activation which initiates an intrinsic myogenic basal tone in the arterial microvessels. This, in turn, induces variable vascular resistance (total peripheral resistance) mainly from the myogenic tone and basically serves to maintain normal arterial pressure at rest. Last, it produces an improved nutritional flow and exchange characterised by blood flow recruitment, capillary recruitment, and adjustments to the capillary perfusion/defusion ratio for optimum exchange of nutrients in a heterogeneous capillary network.[44] This myogenic control seems to initiate and maintain basal vascular tone. In synergism with metabolic vasodilators, it modifies autoregulation of blood flow through the muscle itself. Both the humoral and neurogenic β-adrenergic effects depress myogenic reactivity and counter α-adrenergic constriction.

Nervous control

The direct vasoconstricting activity of the sympathetic nervous system on the muscle blood flow is through the α-adrenergic receptor system. Vasoconstrictor fibres emerge from the ventral roots of the lower thoracic through upper lumbar segments with maximum outflow through L1–L3. In addition, there is cholinergic innervation of the resistance vessels in the muscle bed. This is limited to cholinergic vasodilator fibres from the lumbar region for lower limb innervation. The sympathetic nerves follow the somatic nerves to the vessels innervated and continue along the adventitial surface of the vessels. Only the outer layers of smooth muscle cells within the vessels are in contact with noradrenergic vessels. These axons form varicosities which are demyelinated Schwann cells. Within these varicosities, the vesicles for storage of neurotransmitter substance are situated. At the neuroeffector junction, arterial baroreceptors and chemoreceptors, the cardiopulmonary low pressure mechanoreceptors, the receptors in the skeletal muscle, and those originating from centres in the brain signal alterations in the amount of noradrenaline delivered by the terminal nerves into the junctional clefts near the vascular smooth muscle cells. The actual release of noradrenaline is initiated by action potentials generated within the ganglionic cell body.

Both sympathetic nerve stimulation and exogenous noradrenaline cause vasoconstriction of skeletal muscle resistance vessels. Small amounts of noradrenaline metabolites appear in the venous drainage following nerve stimulation. This indicates that reuptake into the sympathetic nerve terminals must be the main route for terminating action of the released noradrenaline on the muscle vessels. In animal studies, complete ablation of sympathetic activity to a resting limb muscle results in a less than threefold increase in blood flow. Conversely, maximal stimulation of the noradrenergic nerves to the same limb produces a decrease in blood flow of about 75%. Interestingly, simple somatic motor denervation, in the presence of an intact sympathetic innervation of striated muscle, will increase blood flow by 25%. This is thought to be the result of overcoming resting somatic muscle tone which causes relative decompression of the blood supply to the muscle thus opening up flow.[38]

Compared with the local mechanisms regulating muscle blood flow, the noradrenergic nerves control relatively small portions of the maximal flow available to the muscle bed. Nevertheless, because of the great muscle mass within the body, small amounts of variation in flow resistance may permit major changes in total body vascular resistance.[45]

Constriction of the muscle resistance vessels occurs solely by activation of the sympathetic noradrenergic nerves or muscle compression itself. On the other hand, neurogenic vasodilatation can occur either by withdrawal of noradrenergic activity or by release of substances that lead to relaxation of vascular smooth muscle. The most important effectors of this type are sympathetic, cholinergic, and histaminergic systems.

The arteriolar resistance vessels within the muscle vascular bed contain receptors of the β_2 subtype. Activation of these receptors causes relaxation of the smooth muscle which can be prevented by β-adrenergic antagonists. Via this system, adrenaline dilates skeletal resistance vessels. The β_2-adrenoceptors in blood vessels within the muscle respond primarily to adrenaline released from the adrenal medulla rather than to any noradrenaline released from adrenergic nerves. The β_2 activation is an additional mechanism to induce large scale vasodilatation in the working muscle.

Histamine is found in relatively high concentration in the walls of arteries and veins of the muscle bed. Activation of these histamine receptors causes marked vasodilatation of the resistance arterioles similar to that seen with potassium and adenosine. In general, metabolic vasodilators appear to be potassium, hypoxaemia, increased osmolarity, histamine, and nitric oxide.

There are several factors that modify the release of noradrenaline from sympathetic nerve endings. Metabolic acidosis, in addition to relaxing active smooth muscles, depresses the contractile response of blood vessels to sympathomimetic amines and nerve stimulation. Potassium ions in large concentrations cause small vessel vasodilatation via inhibitory effects on neurotransmission and a direct depressant effect on the vascular smooth muscle cell. Hyperosmolarity causes vasodilatation of many vascular beds because of a reduced release of noradrenaline in the sympathetic nerve endings. Adenosine has a relaxing action on the muscle arterioles by a direct effect on vascular smooth muscle and, indirectly, by an inhibitory effect on noradrenergic neurotransmission.

A number of prejunctional receptors have been demonstrated, the activation of which depresses noradrenaline release from sympathetic nerve endings as well. These include specific α_2-adrenoreceptors, muscarinic receptors activated by acetylcholine, histamine, and serotonin (5HT) receptors. In most animals and most probably in humans, there is a cholinergic vasodilator pathway that originates in the motor cortex. The descending pathway has discrete relays in the hypothalamus and continues through the mesencephalon descending via the lateral spinothalamic tract. These cholinergic nerves run in the sympathetic nerves to the muscle vessels and they innervate almost exclusively the small arteries and arterioles. The acetylcholine released on activation of these fibres causes an instant dilatation by activating prejunctional muscarinic receptors, thereby reducing the noradrenaline release from the sympathetic nerve endings. They act on postjunctional muscarinic receptors in the vascular smooth muscle cells which results in dilatation. Cholinergic nerves are generally quiescent. Stimulation of specific hypothalamic areas that produce defence reactions (in times of rage or fear) will, however, increase muscle blood flow by this indirect action without actual muscle activity. In isolated blood vessels from many species, removal of the endothelium abolishes this relaxation induced cholinergic transmitter. Consequently, it is felt that most of this cholinergic reaction may come by way of nitric oxide release.[46] Teleologically the resting vasodilatation caused by this cholinergic mechanism "primes the pump" for subsequent physical activity.

Reflex regulation

Changes in the activity of both the carotid and aortic high pressure mechanoreceptors result in inverse changes in blood flow to the limb muscles via the sympathetic nervous system. Activation of carotid and aortic chemoreflexes leads to constriction of arteriolar resistance vessels which is most pronounced in the skeletal muscle bed. Recent work has shown that the low pressure mechanoreceptors (atriopulmonary receptors) are much less important than previously thought in causing reflex sympathetic activation and vasoconstriction in the human skeletal muscle circulation during stress.[45] Indeed, the high pressure system predominantly controls the resting tone of these resistance arterioles.

Reflexes originate also from receptors in the skeletal muscle. This reflex, via activation of the adrenergic system, may be a prime cause for the rise in blood pressure in an isolated exercising limb. This suggests that intramuscular mechanoreceptors generate part of the reflex drive during induced contractions of the skeletal muscle.[47]

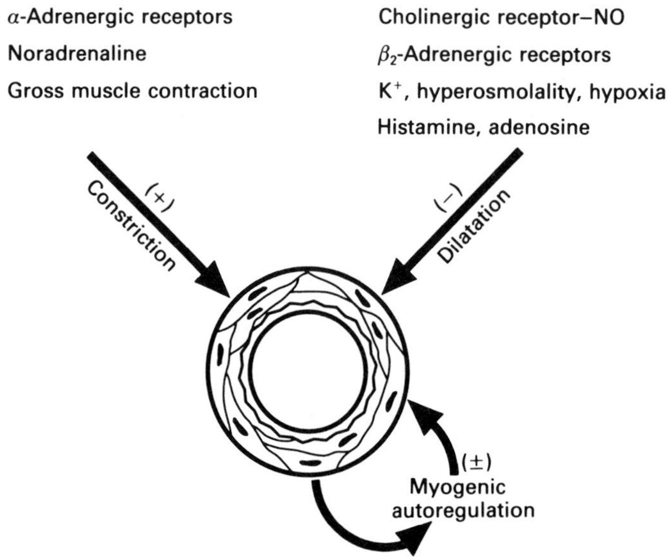

Fig 8.5 Control mechanisms for the circulation through the skeletal muscle.

A summary of factors that influence blood flow in the muscle circulation is illustrated in fig 8.5.

Effects of anaesthetic drugs on muscle blood flow

As was mentioned before, somatic motor denervation of the muscle leads to a 25% decrease in resting vascular tone in the muscle circulation. The use of neuromuscular relaxants in anaesthesia causes the same effect in that patients, supine and with neuromuscular block, demonstrate a fall in calculated vascular resistance compared with their unrelaxed state.

A dual effect by propofol occurs in the muscle bed of humans. An initial increase in blood flow occurs following infusion of propofol which may result, in part, from the direct vasodilating effect of the drug. However, a sustained fall in calculated muscle bed vascular resistance may continue thereafter because of depressed cardiac and muscle sympathetic baroreflex sensitivities. When propofol is used to control the stress response during surgery, the vasodilating effects of the drug override the neural vasoconstriction induced by baroreflex from the surgical stimulation.[48]

Opiates also have a dual effect upon vascular tone in the muscular bed. The direct action of morphine is that of venoconstriction whereas the centrally mediated effects include withdrawal of venous tone in the muscle bed. The short acting synthetic opiates have produced graded dose related decreases in calculated vascular resistance across the muscle bed in animal studies.

Certainly large doses of opiates given acutely may cause marked hypotension through a decrease in calculated vascular resistance.[49] Much of this vascular resistance change occurs in the muscle circulation.

The potent inhalational anaesthetic drugs have a direct vasodilating effect on most skeletal muscle beds. Reflex vasoconstriction from humoral factors such as vasopressin released during the relative hypotension induced by the potent inhalation agents, however, causes an overriding vasoconstriction in many of the beds as well. On the whole there is little change in the skeletal muscle blood flow during most inhaled anaesthesia.

With regional blockade, particularly in segments that involve the sympathetic outflow tract to the lower extremities, blood flow to the muscle beds of the lower limbs increases. This is brought about by a reduction in the resting sympathetic tone to the blood vessels. Active vasodilatation does not take place, but rather myogenic autoregulation limits the amount of dilatation that evolves.

In summary, control of the skeletal muscle vascular resistance involves complex interactions among neurogenic, autoregulatory, and metabolic systems. From the anaesthetic standpoint, resting control by sympathetic innervation, vasopressin levels, and autoregulatory mechanisms makes a significant contribution towards the calculation of total vascular resistance. The redistribution of cardiac output seen in haemorrhage, mild hypothermia, and with anaesthetic drugs is influenced markedly by the striated muscle circulation.

1 Kanwar YS, Venkatachalam MA. Ultrastructure of glomerulus and juxtaglomerular apparatus. In: Windhager EE, ed, *Renal physiology*, Volume 1, *Handbook of physiology*, Section 8. New York: Oxford University Press, 1992: 1–40.

2 Tisher CC, Madsen KM. Anatomy of the kidney. In: Brenner BM, Rector FC Jr, eds, *The kidney*, vol I. Philadelphia: WB Saunders, 1991: 1–75.

3 Dworkin LD, Brenner BM. The renal circulations. In: Brenner BM, Rector FC Jr, eds, *The kidney*, vol I. Philadelphia: WB Saunders, 1991: 164–204.

4 Venkatachalam MA, Kriz W. Anatomy. In: Heptinstall RH, ed, *Pathology of the kidney*, vol I. Boston: Little, Brown & Co., 1992: 1–92.

5 Jones RD, Berne RM. Intrinsic regulation of skeletal muscle blood flow. *Circ Res* 1964; **14**: 126–38.

6 Bayliss WM. On the local reactions of the arterial wall to changes in internal pressure. *J Physiol (Lond)* 1902; **28**: 220–6.

7 Hall JE, Brands MW. The renin–angiotensin–aldosterone systems. Renal mechanisms and circulatory homeostasis. In: Seldin DW, Giebisch B, eds, *The kidney. Physiology and pathophysiology*, vol 2. 1992: 1455–504.

8 Kon V. Neural control of renal circulation. *Miner Electrolyte Metab* 1989; **15**: 33–43.

9 Kien ND, Moore PG, Jaffe RS. Cardiovascular function during induced hypotension by fenoldopam or sodium nitroprusside in anesthetized dogs. *Anesth Analg* 1992; **74**: 72–8.

10 Keeton TK, Campbell WB. The pharmacologic alteration of renin release. *Pharmacol Rev* 1980; **32**(2): 81–227.

11 Venuto R, O'Dorisio CT, Ferris TF, Stein JH. Prostaglandins and renal function II. The effects of prostaglandin inhibition on autoregulation of blood flow in the intact kidney of the dog. *Prostaglandins* 1975; **9**: 817–28.

12 Spielman WS, Thompson CI. A proposed role for adenosine in the regulation of renal hemodynamics and renin release. *Am J Physiol* 1982; **242**: F423–35.

13 Terada Y, Tomita K, Nonoguchi H, Marumo F. Polymerase chain reaction localization of constitutive nitric oxide synthase and soluble guanylate cyclase messenger RNAs in microdissected rat nephrons segments. *J Clin Invest* 1992; **90**: 659–65.

14 Mattson DL, Roman RJ, Cowley AW Jr. Role of nitric oxide in renal papillary blood flow and sodium excretion. *Hypertension* 1992; **19**: 766–9.

15 Tollins JP, Palmer RMJ, Mondada S, Raij L. Role of endothelium-derived relaxing factor in the hemodynamic response to acetylcholine in vivo. *Am J Physiol* 1990; **258**: 665–62.

16 Lüscher TF, Bock HA. The endothelial L-arginine/nitric oxide pathway and the renal circulation. *Klin Wochenschr* 1991; **69**: 603–9.

17 Reilly PM, Bulkley GB. Vasoactive mediators and splanchnic perfusion. *Crit Care Med* 1993; **21**: S55–68.

18 Nishida O, Moriyasu F, Nakamura T, et al. Relationship between splenic and superior mesenteric venous circulation. *Gastroenterology* 1990; **98**: 721–5.

19 Guyton AC. *Textbook of medical physiology*, 7th edn. Philadelphia: WB Saunders, 1986: 340–3.

20 Parks DA, Jacobson ED. Physiology of the splanchnic circulation. *Arch Intern Med* 1985; **145**: 1278–81.

21 Escourrou P, Raffestin B, Papelier Y, Pussard E, Rowell LB. Cardiopulmonary and carotid baroreflex control of splanchnic and forearm circulations. *Am J Physiol* 1993; **264**: H777–82.

22 Stadeager C, Hesse B, Henriksen O, et al. Effects of angiotensin blockade on the splanchnic circulation in normotensive humans. *J Appl Physiol* 1989; **67**(2): 786–91.

23 Holzer P. Peptidergic sensory neurons in the control of vascular functions: mechanisms and significance in the cutaneous and splanchnic vascular beds. *Rev Physiol Biochem Pharmacol* 1992; **121**: 49–146.

24 Gatta A, Merkel C. Clinical pharmacology of splanchnic circulation in cirrhosis. *Pharmacol Res* 1990; **22**(3): 235–52.

25 Tokics L, Brismar B, Hedenstierna G. Splanchnic blood flow during halothane-relaxant anaesthesia in elderly patients. *Acta Anaesthesiol Scand* 1986; **30**: 556–61.

26 Tverskoy M, Gelman S, Fowler KC, Bradley EL. Influence of fentanyl and morphine on intestinal circulation. *Anesth Analg* 1985; **64**: 577–84.

27 Gelman S. Effects of anesthetics on splanchnic circulation. In: Altura BM, Halevy S, eds, *Cardiovascular actions of anesthetics and drugs used in anesthesia*, vol 2. Basel: Karger, 1986: 126–61.

28 Tan OT, Stafford TJ. Cutaneous circulation. In: Fitzpatrick TB, Eisen AZ, Wolff K, Freedberg IM, Austin KF, eds, *Dermatology and general medicine*, 3rd edn. New York: McGraw-Hill, 1987: 357–67.

29 Pavletic MM. Anatomy and circulation of the canine skin. *Microsurgery* 1991; **12**: 103–12.

30 Tripathi A, Mack GW, Nadel ER. Cutaneous vascular reflexes during exercise in the heat. *Med Sci Sports Exerc* 1990; **22**: 796–803.

31 Sessler DI, Rubinstein EH. Letter to the editor. *Anesthesiology* 1989; **70**: 371–2.

32 Johnson JM. Exercise and the cutaneous circulation. *Exerc Sport Sci Rev* 1992; **20**: 59–97.

33 Jager K, Muench R, Seifert H, Beglinger C, Bollinger A, Fischer JA. Calcitonin gene-related peptide (CGRP) causes redistribution of blood flow in humans. *Eur J Clin Pharmacol* 1990; **39**: 491–4.

34 Edfeldt H, Lundvall J. Sympathetic baroreflex control of vascular resistance in comfortably warm man. Analyses of neurogenic constrictor responses in the resting forearm and in its separate skeletal muscle and skin tissue compartments. *Acta Physiol Scand* 1993; **147**: 437–47.

35 Johnson JM, Brengelmann GL, Hales JRS, Vanhoutte PM, Wenger CB. Regulation of the cutaneous circulation. *Fed Proc* 1986; **45**: 2841–50.

36 Kellogg DL Jr, Johnson JM, Kenney WL, Pergola PE, Kosiba WA. Mechanisms of control of skin blood flow during prolonged exercise in humans. *Am J Physiol* 1993; **265**: H562–8.

37 Fruhstorfer H, Wagener G. Effects of intradermal lignocaine and mepivacaine on human cutaneous circulation in areas with histamine-induced neurogenic inflammation. *Br J Anaesth* 1993; **70**: 167–72.

38 Shepherd JT. Circulation to skeletal muscle. In: Shepherd JT, Abboud FM, eds, *Handbook of physiology*, Section 2, *The cardiovascular system*, vol 3, *Peripheral circulation and blood flow*, Part 1. Baltimore: Williams & Wilkins, 1983: 319–70.

39 Carù B, Colombo E, Santoro F, Laporta A, Maslowsky F. Regional flow responses to exercise. *Chest* 1992; **101**: 223S–5S.
40 Sheriff DD, Rowell LB, Scher AM. Is rapid rise of vascular conductance at onset of dynamic exercise due to muscle pump? *Am J Physiol* 1993; **265**: H1227–34.
41 Smith JJ, Porth CJM. Posture and the circulation: the age effect. *Exp Gerontol* 1991; **26**: 141–62.
42 Bevan JA, Laher I. Pressure and flow-dependent vascular tone. *FASEB J* 1991; **5**: 2267–73.
43 Grände PO. Myogenic mechanisms in the skeletal muscle circulation. *J Hypertens* 1989; **7**: S47–53.
44 Mellander S. Functional aspects of myogenic vascular control. *J Hypertens* 1989; **7**: S21–30.
45 Jacobsen TN, Morgan BJ, Scherrer U, *et al*. Relative contributions of cardiopulmonary and sinoaortic baroreflexes in causing sympathetic activation in the human skeletal muscle circulation during orthostatic stress. *Circ Res* 1993; **73**: 367–78.
46 Vane JR, Botting RM. Endothelium-derived vasoactive factors and the control of the circulation. *Semin Perinatol* 1991; **15**(1): 4–10.
47 Longhurst JC, Mitchell JH. Reflex control of the circulation by afferents from skeletal muscle. In: Guyton AC, Young DB, eds, *Cardiovascular physiology III*, vol 18. Baltimore: University Park Press, 1979: 125–48.
48 Sellgren J, Ejnell H, Elam M, Ponten J, Wallin BG. Sympathetic muscle nerve activity, peripheral blood flows, and baroreceptor reflexes in humans during propofol anesthesia and surgery. *Anesthesiology* 1994; **80**: 534–44.
49 White DA, Reitan JA, Kien ND, Thorup SJ. Decrease in vascular resistance in the isolated canine hindlimb after graded doses of alfentanil, fentanyl, and sufentanil. *Anesth Analg* 1990; **71**: 29–34.

9: Microcirculation

JAMES E BAUMGARDNER, DAVID E LONGNECKER

A major concern of modern anaesthesia and critical care practice is the optimal preservation of organs and tissues at risk for ischaemia. The recognition that anaesthetic agents have drug specific differences in preservation of vital organ function is increasingly an influence in the selection of anaesthetic drugs and techniques. Anaesthetic drugs have been shown, in animal models, to influence outcome in several abnormal circulatory conditions which compromise perfusion and tissue delivery of nutrients such as oxygen and glucose. These circulatory pathologies include local organ ischaemia, haemorrhagic shock, and septic shock.

Partial or complete tissue ischaemia presents an obvious compromise of nutrient delivery to tissue. Several anaesthetic drugs have been shown to provide drug specific protective effects for partial ischaemia, or for complete ischaemia followed by reperfusion. Anaesthetic drugs have been shown to differ in their effects on biochemical consequences and histological outcome for incomplete liver ischaemia,[1] for complete liver ischaemia and reperfusion,[2 3] after repeated complete cerebral ischaemic episodes,[4] and after incomplete cerebral ischaemia.[5-7]

Haemorrhagic shock results in selectively reduced blood flow and nutrient delivery to several organs, including the splanchnic, renal, skin, and muscle circulations. Anaesthetic agents have a drug specific effect on outcome in animal models of haemorrhagic shock (induced by controlled haemorrhage for a fixed period of time, followed by reperfusion). Ketamine provided a markedly better survival than halothane or pentobarbitone (pentobarbital) anaesthesia in haemorrhaged rats.[8] This study also reported a reduction in intestinal mucosal lesions with ketamine anaesthesia. More recently, high epidural anaesthesia combined with general anaesthesia in haemorrhaged dogs improved survival compared with general anaesthesia alone,[9] again suggesting that anaesthetic techniques alter outcome from compromised organ perfusion. Anaesthetic specific differences in bacterial translocation and intestinal histological damage were also demonstrated recently in haemorrhaged rats.[10]

The circulatory defects in sepsis and septic shock include a hyperdynamic circulation with high cardiac output, low systemic resistance, and increased oxygen uptake, with proportionally greater increases in oxygen delivery. The resulting decreased oxygen extraction may represent either inadequate nutrient delivery from blood to tissue or impaired biochemical use of oxygen. Anaesthetic drugs have specific effects on oxygen delivery ($\dot{D}o_2$), oxygen uptake ($\dot{V}o_2$), and serum lactate in a dog infused with endotoxin. In a dog model of septic shock, ketamine caused less lactate accumulation than enflurane,[11] and ketamine preserved cardiovascular function better than halothane, isoflurane, or alfentanil.[12] In contrast, enflurane anaesthesia in endotoxaemic rats resulted in significantly less intestinal pathology than ketamine anaesthesia,[13] and halothane improved survival compared with ketamine after reperfusion of ischaemic bowel.[14]

Several mechanisms have been suggested to explain these protective effects of anaesthetic drugs:

- they can suppress tissue metabolic requirements and thereby increase tolerance to reduced nutrient delivery
- they can modulate biochemical and cellular mediators of ischaemic tissue damage and thereby reduce permanent damage after an ischaemic insult
- they are known to have drug specific and dose dependent effects on tissue perfusion which can increase tissue oxygenation during an ischaemic insult.

It is known that most anaesthetic drugs decrease tissue metabolism in many different organs; the degree of this metabolic suppression depends on the specific drug and the specific organ. For example, halothane provides more potent suppression of metabolism in the myocardium than isoflurane, but isoflurane is the more potent inhibitor of metabolism in cerebral tissue. Reduced metabolic requirements may ameliorate the effects of reductions in tissue nutrients, but it is important to understand that these are specific effects of anaesthetic drugs at the tissue level and not a uniform consequence of the general anaesthetic state.

Anaesthetic drugs can also modify the biochemical consequences of tissue hypoxia. The past decade has witnessed a tremendous growth in our knowledge of the role of mediators involved with tissue hypoxia, in the brain in particular. Release of various excitatory neurotransmitters, such as glutamate, increases in intracellular calcium, and expression of free radicals and lipid peroxidation, are all thought to play a role in the permanent tissue damage that follows tissue hypoxia. Anaesthetic drugs can have important effects in modulating these changes after ischaemia. For example, ketamine is an antagonist of the N-methyl-D-aspartate (NMDA) subtype of the glutamate receptor complex. Also, anaesthetic drugs have drug specific and organ specific effects on tissue microcirculation, and these actions can modify organ perfusion and cell viability in response to circulatory insults such as shock, ischaemia, or hypoxaemia.

The primary function of the circulatory system is the delivery of nutrients such as oxygen and glucose, and the removal of waste such as carbon dioxide. The efficient accomplishment of this task depends on the distribution of blood flow within organs, which is regulated primarily by the resistance vessels of the microcirculation, and it also depends on the efficiency of tissue exchange for a given blood flow; this, in turn, depends on the distribution of blood flow within the local microcirculation. The microcirculatory effects of anaesthetic drugs can influence nutrient delivery and the distribution of blood flow in the following:

- in cases of globally impaired perfusion and/or oxygenation, as occurs in haemorrhagic and septic shock
- in cases of incomplete tissue ischaemia as might occur in peripheral vascular disease
- during reperfusion after complete ischaemia such as following arterial occlusion during certain surgical procedures.

This chapter is an introduction to and overview of the microcirculation; it covers anatomy and terminology, the normal function of the microcirculation, physiological control mechanisms, the effects of anaesthetic and other drugs on the microcirculation, and the mechanisms of altered control. The microcirculation has many fascinating biological functions, for example, immune functions, endocrine functions, and solute and water exchange, but the major focus in this chapter will be on the primary tasks of distribution of blood flow, exchange of nutrients, and regulation of vascular capacitance. Wherever possible the effects of anaesthetic drugs will be related to probable roles in improving outcome in abnormal circulatory conditions.

Anatomy

As with larger vascular structures, the microvasculature is described by a series of successive branchings of arterioles, with a decrease in diameter with each branching generation. This arteriolar branching structure culminates in the capillaries, which then coalesce into successively larger branches of venules, finally merging into larger veins. Terminology in the microvasculature follows this branching scheme, with the largest arterioles and venules in a given vital microscopy preparation (a living tissue examined directly under the microscope) designated first order vessels (for example, 1A arterioles and 1V venules) and the next largest integer assigned to each successively smaller generation of vessels (2A, 3A, etc) down to the capillary level. The assignment of typical vessels in a given preparation is somewhat arbitrary, but it is a useful scheme for comparison between preparations, so that a given vessel of a numbered generation may share some features with the same generation of a different sized animal, even though the absolute vessel diameters may not be the same.

The distinction between large arterioles and small arteries is not definitive, but generally arterioles cover a range of sizes from 10 to 150 μm in diameter.

Typically, a microvascular network includes three to five branching orders spanning this size range. The walls of arterioles contain relatively large amounts of vascular smooth muscle which participate in active circulatory regulation; the smallest arterioles—meta-arterioles—contain intermittent bands of vascular smooth muscle.

Capillaries are long thin tubes of endothelium, typically 5–10 μm in diameter and 50–1000 μm in length. They are devoid of vascular smooth muscle except for special bands of muscle at the arteriolar end of the capillary, the precapillary sphincters, which participate in regulation of capillary density. Precapillary sphincters are present in only some tissues, but most small arterioles appear to exhibit sphincter like activity, and thus act as functional sphincters. In addition to active regulation of capillary density in a given tissue, different organs and tissues vary widely in their maximal perfused capillary density, with highly metabolically active tissues generally having a more dense capillary network.

Venules of a given branching order are larger than their equivalent arterioles and have thinner and more distensible walls. As a result, the cross sectional area of a venular generation is larger, and blood flow is slower, than the equivalent arteriolar generation. Larger venules (lower branching orders) tend to pair with adjacent arterioles of the same branch order (fig 9.1). The parallel and countercurrent arrangement of arterioles and venules may provide an opportunity for countercurrent exchange of gases and solutes, most notably in intestinal mucosa.[15]

Quantitative description of even a simple microcirculatory network would require an enormous number of branch lengths, branch diameters, numbers of branches at bifurcations, and branching angles at each bifurcation. Progress has been made recently in fractal descriptions of these networks, reducing the entire description to a single fractal equation with a small number of parameters.[16]

Function

Resistance

Distribution of cardiac output to individual organs is regulated locally by changes in vascular resistance, which is controlled by regulation of vascular diameters. Resistance (defined as pressure decrease across the vascular bed divided by blood flow) in a cylindrical vessel varies approximately with diameter to the fourth power, with the result that small changes in vascular diameter effect large changes in resistance. In skeletal muscle and intestinal circulations, small arterioles (< 100 μm in diameter in the cat) are responsible for nearly all of the vascular resistance to blood flow. Small arterioles make a major contribution to resistance in other circulations as well, but recently it has been recognised that larger arterioles and small arteries make a

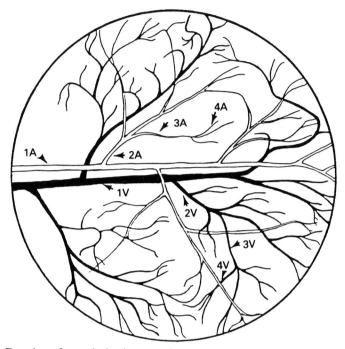

Fig 9.1 Drawing of a typical microvascular network in rat cremaster muscle, with numbering system for vessel generations based on order in branching heirarchy. (Adapted with permission from Hutchins PM, Goldstone J, Wells R. Effects of hemorrhagic shock on the microvasculature of skeletal muscle. *Microvasc Res* 1973; 5: 131.)

significant contribution to resistance in the coronary circulation, and even larger arteries make a significant contribution in the cerebral circulation (fig 9.2).[17 18]

Many organs and tissues regulate local blood flow according to tissue metabolic needs. Autoregulation refers specifically to maintenance of constant tissue blood flow over a range of perfusing pressures, when all other variables (for example, tissue metabolic rate, arterial P_{CO_2} or Pa_{CO_2}, arterial P_{O_2} or Pa_{O_2}, neurohumoral inputs) are constant. This regulation may be mediated by response of vascular smooth muscle to changes in distending pressure (the myogenic hypothesis) or by feedback regulation of local metabolic mediators (the metabolic hypothesis). Although the exact mechanism is unknown, it is evident from microvascular studies that the vessels responsible for autoregulation are the small arterioles, with increasingly less contribution as vessel diameter increases and branching order decreases.[18] Many tissues also vary tissue blood flow in proportion to tissue metabolic rate (again with other variables such as perfusing pressure held constant), a phenomenon known as metabolic regulation. Small arterioles also play the

254

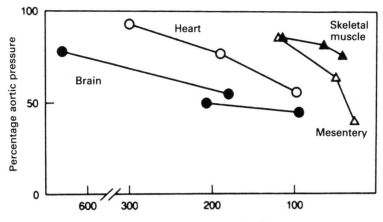

Fig 9.2 Pressure, as percentage of aortic pressure, measured in several sizes of arteries and arterioles of the cat, for brain, heart, mesentery, and skeletal muscle. (Reproduced with permission from Faraci FM, Heistad DD. Regulation of large cerebral arteries and cerebral microvascular pressure. *Circ Res* 1990; **66**: 9.)

major role in this local regulatory response. The mechanism of metabolic regulation is unknown, but recent studies of the cerebral circulation in particular suggest a prominent role for regulation through increased production of nitric oxide (NO) by specific neurons in response to surrounding neuronal activity.[19]

Microvascular studies have led to a growing appreciation that alterations in vascular diameters are usually not uniform and tend to be very site specific. For example, autoregulatory responses do not change all vessel diameters or vessel resistances proportionately, but tend to affect the most distal arterioles. In contrast, changes in vascular diameter from systemic neural inputs alter the larger arterioles and small arteries. Vasoactive drugs and anaesthetic drugs also affect specific branching orders or sizes of arterioles. For example, glyceryl trinitrate (nitroglycerin) produces dose dependent dilatation of coronary arterioles and arteries more than 200 μm in diameter, but causes little change in smaller arteriolar diameters, whereas in contrast nifedipine causes homogeneous dilatation of all coronary microvessels.[18] The functional implications of the specificity of microvascular responses are not yet clear, but may explain in part why a group of vasodilators that produce seemingly equivalent decreases in total resistance can have drug specific differences in protection from tissue ischaemia.

Capacitance

Vascular capacitance refers to the ability of the circulatory system to store variable amounts of blood with minimal changes in central filling pressures.

Regulation of vascular capacitance by neurohumoral mechanisms plays an important role in cardiovascular control in response to haemorrhage and other acute changes in blood volume. About 70% of the blood volume resides in the venous circulation, with most contained in venules in the microcirculation. Neurohumoral regulation controls the diameter of these microcirculatory venules, especially in the splanchnic circulation, whereas large veins function primarily as conduits.[20]

Exchange

The primary function of the microcirculation is the delivery of oxygen to tissue and the removal of carbon dioxide from tissue. Adequate gas exchange depends on tissue blood flow and also on the efficiency with which tissues use blood flow to transfer gases. It is therefore quite possible to have adequate overall perfusion but deficient gas exchange. In septic shock, for example, many tissues receive increased blood flow, but the decreased extraction of oxygen may produce tissue hypoxia from inefficient use of this blood flow.[21]

Capillaries, and probably also smaller arterioles and venules, are the main vessels of gas exchange. Convective transport involves delivery of gases dissolved in blood to tissue vascular beds. Thereafter, the gases must diffuse into the tissue from the microcirculation. Effective diffusion requires an adequate surface area for diffusion and adequate time for diffusion, both of which change with capillary density. At a fixed blood flow, increases in the number of open capillaries cause a larger area for diffusive transport. Increases in the number of open capillaries also increase total capillary cross sectional area, which leads to lesser flow velocities and longer transit times, and therefore more time for diffusion. Overall efficiency of gas exchange also depends on the distribution of blood flow within a vessel network, with most efficient exchange taking place when blood flow and metabolism are evenly matched. For example, a large blood flow through capillaries surrounded by poorly metabolising tissue will behave functionally as a shunt, decreasing the overall efficiency with which that tissue can exchange gases.[22]

Efficient tissue gas exchange, then, depends on the total number of open vessels in a microvascular network, and on the distribution of blood flow within those vessels. Both of these variables can be regulated by the precapillary sphincters, which may be distinct anatomical entities or functional entities, depending on the specific organ. Anaesthetic drugs and other vasoactive drugs that act at vascular smooth muscle probably influence the efficiency of gas exchange by these mechanisms, although experimental studies at this level have been limited. It is known that, in normal tissue, gas exchange is very efficient and blood flow can be dramatically reduced (by anaesthetic drugs or other mechanisms) in most organs before the onset of cellular hypoxia. In circulatory pathologies that compromise tissue oxygenation, however, the microvascular effects of anaesthetic drugs may have an important impact on tissue oxygenation by these mechanisms.

Control of the microcirculation

The contractile activity of smooth muscle in the walls of arteries, arterioles, venules, and veins is controlled by multiple mechanisms. Vascular smooth muscle tone is influenced by remote (or centrally mediated) control mechanisms and local control mechanisms. Remote control mechanisms can be further divided into neural control and humoral control. Alterations in arteriolar smooth muscle contraction, resulting from these influences, is responsible for the changes in resistance that determine the distribution of cardiac output. There is a remarkable variation of basal vascular tone and resistance from organ to organ. Renal arterioles, for example, have a very low resting vascular tone and can constrict markedly in response to stimuli such as hypovolaemia, but they have little capacity to dilate. In contrast, arterioles in the skin have a high resting tone and can both dilate and constrict in response to thermoregulatory stimuli.

Neural control

Arteries and arterioles are innervated by sympathetic fibres terminating in the blood vessel walls. The extent of sympathetic innervation varies from organ to organ. For example, renal vessels and mesenteric vessels receive dense innervation by adrenergic neurons, although the cerebral and coronary vessels receive fairly sparse adrenergic innervation. Accordingly, organs with a rich supply of adrenergic neurons exhibit a much greater constrictor response to sympathetic neural stimulation than the cerebral and coronary circulations. Similarly, neuronal supply along the generations of the vascular tree is not uniform, but generally tends to be more dense in the larger vessels with a decreasing neuronal supply in the more distal generations. Consequently, vasoconstrictor fibre stimulation results not only in a change in organ vascular resistance, but also in a change in the distribution of organ vascular resistance, with an increased contribution by larger arterioles and arteries.[17][18] Autonomic innervation plays an important regulatory role in coordination of the vascular response to any stimuli that activate the sympathoadrenal axis, such as hypovolaemia, hypoxia, hypercapnia, tissue trauma, and pain. Sympathetic innervation probably plays a minimal role in more local control such as local regulation of blood flow in response to increased organ metabolism.

Systemic humoral control

An enormous number of endogenously produced mediators have been shown to constrict or dilate vascular smooth muscle. Intravascularly administered adrenaline, noradrenaline, angiotensin II, vasopressin, endothelin, prostaglandin $PGF_{2\alpha}$, and thromboxane cause dose dependent, organ specific, and site specific vasoconstriction. Intravascularly administered acetylcholine, atrial natriuretic peptide, bradykinin, serotonin (5-hydroxytryptamine), adenosine, prostacyclin (PGI_2), and PGE_2 cause dose dependent, organ specific, and site specific vasodilatation.[18][23][24] Dose–response curves for vasoactive substances are often constructed by administering high concentrations of agonist intravascularly in isolated perfused tissues, thereby avoiding the confounding influence of systemic effects, or by topical application of the agonist to exposed tissue. There is no doubt that many of these substances play a role in local humoral regulation of vascular smooth muscle tone. Their role in remote humoral control is, however, less certain. Clearly, intravascular concentrations beyond the range of normal endogenous concentrations reflect pharmacological, not physiological, effects. Topical or abluminal application, on the other hand, may mimic actions in local control, where locally secreted mediators can diffuse through tissue to interact directly with vascular smooth muscle. The relationship of abluminal effects of topically applied mediators to the effects from mediators applied to the vascular lumen is not, however, direct. During the last decade there has been a tremendous growth in our understanding of the role of vascular endothelium in mediating intraluminal effects of vasoactive drugs. For example, acetylcholine administered intraluminally dilates arterioles, an effect now known to be mediated by endothelial secretion of NO. In contrast, acetylcholine administered abluminally constricts arterioles.[25] Although our knowledge of the complexities of endogenous mediators in vascular control is growing rapidly, the role of endogenous mediators in remote humoral control remains uncertain.

Local control—vascular endothelium

Our understanding of local microvascular control mechanisms has increased tremendously in recent years, principally through the discovery[26] that NO (then called "endothelium derived relaxing factor" or EDRF) functions as an important mediator of vasodilatation. NO is produced by the conversion of arginine and oxygen into NO and citrulline, a reaction that is catalysed by the enzyme nitric oxide synthase (NO synthase). Although many forms of NO synthase have been identified, they may be classified into constitutive forms, found in endothelial cells and neurons, and inducible forms which predominate in macrophages and hepatocytes.

The multiple locations of these isoforms of nitric oxide synthase imply multiple functions for the gaseous transmitter, and it is now evident that NO is involved in a variety of biological functions, including local cardiovascular control, neuronal transmission, immune function, and the control of pathogens (for example, bacteria). This discussion will focus only on microvascular control functions of NO, but concise reviews are available which describe its other biological functions.[27]

The actions of NO on the peripheral circulation can be evaluated by the infusion of an inhibitor ($N_\omega$monomethyl-L-arginine or L-NMMA) into intact animals, and recording the changes in cardiovascular function that result. We have used this approach to determine the actions of NO on blood pressure, cardiac output, and regional blood flows in conscious rats, by injecting radioactively labelled microspheres into the circulation before and during the infusion of L-NMMA (and again after the infusion of L-arginine, to demonstrate that the changes observed in response to L-NMMA were reversible by providing more substrate for NO production).[28] Inhibition of NO produced major changes in blood pressure regulation and peripheral circulatory control. The general circulatory effects are summarised in table 9.1.

Table 9.1 Effects of EDRF/NO inhibition by L-NMMA and reversal of inhibition by L-arginine on systemic haemodynamics.

Parameter	Control	Treatment	
		L-NMMA	L-Arginine
CO (ml/min)	90 ± 5	52 ± 5	68 ± 6
HR (beats/min)	441 ± 13	404 ± 17	430 ± 16
MAP (mm Hg)	129 ± 5	145 ± 5	134 ± 4
SVR (mm Hg $\times$ min $\times$ g/ml)	$1\cdot5 \pm 0\cdot1$	$3\cdot0 \pm 0\cdot3$	$2\cdot1 \pm 0\cdot2$

Reproduced with permission from Greenblatt et al.[28]
CO, cardiac output; HR, heart rate; MAP, mean arterial pressure; SVR, systemic vascular resistance.

In brief, inhibition of NO caused a doubling of systemic vascular resistance and increased arterial pressure, accompanied by decreases in heart rate and cardiac output.

Inhibition of NO by L-NMMA decreased local blood flow in the cerebrum, heart, kidneys, spleen, gastrointestinal tract, portal vein, liver (total flow), skin, ear, and white fat, whereas flow increased in the hepatic artery (presumably in response to the decrease in portal and total hepatic blood flow). Vascular resistances increased in every tissue studied, although the magnitude of the response was variable among organs and tissues, indicating that the relative importance of this system depends on local factors (fig 9.3).

Similar results have been observed in numerous studies in isolated blood vessels or local microvascular networks, suggesting that the results obtained above can be attributed to inhibition of NO in the vascular endothelium, although the possibility of remote effects cannot be ruled out whenever inhibitors of NO are administered systemically. These studies provide clear evidence that NO is a profound and ubiquitous controller of the peripheral

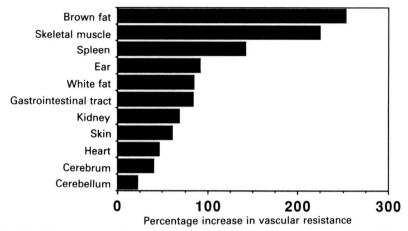

Fig 9.3 The percentage increase in mean regional vascular resistances induced by L-NMMA in conscious rats, reflecting the heterogeneity of the contribution of EDRF/NO to regional vascular control. (Reproduced with permission from Greenblatt EP, Loeb AL, Longnecker DE.[28] Marked regional heterogeneity in the magnitude of EDRF/NO-mediated vascular tone in awake rats. *J Cardiovasc Pharmacol* 1993; **21**: 237.)

circulation. However, it is clear that NO is not the only controller of the peripheral circulation, and it is impossible to attribute either physiological or pharmacological effects in the microcirculation to a single mechanism, because multiple mechanisms are involved in the control of vascular tone.

Effects of anaesthetic drugs on the microcirculation

This section will not present a comprehensive review of the effects of each anaesthetic agent on each individual tissue, but will focus instead on a few illustrative studies of the differences in peripheral circulatory effects of anaesthetic drugs. Wherever possible, comparison will be made between the effects of two anaesthetic drugs in the same study, using the same protocol.

Isoflurane versus halothane

Comparison of the effects of isoflurane with those of halothane emphatically illustrates the point that two anaesthetic drugs that appear similar on a superficial level can be quite distinctive on more detailed investigation. When delivered in equal MACs (minimum alveolar concentrations), these two agents produce approximately equal decreases in mean arterial blood pressure. When cardiac output and systemic vascular resistance are also measured, however, it becomes apparent that halothane achieves these changes in blood pressure primarily by decreases in cardiac output, in contrast to isoflurane, which primarily decreases systemic vascular resistance.[29–31] Further differences between these two agents are evident on more detailed investigation of individual organ blood flow and microcirculatory vascular diameters. In general, isoflurane is the more potent vasodilator, although the relative decreases in vascular resistance for these agents are organ specific, and the extent of dilatation also tends to be specific for vessel branching order within a tissue.

Organ resistances and blood flows

Anaesthetic drugs mediate changes in organ blood flow by changes in vascular diameter and resistance. Resistance is equal to pressure divided by flow, and therefore measurements of systemic pressure and local (organ or tissue) blood flow can be used to calculate changes in local resistance. Several techniques are available to measure organ blood flow in laboratory and clinical studies. Radioactive microspheres, which distribute to organs in proportion to blood flow, provide a quantitative and absolute measure of tissue blood flow, but require destruction of the tissue sample for counting and weighing for the most accuracy, and therefore are limited to laboratory studies. Indicator dilution techniques (for example, thermal dilution or indocyanine green) also provide absolute and quantitative blood flow measurements. These techniques require venous outflow sampling, but are applicable in some clinical studies when an appropriate venous catheter can be placed. Large vessel flow probes (for example, electromagnetic or Doppler probes) require invasive placement but can be implanted for chronic use. Some thermal and inert tracer clearance methods are highly invasive (for example, hydrogen clearance by implantation of hydrogen microelectrodes); some are non-invasive and are used clinically, for example, radioactive xenon (^{133}Xe) wash-out. More recently, laser Doppler velocimetry (LDV) has been used in both laboratory and clinical studies. This technique measures relative changes in blood flow quantitatively and continuously.

In dogs receiving an opiate general anaesthetic drug, either halothane or isoflurane was added and titrated to decrease mean arterial pressure to 60 mm Hg.[32] Inspired isoflurane 1·5% maintained myocardial blood flow (measured by radioactive microspheres) and decreased coronary vascular resistance by 40%. In contrast, 1·1% inspired halothane decreased myocardial blood flow by 35% and decreased coronary resistance by 13%.

Debaene *et al*[33] induced cirrhosis in rats by bile duct ligation and then compared the influence of anaesthetic drugs on liver blood flow during mild haemorrhage (removal of 20% of estimated blood volume). One MAC (1·3% inspired in rats) isoflurane anaesthesia maintained hepatic arterial flow (measured by radioactive microspheres) at prehaemorrhage values. One MAC (1·0% inspired in rats) halothane anaesthesia caused a significant decrease in hepatic arterial flow during haemorrhage.

Frink *et al*[1] studied portal venous and hepatic arterial blood flows by means of chronically implanted probes in healthy dogs. They measured the effects of four different anaesthetic drugs on portal venous and hepatic arterial blood flow, compared with conscious controls, for three different doses of anaesthetics (1·0, 1·5, and 2·0 MAC). Halothane reduced hepatic arterial blood flow in a dose dependent fashion and increased hepatic arterial vascular resistance. In contrast, isoflurane maintained hepatic arterial flow at all doses. Isoflurane reduced portal venous flow at the higher doses. Halothane caused greater decreases in portal venous flow at all doses.

Vollmar et al[34] studied liver and pancreatic blood flows (by microspheres) and tissue oxygen tensions (by multiwire surface electrodes) in rats. Isoflurane and halothane were titrated to reduce mean arterial pressure to 50 mm Hg (2·3% inspired isoflurane and 1·0% inspired halothane). Isoflurane and halothane both caused similar reductions in portal venous and hepatic arterial blood flows (by radioactive microspheres) compared with chloralose anaesthetised controls; however, isoflurane reduced mean tissue Po_2 from 4·08 kPa to 2·33 kPa, whereas halothane caused greater reductions to a mean tissue Po_2 of 1·53 kPa. Halothane maintained pancreatic blood flow and tissue oxygen tension compared with a control. In contrast, isoflurane increased pancreatic blood flow and tissue oxygen tension.

Jacob et al[35] studied arterial blood flow (by means of implanted Doppler probes) supplying an ileocolic graft following oesophageal reconstruction in humans. Fentanyl infusions of 300 μg/h which were established intraoperatively were maintained immediately postoperatively and then 0·65 MAC isoflurane or halothane was administered in a crossover design. Halothane did not change mesenteric blood flow, and isoflurane increased mesenteric blood flow by 38%.

Hansen et al[36] studied the distribution of cerebral blood flow in rats at 1 MAC of either isoflurane or halothane. Blood flows to the subcortex were not significantly different between halothane and isoflurane, but halothane caused significantly greater blood flows in the neocortex.

Vessel diameters

Vessel diameters can be studied in intact tissue under direct microscopic visualisation (vital microscopy) by means of either transillumination for a suitably thin tissue or by epi-illumination of a tissue surface. This invasive technique has been applied primarily in anaesthetised animals. Some vascular networks have been examined microscopically in humans (for example, the nail fold),[37] but these are fairly specialised circulations and it is difficult to extrapolate results to other organs of interest. Direct microscopic visualisation has the unique advantage of providing information about the specific vessels and branching orders which are influenced by anaesthetic drugs. The studies are, however, technically demanding and there have been fewer reports of the comparative effects of anaesthetic drugs studied by these techniques.

Conzen *et al*[32] studied the microcirculation of the epicardial surface of the left ventricle in intact, beating, dog hearts by means of epi-illumination. The dogs were anaesthetised with opiate infusions and then received isoflurane or halothane titrated to reduce mean arterial pressure to 60 mm Hg (1·1% inspired halothane, 1·5% inspired isoflurane). Isoflurane caused larger increases in arteriolar diameters than halothane. Both agents dilated 20–200 μm vessels specifically, and had no effects on larger arterioles or on precapillary sphincters.

Leon *et al*[38] studied rat diaphragm arteriolar diameters and functional capillary density by vital microscopy. All rats received pentobarbitone (pentobarbital) anaesthesia, followed by three concentrations (0·50, 0·75, and 1·0 MAC) of either halothane or isoflurane. Halothane administration caused dose dependent constriction specifically in the A4 arterioles of the diaphragm, leaving A2 and A3 arterioles unchanged, and also decreased capillary density in a dose dependent manner. Administration of isoflurane caused no significant changes in arteriolar diameter or capillary density.

Summary

This brief and selective review of recent studies of organ resistances and blood flows demonstrates the different effects of isoflurane and halothane for heart, liver, pancreas, mesentery, and brain, and also different effects on specific regions within an organ. In the case of liver and pancreas, these agent specific microcirculatory effects have been associated with changes in tissue oxygen tension. The vital microscopy studies in cardiac and skeletal muscle demonstrate the specificity of the circulatory effects of anaesthetic drugs for vessels of a particular size and branching order. Further studies will be required to connect the specificity of these changes to the specific influence of anaesthetic drugs on delivery of nutrients to tissue. In general, isoflurane tends to be a more potent vasodilator than halothane, and as a result tends to maintain tissue blood flow, although there are exceptions for selected tissues and for specific pathologies. The clinical importance is that, in patients with circulatory pathology and compromised tissue oxygenation, the microcirculatory effects of anaesthetic drugs have the potential to influence tissue preservation in the perioperative period.

Parenteral anaesthetic drugs

Compared to the inhalational anaesthetic drugs, considerably fewer studies of the effects of parenteral anaesthetic agents on organ blood flows and microvascular diameters have been reported. Data are particularly scarce for direct comparisons of two or more parenteral anaesthetic techniques, for example, high dose opiate anaesthesia compared with propofol infusion. There have, however, been several microvascular studies comparing ketamine with other anaesthetic techniques, and a selective review of these reports further supports the concept of drug specific effects on organ blood flows and branching generations. Interest in ketamine arises in part because it is a commonly used anaesthetic in the laboratory, but also because of its unique beneficial properties in haemorrhagic shock.[8 39] Ketamine may also be uniquely beneficial in septic shock,[12 40] although the data in this area are more conflicting.[13 14]

Organ resistances and blood flows

Debaene *et al*[33] compared the effects of several anaesthetic drugs, including ketamine and enflurane, on portal venous blood flow and hepatic arterial blood flow during mild haemorrhage (removal of 20% of estimated blood volume) in cirrhotic rats.[33] During haemorrhage, enflurane (2·2% inspired) decreased portal venous flow more than ketamine (1·5 mg/kg per min intravenously (i.v.)), but after reinfusion of the shed blood the portal venous blood flows were similar. During haemorrhage, enflurane decreased hepatic arterial blood flow and ketamine resulted in an unchanged hepatic arterial blood flow.

In isolated intestinal loops in dogs, Tverskoy *et al*[41] found that ketamine (both 8 and 16 mg/kg i.v.) caused increased vascular resistance and decreased blood flow compared with pentobarbitone.

Seyde and Longnecker[42] studied the effects of four anaesthetic drugs (ketamine 1 mg/kg per min i.v., halothane 1·2% inspired, isoflurane 1·4% inspired, and enflurane 2.2% inspired) on organ blood flows (measured by microspheres) and organ vascular resistances in rats, compared with conscious controls, for both normovolaemia and during moderate haemorrhage (removal of 30% of estimated blood volume).[42] Before haemorrhage, ketamine maintained cerebral blood flow at conscious values, whereas the inhaled agents increased cerebral blood flow. After haemorrhage, ketamine, enflurane, and halothane reduced cerebral blood flow significantly, compared with conscious animals, although isoflurane did not. At baseline, isoflurane maintained myocardial blood flow at conscious values, and ketamine, enflurane, and halothane progressively reduced myocardial blood flow. After haemorrhage, myocardial blood flow increased in conscious animals, did not change under isoflurane or halothane anaesthesia, and decreased under ketamine or enflurane anaesthesia. Before haemorrhage, portal venous flow was increased, compared with conscious animals, by ketamine anaesthesia and was reduced compared with controls by halothane anaesthesia; portal flow was decreased in all groups after haemorrhage. Hepatic arterial blood flow after haemorrhage was greatest in animals receiving isoflurane anaesthesia, although in the ketamine group haemorrhage resulted in an increase in hepatic arterial blood flow, compared with normovolaemia. Several other organ blood flows were studied, and the study demonstrates the drug specific effects of the anaesthetic drugs on organ vascular resistances, as well as the unique properties of ketamine.

Miller et al[43] compared the distribution of cardiac output of conscious rats with the distribution of cardiac output during halothane, enflurane, or ketamine anaesthesia. Halothane, 1·3% inspired, decreased cardiac output and increased the percentage of cardiac output going to brain, kidney, liver, and large intestine. Enflurane, 2·2% inspired, also increased the percentage of cardiac output going to the liver, spleen, and large intestine, although the cardiac output did not decrease compared with the conscious state. Intramuscular (i.m.) ketamine 125 mg/kg tended to decrease cardiac output (although not significantly), and the percentage of cardiac output going to the brain increased, whereas the percentage of cardiac output going to muscle decreased, and the percentage of cardiac output going to the heart, intestine, liver, and kidneys did not change.

In rats haemorrhaged to a mean arterial pressure of 60 mm Hg, ketamine anaesthesia (1·5 mg/kg per min i.v.) resulted in increased blood flow to brain heart, kidneys, intestine, and liver, compared with pentobarbitone anaesthesia (6 mg/kg per h i.v.).[44]

Gaab et al[45] used multiwire surface microelectrodes on the surface of rat cerebral cortex to measure tissue P_{O_2} profiles, local blood flow profiles (by means of hydrogen clearance), and local metabolism (by means of rate of oxygen depletion during carotid occlusion). Intraperitoneal (i.p.) ketamine 320 mg/kg and pentobarbitone 65 mg/kg i.p. were found to result in almost identical tissue P_{O_2} profiles, but very different local blood flow profiles. Ketamine anaesthesia resulted in higher mean blood flows compared with pentobarbitone anaesthesia. Ketamine also resulted in greater tissue metabolism compared with pentobarbitone anaesthesia.

Dempsey et al[46] measured cerebral blood flow in cats after release of middle cerebral artery occlusion. In cats anaesthetised by pentobarbitone, pre-treatment with indomethacin resulted in increased postischaemic cerebral blood flow compared with cats that did not receive indomethacin pre-treatment. In cats anaesthetised by ketamine, pre-treatment with indomethacin did not affect postischaemic cerebral blood flow.

Vessel diameters

Longnecker et al[47] measured arteriolar diameters microscopically in rat cremaster muscle during haemorrhage and compared the effects of enflurane anaesthesia and ketamine anaesthesia. They also measured tissue P_{O_2} with oxygen microelectrodes. Severe haemorrhage (removal of blood to decrease mean arterial pressure to 35 mm Hg for 30 minutes) during enflurane anaesthesia (2·2 vol% inspired) resulted in constriction in 1A, 3A, and 4A arterioles and decreased tissue P_{O_2} in skeletal muscle. Haemorrhage during ketamine anaesthesia (125 mg/kg i.m. with supplements of 30 mg/kg i.m. as needed) resulted in less constriction of the larger arterioles and increases in diameter in the 4A arterioles, and no significant decreases in tissue P_{O_2}.

Longnecker and Harris reported changes in arteriolar and venular diameters in bat wing, a mammalian skin microvasculature, and compared the conscious state with the anaesthetised state for ketamine and halothane.[48 49] An anaesthetic dose of ketamine (120 mg/kg i.m.) produced dilatation of the small arterioles (30–65 μm) and no change in diameters of the venules, compared with conscious controls. A smaller dose of ketamine, 40 mg/kg i.m., did not change arteriolar or venular diameters. In contrast, 0·71 MAC of halothane (0·81% inspired) caused arteriolar dilatation and no change in diameters of venules, and 1·25 MAC of halothane (1·42% inspired) in more dilatation of the arterioles and also dilatation of the venules.

Summary
There have been relatively few studies of the microcirculatory effects of parenteral anaesthetic drugs, and generalisations about their effects are therefore difficult. It is clear, however, from the studies on organ blood flows and vessel diameters reviewed here that the effects of parenteral anaesthetic drugs are agent specific, organ specific, pathology specific (for example, haemorrhaged versus non-haemorrhaged) and vessel generation specific (for example, 4A arterioles versus 1A and 2A arterioles). Further studies will be required to connect the specificity of these changes to the specific influence of anaesthetic drugs on delivery of nutrients to tissue.

Mechanisms of anaesthetic effects on the microcirculation

The microcirculation is controlled by a number of remote (neural, humoral, and hormonal) and local (metabolic, endothelial, and myogenic) regulatory mechanisms, and it is the summation of these actions that result in overall microcirculatory control. Similarly, the anaesthetic drugs alter numerous biological functions, including cellular metabolism, neuronal activity and transmission, humoral and hormonal control, and direct actions on vascular smooth muscle. It is, however, possible to demonstrate the effects of anaesthetic drugs on specific microvascular control systems in some situations, and these at least enhance the logic of the argument that the peripheral vascular actions of the anaesthetic drugs can be explained by actions on physiological systems that control the microcirculation. The actions of nitrous oxide, halothane, and isoflurane will be used as examples here.

Nitrous oxide (N_2O) has been shown to activate the sympathetic nervous system, as evidenced by increased splanchnic nerve activity when nitrous oxide was administered to cats receiving halothane anaesthesia.[50] We studied the peripheral circulatory actions of nitrous oxide, when added to a halothane anaesthesia in rats, to determine whether the reported changes in sympathetic activity in the splanchnic nerve were associated with changes in blood flow and vascular resistance in the splanchnic viscera.[51] Blood flows were measured using the radiolabelled microsphere method. Nitrous oxide, when substituted for nitrogen in the breathing mixture, caused increased vascular resistance in the kidneys, small bowel, and spleen, and decreased blood flow in the kidneys, small bowel, spleen, and liver. Cardiac output decreased in response to nitrous oxide and the cerebral blood flow increased subsequent to cerebral vasodilatation. The increase in vascular resistance and the decrease in blood flow to the splanchnic viscera are consistent with the increase in sympathetic nerve activity seen in the splanchnic nerve of cats, and suggests that the effects of N_2O in the splanchnic viscera can be attributed to an action of sympathetic nerves. (This mechanism does not, of course, explain the actions of N_2O on the cerebral circulation, and serves to emphasise the diverse actions of anaesthetic drugs on various peripheral vascular circulations.)

Although both halothane and isoflurane produce arterial hypotension in humans and animals, the mechanism(s) of this effect differ considerably. Halothane decreases blood pressure primarily by decreasing cardiac output,[30 42] whereas isoflurane acts primarily as a periopheral vasodilator.[31 42] We reasoned that the peripheral vascular actions of isoflurane might result from its actions on the nitric oxide system, and tested this hypothesis by administering NMMA, in the presence of either halothane or isoflurane anaesthesia.[52] Systemic and regional haemodynamics were measured with the radioactively labelled microsphere technique.

Blockade of NO by L-NMMA produced greater increases in arterial blood pressure and systemic vascular resistance in animals anaesthetised with isoflurane, indicating that the NO pathway was more prominent under isoflurane anaesthesia (fig 9.4).

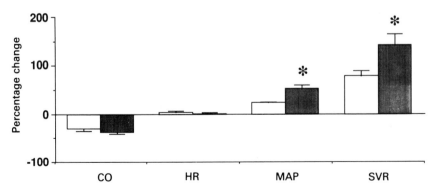

Fig 9.4 Comparison of changes in systemic haemodynamics induced by L-NMMA during 1 MAC of halothane anesthesia (open columns) versus 1 MAC of isoflurane anaesthesia (filled columns), in rats. (CO, cardiac output; HR, heart rate; MAP, mean arterial pressure; SVR, systemic vascular resistance. (Reproduced with permission from Greenblatt and Loeb.[52])

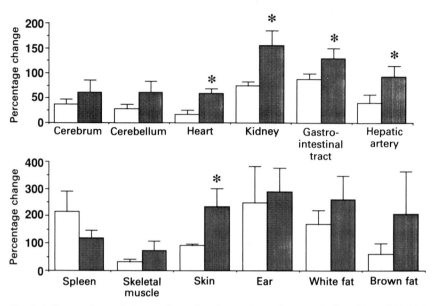

Fig 9.5 Comparison of changes in regional vascular resistances induced by L-NMMA during 1 MAC of halothane (open columns) versus 1 MAC of isoflurane (filled columns) in rats. (Reproduced with permission from Greenblatt and Loeb.[52])

Similarly, blockade of the NO system produced greater increases in vascular resistance in the heart, kidneys, gastrointestinal tract, hepatic artery, and skin in those receiving isoflurane anaesthesia (fig 9.5).

These results provide evidence that the NO pathway acts during both halothane and isoflurane anaesthesia to produce vasodilatation, but the system is much more active during isoflurane anaesthesia and this mechanism contributes at least in part to the vasodilatation that is observed during isoflurane anaesthesia.

Together, these results for nitrous oxide (sympathetic activation and vasoconstriction in the splanchnic viscera) and for isoflurane (activation of nitric oxide and peripheral vasodilatation) indicate that the anaesthetic drugs act on at least some of the known peripheral circulatory control mechanisms to produce their effects on organ blood flows and vascular resistances. They do not, however, imply that the mechanisms described here are the only mechanisms that may be active during anaesthesia. For example, peripheral vasoconstriction may occur during hypovolaemia under anaesthesia,[42] and presumably other remote or local factors may predominate under other circumstances. The results with the inhalational anaesthetic drugs illustrate, however, that an understanding of microcirculatory control mechanisms, combined with an understanding of the actions of the anaesthetic drugs, allows reasonable assumptions to be made about the mechanisms that may explain the peripheral circulatory actions of the anaesthetic drugs.

1 Frink EJ, Morgan SE, Coetzee A, Conzen PF, Brown BR. The effects of sevoflurane, halothane, enflurane, and isoflurane on hepatic blood flow and oxygenation in chronically instrumented greyhound dogs. *Anesthesiology* 1992; **76**: 85–90.
2 Nordstrom G, Winso O, Biber B, Hasselgren PO. Influence of pentobarbital and chloralose on metabolic and hemodynamic changes in liver ischemia. *Ann Surg* 1990; **212**: 23–9.
3 Nagano K, Gelman S, Parks D, Bradley EL. Hepatic circulation and oxygen supply-uptake relationships after hepatic ischemic insult during anesthesia with volatile anesthetics and fentanyl in miniature pigs. *Anesth Analg* 1990; **70**: 53–62.
4 Holder DS. Effects of urethane, alphaxolone/alphadolone, or halothane with or without neuromuscular blockade on survival during repeated episodes of global cerebral ischemia in the rat. *Lab Anim* 1992; **26**: 107–13.
5 Rasool N, Faroqui M, Rubenstein EH. Lidocaine accelerates neuroelectrical recovery after incomplete global ischemia in rabbits. *Stroke* 1990; **21**: 929–35.
6 Helfaer MA, Kirsch JR, Traystman RJ. Anesthetic modulation of cerebral hemodynamic and evoked responses to transient middle cerebral artery occlusion in cats. *Stroke* 1990; **21**: 795–800.
7 Sano T, Patel PM, Drummond JC, Cole DJ. A comparison of the cerebral protective effects of etomidate, thiopental, and isoflurane in a model of forebrain ischemia in the rat. *Anesth Analg* 1993; **76**: 990–7.
8 Longnecker DE, Sturgill BC. Influence of anesthetic agent on survival following hemorrhage. *Anesthesiology* 1976; **45**: 516–21.
9 Shibata K, Yamamoto Y, Murakami S. Effects of epidural anesthesia on cardiovascular response and survival in experimental hemorrhagic shock in dogs. *Anesthesiology* 1989; **71**: 953–9.
10 LaRocco MT, Rodriguez LF, Chen CY, *et al.* Reevaluation of the linkage between acute hemorrhagic shock and bacterial translocation in the rat. *Circ Shock* 1993; **40**: 212–20.
11 VanderLinden P, Gilbart E, Engleman E, deRood M, Vincent JL. Adrenergic support during anesthesia in experimental endotoxin shock: norepinephrine versus dobutamine. *Acta Anaesthesiol Scand* 1991; **35**: 134–40.
12 VanderLinden P, Gilbart E, Engelman E, Schmartz D, deRood M, Vincent JL. Comparison of halothane, isoflurane, alfentanil, and ketamine in experimental septic shock. *Anesth Analg* 1990; **70**: 608–17.
13 Schaefer CF, Brackett DJ, Tompkins P, Wilson MF. Choice of anesthetic alters the circulatory shock pattern as gauge by conscious rat endotoxemia. *Acta Anaesthesiol Scand* 1987; **31**: 550–6.
14 Bavister PH, Longnecker DE. Influence of anaesthetic agents on the survival of rats following acute ischaemia of the bowel. *Br J Anaesth* 1979; **51**: 921–5.
15 Lundgren O, Haglund U. The pathophysiology of the intestinal countercurrent exchanger. *Life Sci* 1978; **23**: 1411–22.
16 Glenny RW, Robertson HT, Yamashiro S, Bassingthwaighte JB. Applications of fractal analysis to physiology. *J Appl Physiol* 1991; **70**: 2351–67.
17 Faraci FM, Heistad DD. Regulation of large cerebral arteries and cerebral microvascular pressure. *Circ Res* 1990; **66**: 8–17.
18 Marcus ML, Chilian WM, Kanatsuka H, Dellsperger KC, Eastham CL, Lamping KG. Understanding the coronary circulation through studies at the microvascular level. *Circulation* 1990; **82**: 1–7.
19 Iadecola C. Regulation of the cerebral microcirculation during neural activity: is nitric oxide the missing link? *Trends Neurol Sci* 1993; **16**: 206–14.
20 Hainsworth R. The importance of vascular capacitance in cardiovascular control. *News Physiol Sci* 1990; **5**: 250–4.
21 Nelson DP, King CE, Dodd SL, Schumacker PT, Cain SM. Systemic and intestinal limits of O_2 extraction in the dog. *J Appl Physiol* 1987; **63**: 387–94.
22 Piiper J, Pendergast DR, Marconi C, Meyer M, Heisler N, Cerretelli P. Blood flow distribution in dog gastrocnemius muscle at rest and during stimulation. *J Appl Physiol* 1985; **586**: 2068–74.

23 Carmines PK, Fleming JT. Control of the renal microvasculature by vasoactive peptides. *FASEB J* 1990; **4**: 3300–9.

24 Vanlersberghe C, Lauwers MH, Camu F. Prostaglandin synthetase inhibitor treatment and the regulatory role of prostaglandins on organ perfusion. *Acta Anesthesiol Belg* 1992; **43**: 211–25.

25 Furchgott RF. The role of endothelium in the responses of vascular smooth muscle to drugs. *Ann Rev Pharm Toxicol* 1984; **24**: 175–97.

26 Furchgott RF, Zawadzki JV. The obligatory role of endothelial cells in the relaxation of arterial smooth muscle by acetylcholine. *Nature* 1980; **288**: 373–6.

27 Lowenstein CJ, Dinerman JL, Snyder SH. Nitric oxide: a physiologic messenger. *Ann Intern Med* 1994; **120**: 227–37.

28 Greenblatt EP, Loeb AL, Longnecker DE. Marked regional heterogeneity in the magnitude of EDRF/NO-mediated vascular tone in awake rats. *J Cardiovasc Pharmacol* 1993; **21**: 235–40.

29 Longnecker DE. Effects of general anesthetics on the microcirculation. *Microcirculation Endothelium Lymphatics* 1984; **1**: 129–50.

30 Eger EI II, Smith NT, Cullen DJ, Cullen BF, Gregory GA. A comparison of the cardiovascular effects of halothane, fluroxene, ether, and cyclopropane in man: a resumé. *Anesthesiology* 1971; **34**: 25–41.

31 Stevens WC, Cromwell TH, Halsey MJ, Eger EI II, Shakespeare TF, Bahlman SH. The cardiovascular effects of a new inhalation anesthetic, Forane, in human volunteers at arterial carbon dioxide tension. *Anesthesiology* 1971; **35**: 8–16.

32 Conzen PF, Habazettl H, Vollmar B, Christ M, Baier H, Peter K. Coronary microcirculation during halothane, enflurane, isoflurane, and adenosine in dogs. *Anesthesiology* 1992; **76**: 261–70.

33 Debaene B, Goldfarb G, Braillon A, Jolis P, Lebrec D. Effects of ketamine, halothane, enflurane, and isoflurane on systemic and splanchnic hemodynamics in normovolemic and hypovolemic cirrhotic rats. *Anesthesiology* 1990; **73**: 118–24.

34 Vollmar B, Conzen PF, Kerner T, *et al*. Blood flow and tissue oxygen pressures of liver and pancreas in rats: Effects of volatile anesthetics and of hemorrhage. *Anesth Analg* 1992; **75**: 421–30.

35 Jacob L, Boudaoud S, Payen D, *et al*. Isoflurane, and not halothane, increases mesenteric blood flow supplying esophageal ileocoloplasty. *Anesthesiology* 1991; **74**: 699–704.

36 Hansen TD, Warner DS, Todd MM, Vust LJ, Trawick DC. Distribution of cerebral blood flow during halothane versus isoflurane anesthesia in rats. *Anesthesiology* 1988; **69**: 332–37.

37 Fagrell B, Fronek A, Intaglietta M. A microscope-television system for studying flow velocity in human skin capillaries. *Am J Physiol* 1977; **233**: H318–21.

38 Leon A, Boczkowski J, Dureuil B, Vicaut E, Aubier M, Desmonts J. Diaphragmatic microcirculation during halothane and isoflurane exposure in pentobarbital-anesthetized rats. *J Appl Physiol* 1992; **73**: 1614–18.

39 Longnecker DE, McCoy S, Drucker WR. Anesthetic influence on response to hemorrhage in rats. *Circ Shock* 1979; **6**: 55–60.

40 Worek FS, Blumel G, Zeravik J, Zimmermann GJ, Pfeiffer UJ. Comparison of ketamine and pentobarbital anesthesia with the conscious state in a porcine model of *Pseudomonas aeruginosa* septicemia. *Acta Anaesthesiol Scand* 1988; **32**: 509–15.

41 Tverskoy M, Gelman S, Fowler KC, Bradley EL. Effects of anaesthesia induction drugs on circulation in denervated intestinal loop preparation. *Can Anaesth Soc J* 1985; **32**: 516–24.

42 Seyde WC, Longnecker DE. Anesthetic influences on regional hemodynamics in normal and hemorrhaged rats. *Anesthesiology* 1984; **61**: 686–98.

43 Miller ED, Kistner JR, Epstein RM. Whole-body distribution of radioactively labelled microspheres in the rat during anesthesia with halothane, enflurane, or ketamine. *Anesthesiology* 1980; **52**: 296–302.

44 Idvall J. Influence of ketamine anesthesia on cardiac output and tissue perfusion in rats subjected to hemorrhage. *Anesthesiology* 1981; **55**: 297–304.

45 Gaab MR, Poch B, Heller V. Oxygen tension, oxygen metabolism, and microcirculation in vasogenic brain edema. *Adv Neurol* 1990; **52**: 247–56.

46 Dempsey RJ, Roy MW, Meyer KL, Donaldson DL. Indomethacin-mediated improvement following middle cerebral artery occlusion in cats. *J Neurosurg* 1985; **62**: 874–81.

270

47 Longnecker DE, Ross DC, Silver IA. Anesthetic influence on arteriolar diameters and tissue oxygen tension in hemorrhaged rats. *Anesthesiology* 1982; **57**: 177–82.
48 Longnecker DE, Miller FN, Harris PD. Small artery and vein response to ketamine HCl in the bat wing. *Anesth Analg* 1974; **53**: 64–8.
49 Longnecker DE, Harris PD. Dilation of small arteries and veins in the bat during halothane anesthesia. *Anesthesiology* 1972; **37**: 423–9.
50 Fukunaga AF, Epstein RM. Sympathetic excitation during nitrous oxide–halothane anesthesia in the cat. *Anesthesiology* 1973; **39**: 23–36.
51 Seyde WC, Ellis JE, Longnecker DE. The addition of nitrous oxide to halothane decreases renal and splanchnic flow and increases cerebral blood flow in rats. *Br J Anaesth* 1986; **58**: 63–8.
52 Greenblatt EP, Loeb AL, Longnecker E. Endothelium-dependent circulatory control – a mechanism for the differing peripheral vascular effects of isoflurane versus halothane. *Anesthesiology* 1992; **77**: 1178–85.

10: Anaesthesia and the cardiovascular system

ANDREAS HOEFT, WOLFGANG BUHRE

The objective of anaesthesia is to provide analgesia, unconsciousness, suppression of reflex responses to surgical stimuli, and muscular relaxation, if required. In general this goal is achieved by administering a combination of various agents, such as volatile and intravenous anaesthetic drugs, opiates, benzodiazepines, and muscle relaxants. In principle all drugs used in anaesthetic practice affect the performance of the cardiovascular system, either by direct effects on the heart and the vessels or indirectly by altering neurohumoral control of the circulation. As a result of the interaction of direct and indirect effects, it is very difficult to obtain a clear pharmacodynamic profile of an anaesthetic drug under conditions in vivo. As most anaesthetic drugs alter both vascular tone and myocardial performance it is difficult to distinguish whether a decrease in blood pressure and/or stroke volume is the result of changes in myocardial loading conditions or of direct inotropic effects of the agent. In vitro studies with isolated heart and vessel preparations, in which loading conditions can be carefully controlled, are therefore a rational approach to investigate anaesthetic agents. It has been shown by studies of this type that most of the volatile and many of the intravenous anaesthetic agents exert direct negative inotropic effects on the myocardium and some of them cause systemic vasodilatation. The isolated models are, however, relatively artificial and the experimental results are not always in accordance with clinical observations. For instance, opiates as well as benzodiazepines are thought to be more or less haemodynamically inert, that is, they elicit no negative inotropic effects on the myocardium or cause no significant vasodilatation.[1-5] In some patients, however, induction of anaesthesia with these drugs leads to dramatic hypotension, even if small doses are given.[6] Conversely, patients with definitely compromised myocardial function and documented low ejection fractions often tolerate anaesthetic agents with known negative inotropic properties, such as halothane, surprisingly well. Thus, clinical experience suggests that, at least in some patients, centrally mediated indirect effects of anaesthesia, in particular the depression of the sympathetic drive, may be much more important than direct effects of the anaesthetic agents on the myocardium or vascular smooth muscle.

In fact, the interaction of anaesthesia with central control mechanisms of the circulation seems to be an intrinsic dilemma of anaesthesia. Even if an ideal anaesthetic drug with no adverse effects on the myocardium or vascular smooth muscle could be found, it is questionable whether the centrally mediated effects of anaesthesia on autonomic control of the cardiovascular system can be separated from the desired goals of anaesthesia, that is, unconsciousness, muscle relaxation, and suppression of reflex responses to surgical stimuli. Basically (with the possible exception of ketamine), centrally mediated depression of cardiovascular performance is more or less common to all anaesthetic techniques, regardless of whether volatile anaesthetic agents, opiates, or other intravenous anaesthetic agents are employed.

Effects of anaesthesia on the sympathetic system

Cardiovascular homoeostasis is in large part controlled by the autonomic nervous system, which controls heart rate, myocardial contractility, vascular resistance, and the tone of the venous capacitance vessels. Anaesthesia alters basic sympathetic tone as well as the sympathetic response to painful (surgical) stimuli. It is essential for the anaesthetist to be familiar with the interaction of anaesthesia with the autonomic nervous system to evaluate and manage haemodynamic disorders during anaesthesia. Current knowledge about the interaction of anaesthetic agents with the sympathetic nervous system is based mainly on studies of plasma catecholamine levels and assessment of baroreceptor reflex response before and during anaesthesia. More recently, direct recordings of sympathetic nerve activity in patients have been employed to investigate the effects of anaesthetic agents on the sympathetic system.[7-12]

Sympathetic nerve activity

Measurements of sympathetic nerve activity can be recorded from the peroneal nerve. A very thin epoxy coated needle (0·2 mm) with a small tip (5 μm) is placed within the peroneal nerve below the bony prominence at the head of the fibula. Using a reference electrode and a special set up with a differential preamplifier and a bandpass filter, identification of characteristic muscle sympathetic bursts is possible (fig 10.1). Sympathetic activity is quantified by the number of bursts per minute, number of bursts per 100 cardiac cycles, or as total activity calculated from the product of bursts per minute and mean burst amplitude. Efferent bursts frequently occur in pulse synchronous groupings and are often phase locked to late expiration and early inspiration efforts.[7] This pattern is thought to be caused by baroreceptor modulation.[10]

Effects of induction of anaesthesia on sympathetic nerve activity

There are a number of reports on the effects of induction of anaesthesia,

273

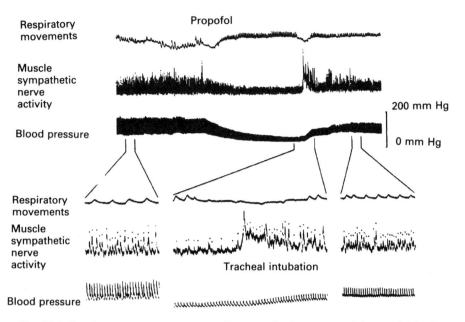

Fig 10.1 Respiratory movements, muscle sympathetic nerve activity, and blood pressure in a patient undergoing induction of anaesthesia with propofol. The upper panel shows condensed recordings; the lower panel depicts selected periods in an enlarged time scale. Induction of anaesthesia with propofol decreases muscle sympathetic nerve activity and blood pressure (upper panel). Tracheal intubation causes a dramatic increase in muscle sympathetic nerve activity. (Modified from Sellgren et al.[11])

tracheal intubation, and surgical stimulation on muscle sympathetic nerve activity. Most of the work has been performed by the groups of Ebert et al and Sellgren et al.[7 9–12] Induction of anaesthesia decreased sympathetic outflow as evaluated by direct recordings of sympathetic nerve activity (fig 10.2). Propofol and thiopentone had the most pronounced effects,[7 10 11] whereas etomidate preserved muscle sympathetic nerve activity[7] (fig 10.2). Moreover, it has been observed that the decrease of muscle sympathetic nerve activity after propofol is more pronounced in unpremedicated patients than in those who received preoperative benzodiazepines.[7 11] Hence, baseline sympathetic drive seems to be a significant factor for the impact of anaesthesia on sympathetic outflow and the resulting haemodynamics. These findings are in line with the clinical observation that propofol is occasionally associated with severe hypotension, in particular in patients who presumably are under an increased sympathetic drive in the conscious state, that is, patients with borderline hypovolaemia or compensated myocardial failure. Induction of anaesthesia with methohexitone has also been reported to decrease muscle sympathetic nervous activity.[10] Thus, it seems to be justified

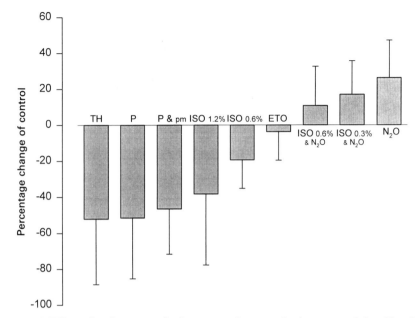

Fig 10.2 Effect of various anaesthetics on muscle sympathetic nerve activity. Muscle sympathetic nerve activity is given as bursts per minute and percentage change of baseline values. Induction of anaesthesia with thiopentone (TH, 4 mg/kg), propofol (P, 2·5 mg/kg), and propofol following premedication with diazepam (P & pm, 2–2·5 mg/kg and 0·25 mg/kg, respectively), is associated with a significant decrease in muscle sympathetic nerve activity, whereas etomidate (ETO, 0·3 mg/kg) exerts only minor effects. Isoflurane alone (ISO 1·2 vol% and ISO 0·6 vol%) also inhibit muscle sympathetic nerve activity. In contrast, nitrous oxide (N_2O, 70%) causes sympathetic hyperactivity, which is counterbalanced by combination with isoflurane (ISO 0·6 vol% and N_2O 70%, ISO 0·3 vol% and N_2O 70%). (Data from Ebert et al[7 12] and Sellgren et al.[10])

that etomidate is considered by most clinicians as the induction anaesthetic drug of choice for patients with compromised cardiovascular performance and compensatory increased sympathetic drive.

Laryngoscopy as well as surgical stimulation are associated with an immediate and often dramatic increase of sympathetic activity (fig 10.1). Sellgren reported that, under these conditions, in some patients the pulse synchronous rhythmicity is lost and a more continuous activity pattern is observed.[11] No systematic studies are available yet about how this sympathetic response can be influenced by specific anaesthetics or adjuvant interventions, for instance β blockade or α_2 agonists.

Effects of maintenance of anaesthesia on sympathetic nerve activity

As maintenance of anaesthesia is inevitably associated with suppression of cerebral activity, it can be anticipated that all maintenance anaesthetic agents that non-specifically inhibit nervous activity will also decrease sympathetic outflow. This has been demonstrated for those general anaesthetic agents for which data are available[10][11] (propofol, isoflurane, halothane) (fig 10.2). Fentanyl (3 μg/kg) given before induction of anaesthesia, to a spontaneously breathing patient, induces a temporary slight increase in muscle sympathetic nerve activity,[10] possibly because of associated hypercapnia. Data for sufentanil or alfentanil are currently not available.

Nitrous oxide seems to be an exception. Ebert and Kampine[9] observed in healthy volunteers a progressive large increase in muscle sympathetic nerve activity when low doses of nitrous oxide (25% and 40%) were inhaled via a facemask. These changes were associated with a significant increase in blood pressure. Sellgren et al[11] also found that sympathetic nervous activity is enhanced by nitrous oxide in comparison with the conscious state. In addition, he demonstrated that the combination of isoflurane and nitrous oxide increases sympathetic nervous activity compared with isoflurane alone (fig 10.2). In this study total sympathetic nerve activity was 45% of baseline when 1·2% isoflurane was administered as the sole anaesthetic agent.

Plasma catecholamines

Several studies have measured plasma catecholamine levels during anaesthesia.[13] Noradrenaline is believed to correlate more or less with overall sympathetic nervous activity,[14] whereas adrenaline plasma levels mainly result from adrenal release.[15] Interpretation of circulating plasma catecholamine levels is, however, hampered by the fact that measurable circulating noradrenaline is the result of an "overspill" phenomenon at the nerve ending, that is, the net effect of release and reuptake mechanisms.[15][16] Furthermore, in earlier studies determinations of plasma catecholamine levels have to be interpreted cautiously from the methodological point of view.[15] Baseline levels of adrenaline and noradrenaline were barely in the range of the methodological sensitivity. In spite of these objections, however, changes in plasma noradrenaline levels seem to correlate well with muscle sympathetic nerve activity in healthy volunteers.[17]

In accordance with muscle nerve sympathetic activity, induction of anaesthesia is associated with a decrease in plasma catecholamine levels. This has been shown for various anaesthetic agents.[18] A complete protection against noxious stimuli is, however, difficult to achieve, even with very high doses of opiates. Philbin et al measured plasma catecholamine levels in the conscious state, after intubation, and during sternotomy in patients undergoing coronary artery bypass surgery.[19] Neither high doses of fentanyl (50 μg/kg or 100 μg/kg) nor high doses of sufentanil (10, 20, or 30 μg/kg) prevented increases in plasma catecholamines during sternotomy. This study confirmed earlier results of Sonntag et al[20] who showed that neither high doses of

276

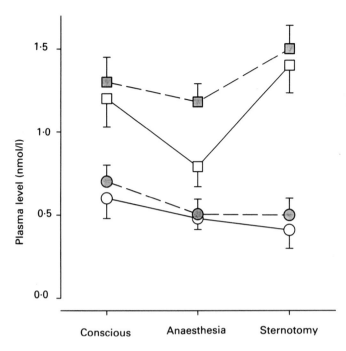

Fig 10.3 Plasma levels of adrenaline and noradrenaline in patients undergoing cardiac surgery with sufentanil anaesthesia. Neither high dose sufentanil (10 μg/kg + 0·10 μg/kg per min) norsufentanil–nitrous oxide anaesthesia (1 μg/kg + 0·015 μg/kg per min in 30% O_2/70% N_2O) are able to prevent the noradrenaline response to surgical stimulation (sternotomy). No additional hypnotics were used in this study. ▣ Noradrenaline : sufentanil–nitrous oxide; □ noradrenaline : high dose sufentanil; ◍ adrenaline : sufentanil–nitrous oxide; ○ adrenaline : high dose sufentanil. (Data from Sonntag et al.[20])

sufentanil (10 μg/kg and 0·15 μg/kg per min) nor moderate doses of sufentanil (1 μg/kg and 0·015 μg/kg per min) in combination with nitrous oxide (30% O_2/70% N_2O) prevented a response to surgical stimuli in terms of blood pressure increase and noradrenaline plasma levels (fig 10.3). Interestingly, in spite of significant increases in circulating noradrenaline levels, no concomitant change in adrenaline plasma levels was observed.[20] Similar results were obtained in a more recent study performed by Liem et al.[21] In patients anaesthetised with sufentanil and midazolam, a significant increase in noradrenaline levels occurred during sternotomy whereas adrenaline levels remained unchanged. In the same study thoracic epidural anaesthesia in combination with light general anaesthesia (nitrous oxide and midazolam) was investigated. In fact, thoracic epidural analgesia was able to block the haemodynamic and humoral (norepinephrine) response to sternotomy. Moreover, compared with general anaesthesia, lower levels of

277

norepinephrine and epinephrine were observed during bypass. Possibly, thoracic epidural anaesthesia is an appropriate measure to block the sympathetic response to surgical stimuli.[21]

In summary, induction and maintenance of anaesthesia with volatile and intravenous anaesthetic agents are associated with sympathetic depression and decreased catecholamine levels. A rapid increase in inspired isoflurane or desflurane to high concentrations has, however, been shown to cause sympathetic hyperactivity, possibly because of a response initiated by airway irritation.[22 23]

Baroreceptor reflex

Baroreflex control of the heart can be studied in conscious and anaesthetised subjects by intravenous administration of vasoactive drugs, such as phenylephrine (pressor test) and sodium nitroprusside (depressor test). A bolus of phenylephrine (about 150 μg) is administered preferably via a central venous catheter. As a result of the baroreceptor reflex, the increase in blood pressure results in a reflex slowing of heart rate. Baroreceptor sensitivity is defined as the slope of arterial pressure change divided by the R–R interval change in the ECG. In a similar way baroreceptor reflex, following an abrupt decline in blood pressure, can be determined. Most commonly, boluses of sodium nitroprusside (100 μg) are used. Pressor and depressor tests are affected to a different degree by anaesthetic agents.[24]

The effect of propofol, etomidate, and thiopentone on baroreceptor reflex has recently been studied by Ebert et al[7] in healthy volunteers. They found that etomidate had the least effect on the depressor test of baroreceptor reflux function, followed by propofol and thiopentone (fig 10.4). Thiopentone almost abolished baroreceptor response when given in equipotent doses. Methohexitone also inhibits the baroreceptor reflex in the experimental animal.[25]

Inhalational anaesthetic agents have been shown to depress the arterial baroreceptor reflex in both humans and animals. A number of studies have been published which describe the alteration of baroreceptor reflexes by halothane, halothane with nitrous oxide, enflurane, enflurane with nitrous oxide, and isoflurane.[24 26] The depression of the baroreflex response caused by isoflurane is less pronounced than that caused by equipotent doses of halothane or enflurane.[24] The effect of desflurane seems to be similar to that of isoflurane.

Effects of anaesthesia on the heart

The effect of anaesthetic agents on the myocardium has been the subject of numerous experimental and clinical investigations. As outlined above, it is

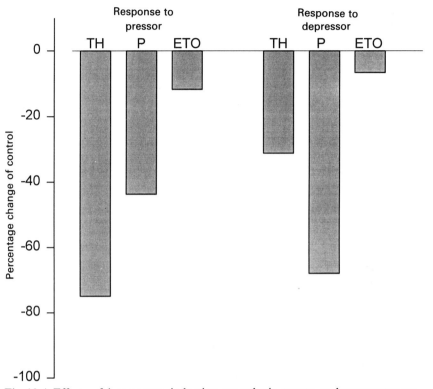

Fig 10.4 Effects of intravenous induction anaesthetic agents on baroreceptor response. Baroreceptor response to pressor (phenylephrine 150 μg) and depressor
stimulus (sodium nitroprusside 100 μg) is assessed by cardiac baroslopes, that is, the
ratios of R–R interval change to systolic blood pressure changes. Induction of
anaesthesia with thiopentone (TP, 4 mg/kg) and propofol (P, 2·5 mg/kg) significantly
inhibits baroreceptor response whereas etomidate (ETO, 0·3 mg/kg) preserves the
activity of the baroreceptor reflex. (Data from Ebert et al.[7][12])

very difficult to differentiate, under in vivo conditions, direct myocardial
effects of anaesthetic agents, direct vascular effects, and indirect effects
mediated via the autonomic nervous system. A reasonable approach is to
investigate the influence of anaesthetic agents on myocardial contractility in
isolated in vitro models, such as cultured myocytes, papillary muscles, or
isolated working heart preparations. Preload and afterload can be very well
controlled in these preparations, and any interference with sympathetic or
parasympathetic innervation is avoided. For the same reasons it is, however,
difficult to extrapolate from results obtained from in vitro models to the
clinical situation. Basically, the more isolated a preparation the more artificial
is the functional environment for the myocardium (or myocytes). For
instance, isolated working heart preparations are deprived of any basic

sympathetic drive, and coronary oxygen supply is often limited because of asanguineous crystalloid perfusion. Papillary muscle preparations are devoid of blood supply, and the experiments are often performed at room temperature to decrease metabolic rate and to facilitate sufficient oxygen supply by diffusion. Cultured myocytes or skinned muscle fibres are obviously artificial models, far from clinical reality.

Myocardial contractility

Nevertheless, isolated models can be useful to identify the pure effect of substances on the myocardium itself. Several induction agents have been shown to elicit negative inotropic properties in papillary muscle experiments or isolated working heart models.[27–39] Most recently Stowe and co-workers[32] investigated the effects of etomidate, ketamine, midazolam, propofol, and thiopentone (thiopental) on cardiac function and metabolism in an isolated guinea pig heart model at equimolar doses. In principle all induction agents (including midazolam and etomidate) produce a dose dependent decrease in myocardial contractility (fig 10.5). On a molar basis, propofol (less so midazolam and etomidate) depresses cardiac function moderately more than thiopentone and ketamine. The peak concentrations required for induction of anaesthesia are, however, quite different from one agent to another. Peak plasma concentrations during induction of anaesthesia have been reported to be about 0·5 μmol/l for midazolam, 3 μmol/l for etomidate, 60 μmol/l for ketamine, 50 μmol/l for propofol, and 100 μmol/l for thiopentone (fig 10.5). Thus, under clinical conditions midazolam and etomidate are basically not cardiodepressive, whereas thiopentone and propofol exert significant direct negative inotropic action.

In contrast to volatile anaesthetic agents, which have been extensively investigated,[34] only little is known about the molecular mechanisms responsible for the direct negative inotropic properties of intravenous induction agents. Initial controversial results about the direct action of ketamine on the myocardium prompted some more detailed investigations. Ketamine has been shown to exert myocardial depression in intact dogs, isolated dog heart preparations, and in isolated rabbit hearts.[35 36] Riou et al[35] have demonstrated that ketamine has a dual opposing effect on the myocardium:

1 A positive inotropic effect associated with increased Ca^{2+} influx
2 A negative inotropic effect possibly because of an impaired function of the sarcoplasmic reticulum.[37]

In an isolated ferret ventricular papillary muscle model the positive inotropic effects of ketamine could be blocked by bupranolol, indicating involvement of β receptors.[36] Moreover, depletion of noradrenaline stores by reserpine also abolished the positive inotropic action of ketamine. It was concluded that inhibition of neuronal catecholamine uptake is the predomi-

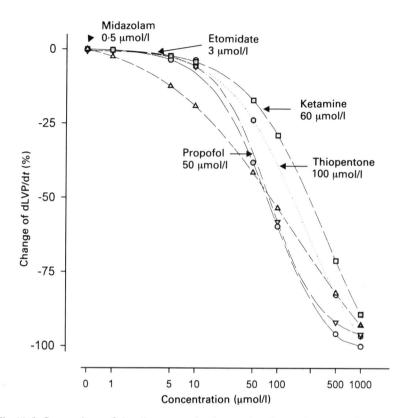

Fig 10.5 Comparison of the direct negative inotropic effects of common intravenous induction anaesthetic agents in an isolated working heart model. The effects of etomidate, ketamine, midazolam, propofol, and thiopentone were studied in an isolated working heart model. Percentage change in the peak positive derivative of left ventricular pressure ($dLVP/dt_{max}$) are shown. A wide range of concentrations from 0·5 to 1000 μmol/l was investigated. All induction anaesthetic agents (including midazolam and etomidate) produce a dose dependent depression of myocardial contractility. However, in doses, which are equivalent to peak plasma levels during induction of anaesthesia (marked by arrows for each anaesthetic agent), propofol (60 μmol/l peak plasma concentration corresponds to an induction dose of 2·5 mg/kg) and thiopentone (100 μmol/l peak plasma concentration ≅ 3·5 mg/kg) appear to depress cardiac function more than ketamine (60 μm ≅ 2 mg/kg), etomidate (3 μmol/l ≅ 0·3 mg/kg), and midazolam (0·5 μm ≅ 0·2 mg/kg). -- ▲--, Midazolam; ·-◉-·, etomidate; ·-▣-·, ketamine; ··· ▽ ··, propofol; ··· ◉ ···, thiopentone. (Data from Stowe et al.[32])

nant mechanism of ketamine's positive inotropic effect.[36] The negative inotropic effect of ketamine was recently elucidated by Kongsayreepong et al[37] using measurements of intracellular Ca^{2+} transients with aequorin. Ketamine decreased intracellular calcium availability, which also occurred when the sarcoplasmic reticulum was blocked by ryanodine.

281

The influence of volatile anaesthetic agents on myocardial contractility has been extensively investigated in papillary muscle experiments and working heart models.[34] Myocardial contractility is decreased by all volatile anaesthetic agents in a dose dependent manner.[40-45] Isoflurane seems to be less negatively inotropic than enflurane and halothane[45] (fig 10.6). The cardio-depressive effect of volatile anaesthetic agents is caused by an alteration of calcium transients involving sarcolemmal calcium exchange processes as well as uptake and release of calcium by the sarcoplasmic reticulum.[44] It has been suggested that halothane and isoflurane depress cardiac function by different mechanisms.[44] Nitrous oxide has been demonstrated in papillary muscle experiments to exert moderately negative inotropic effects (5–15% depression of contractility).[46]

The effects of opiates on cardiac muscle have been investigated in only a few isolated papillary muscle experiments. Negative inotropic action has been demonstrated for morphine, pethidine (meperidine), fentanyl, and alfentanil. These effects occurred, however, at concentrations one hundred to several thousand times above the clinically used doses.[5 47]

Assessment of myocardial contractility in intact animals or in patients

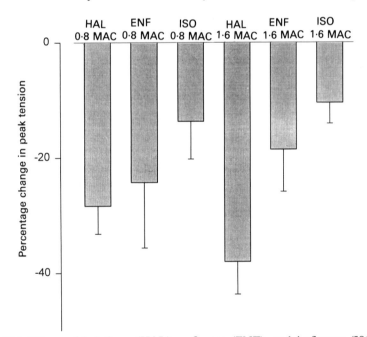

Fig 10.6 Effects of halothane (HAL), enflurane (ENF), and isoflurane (ISO) on myocardial contractility in isolated papillary muscles. All volatile anaesthetic agents exert a dose dependent negative inotropic effect shown as percentage depression of peak developed tension. Halothane was found to be significantly more depressant than isoflurane at 1·6 MAC, wheras enflurane caused intermediate depression. (Data from Lynch and Frazer.[40])

requires considerable methodological efforts. The effect of anaesthesia on blood pressure, left ventricular pressure, stroke volume index, and stroke work, as well as on maximal velocity of rise in left ventricular pressure (dP/dt_{max}) are considered unreliable measures of myocardial contractility. The essential question is whether an observed decline in blood pressure or stroke volume after application of an anaesthetic drug is the result of decreased contractility or merely of changes in loading conditions. Several contractility indices have been suggested in the literature. Currently, the "end systolic elastance" index described by Sagawa[48] is considered to be relatively load independent. End systolic elastance is determined from measurements of instantaneous pressure–volume loops during variation of preload or afterload. As already described by Frank in 1895[49] a decline in preload is associated with a decrease of stroke volume and blood pressure, a phenomenon which is well known as the "Frank–Starling" effect. Since then, Frank, who carried out studies on isolated frog hearts, was also the first to construct a curve through the end systolic pressure–volume relationship (fig 10.7). He named the resultant curve "*Unterstützungszuckungskurve*".* Almost a century later Sagawa conducted a series of experiments in an isolated dog working heart model in which he also investigated the end systolic pressure–volume relationship. He found that the end systolic pressure volume relationship ("*Unterstützungszuckungskurve*") is linear under a variety of afterload conditions. Sagawa proposed that the slope of the respective regression line through the end systolic pressure–volume points (end systolic elastance) is a load insensitive measure of myocardial contractility. The concept of the end systolic pressure–volume relationship has been used extensively in animal experiments. In intact animals, preload variation is usually accomplished by vena caval obstruction. Often the autonomic nervous system is pharmacologically blocked (for instance with propanolol 2 mg/kg, atropine methylnitrate 3 mg/kg, and hexamethonium 20 mg/kg) to exclude baroreceptor reflex interference with the measurements.[50] In animals left ventricular dimensions are most commonly measured by sonomicrometry.

The end systolic elastance concept has also been applied in various clinical studies.[51-54] In patients variation of loading conditions can be performed by bolus injections of glyceryl trinitrate (nitroglycerin) or phenylephrine.[51-54] Left ventricular volume measurements can be performed by echocardiography, preferably by the transoesophageal route.[51] Under clinical conditions it might be justified to substitute end systolic left ventricular pressure (which requires a left ventricular catheter tip manometer) by aortic peak systolic pressure.

---

* Literal translation of "*Unterstützungszuckungskurve*" is "support twitch curve." Frank had chosen this term for the auxotonic form of muscle contraction in analogy to muscle strip experiments, where a weight is attached to the muscle and supported in the relaxed position.

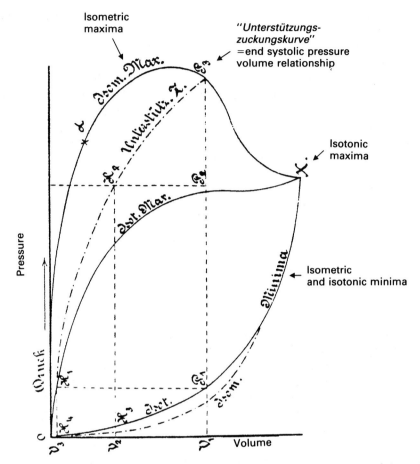

Fig 10.7 Original pressure–volume diagram from O Frank. The concept of the end systolic pressure–volume relationship was first described by O Frank in 1895.[49] The diagram demonstrates the end points of isometric contractions (isometric maxima), isotonic contractions (isotonic maxima), and contractions with normal ejection (*Unterstützungszuckungskurve* = end systolic pressure–volume relationship). Sagawa described in 1974 that the end systolic pressure–volume relationship is linear in the physiological range, and the slope of this relationship can be used as a load independent index of myocardial contractility. (Modified from Frank.[49])

An alternative approach for load independent assessment of myocardial contractility is the determination of preload recruitable stroke work.[55] Similar to end systolic elastance measurements, loading conditions are varied by appropriate pharmacological or mechanical interventions, and pressure–volume loops are constructed. In a second step, stroke work (the area under the pressure–volume loop) is plotted versus end diastolic dimensions of the left ventricle (end diastolic volume or segment length). The slopes of the respective regression lines have been suggested to be even less dependent on myocardial loading conditions than end systolic elastance index.[55-57]

Yet, there is a paucity of clinical studies in which myocardial effects of anaesthetic agents are characterised based on end systolic elastance or preload recruitable stroke work. A reason might be that transoesophageal echocardiography has only recently become available as a research tool in anaesthesia. A very interesting clinical study of this type has been performed by Mulier *et al*,[52] in which the haemodynamic effects of thiopentone and propofol were compared. In contrast to previous studies it could be demonstrated clearly in patients that propofol significantly decreases myocardial contractility and (in accordance with the in vitro results of Stowe *et al*[32]) in vivo is at least as negatively inotropic as thiopentone. The authors even suggest that the negative inotropic properties of propofol are more pronounced and more prolonged than those of equipotent doses of thiopentone.[52] The differences were, however, only marginal and barely statistically significant. It is questionable whether the observation of Mulier *et al*[52] is the result of direct negative inotropic effects of propofol alone. An alternative explanation could be a marked decrease in sympathetic outflow, which has been demonstrated during propofol anaesthesia[7] (case fig 10.2). As in other studies, the induction agent with the least negative inotropic effects was probably etomidate.

As expected from results in isolated models, volatile anaesthetic agents act as cardiodepressors in intact animals and patients as well.[50 51 55-58] Pagel *et al*[57] demonstrated, in chronically instrumented dogs with autonomic blockade, that isoflurane and desflurane produced less depression of myocardial contractility than halothane or enflurane. Without autonomic blockade, however, desflurane preserved mean arterial pressure and cardiac output to a greater degree than equipotent doses of isoflurane, especially at higher concentrations.[57] The authors concluded that desflurane has less depressant effect on autonomic activity than other volatile anaesthetic agents.[57] In fact, Ebert and Muzi[22] demonstrated sympathetic hyperactivity during desflurane anaesthesia in healthy volunteers, possibly as a result of airway irritation.

The in vivo effects of nitrous oxide are very complex. As outlined above, nitrous oxide increases sympathetic activity and in some patients increases blood pressure.[9 11 12] The weight of currently available evidence, however, demonstrates that nitrous oxide is a myocardial depressant[46] when used as a supplement during anaesthesia. Pagel *et al*[56] investigated the effects of nitrous oxide in chronically instrumented dogs in the presence of pharmacological blockade of the autonomic nervous system. Based on preload recruitable stroke work, myocardial contractility significantly decreased when nitrous oxide was added to a baseline anaesthesia with isoflurane or sufentanil (fig 10.8). The evidence for a myocardial depressant effect of nitrous oxide is strong in patients with compromised myocardial function, that is, in those patients in whom the cardiovascular properties of anaesthetic agents are clinically relevant. In summary, nitrous oxide has a weak direct myocardial

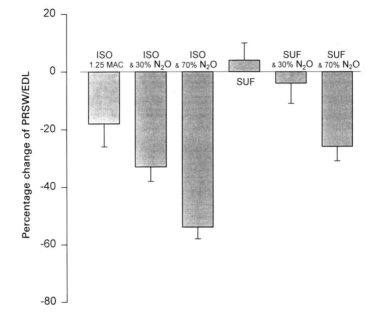

Fig 10.8 Influence of nitrous oxide (N_2O) on myocardial contractility in chronically instrumented dogs. Two sets of experiments were performed in chronically instrumented dogs with pharmacological blockade of the autonomic nervous system. Basic anaesthesia was performed with isoflurane (ISO 1·25 MAC) or sufentanil (SUF, 100–150 mg/kg per h). Myocardial contractility was evaluated by the relationship of preload recruitable stroke work (PRSW) to end diastolic length (EDL). The addition of nitrous oxide (N_2O 30% and N_2O 70%) results in a decrease in myocardial contractility in both groups. (Data from Pagel et al.[56])

depressant effect, which in intact animals and healthy patients may be counterbalanced by an intrinsic increase in sympathetic activity by nitrous oxide.[58]

Myocardial metabolism

The rate of myocardial oxygen and substrate turnover depends on the mechanical activity of the heart. Under aerobic conditions glucose, free fatty acids, and lactate are oxidised for energy production. Compared with oxygen, substrate availability is not critical in cases of limited coronary blood supply because the arteriocoronary venous extraction ratios for free fatty acids, lactate, and glucose are much smaller (40, 25, and 3%, respectively) than that of oxygen (70%). Glucose is converted to lactate under anaerobic conditions for energy production, and mainly intracellular glycogen is used as a glucose source.[59]

Measurement of myocardial blood flow and myocardial oxygen uptake

In animal experiments as well as in clinical research, measurements of myocardial blood flow are essential to investigate myocardial metabolism. Determinations of myocardial oxygen consumption are based on the Fick principle, that is, on the product of myocardial blood flow and arterio-coronary venous oxygen content difference. Various techniques have been developed for experimental coronary blood flow measurements, such as electromagnetic flowmeters, ultrasonic devices, microspheres, and miscellaneous tracer methodologies. Most of these methods cannot, however, be applied in humans because of their invasiveness.[60] Measurement of coronary blood flow in patients is most commonly performed by local coronary sinus thermodilution: a catheter is placed in the coronary sinus under fluoroscopic control deep into the great cardiac vein. A cold solution is infused continuously via the distal lumen and coronary sinus outflow is calculated from downstream measurements of coronary sinus blood temperature. Besides some methodological problems (in particular mixing of the indicator with the laminar blood flow in the coronary sinus), a basic disadvantage of this technique is that coronary sinus outflow is measured in absolute terms. Thus, only *intraindividual* relative changes of blood flow and oxygen consumption can be assessed with the coronary sinus thermodilution technique, because normalisation to blood flow per 100 g tissue is essential for *interindividual* comparison of myocardial blood flow and myocardial oxygen uptake. A more laborious method, but the only one currently available for clinical measurements of weight normalised blood flows, is the Kety–Schmidt technique[61] and their subsequent modifications.[62-66] An inert gas, usually argon, is inhaled during spontaneous breathing or controlled ventilation, and the transit time of the diffusible tracer through the myocardium is determined from arterial and coronary sinus blood samples. Based on the blood/tissue partition coefficient myocardial blood flow per 100 g tissue can be calculated. This method was used in a few studies in which the effects of anaesthesia on myocardial oxygen consumption and myocardial blood flow were investigated.[67-73]

Estimation of myocardial oxygen consumption

As outlined above, measurements of myocardial blood flow and myocardial oxygen consumption in patients are very cumbersome and can therefore be performed only for investigational purposes. An estimate of myocardial oxygen demand from haemodynamic parameters, for instance, for evaluation of myocardial oxygen demand during anaesthesia or (more important) during recovery from anaesthesia, would therefore be desirable. The major determinants of myocardial oxygen demand comprise the energy required for development and maintenance of systolic wall tension. As reliable measures of wall tension are difficult to obtain, several derived indices of myocardial oxygen demand have been suggested in the literature.[74] Intuitively, most

287

clinicians believe that both an increase in heart rate and an increase in blood pressure will increase myocardial oxygen demand. This belief forms the rationale for using the pressure rate product (PRP), which was first suggested by Rhode[75] and which is still widely used as an index of myocardial oxygen demand. In animals as well as in patients, however, only a poor correlation is found between pressure–rate product and myocardial oxygen uptake.[74 76] Similarly, the tension time index does not correlate well with measured myocardial oxygen uptake.[74 76] A clinically useful alternative is the pressure work index, which was first suggested by Rooke and Feigl.[77 78] In addition to blood pressure and heart rate this index requires only measurements of cardiac output, which is routinely performed in many critically ill patients. As with all other haemodynamic indices of myocardial oxygen demand species, however, specific differences exist between animals and humans. The empirical constants derived by Rooke and Feigl for dogs can therefore not be used for estimation of myocardial oxygen demand in humans.[74] A modification of the pressure work index was therefore developed by Hoeft et al[74] and validated based on human data from measurements of myocardial blood flow and myocardial oxygen uptake in patients using a modified Kety–Schmidt technique (fig 10.9). Currently the modified pressure work index seems to be the best alternative for clinical estimation of myocardial oxygen demand. This estimate seems to be applicable during the conscious state as well as during anaesthesia.[74 77]

Effects of anaesthetic agents on myocardial oxygen consumption

Theoretically, it could be possible that anaesthesia is associated with specific metabolic effects such as uncoupling of oxidative phosphorylation or uncoupling of myocardial energy turnover from myocardial haemodynamic performance. Myocardial oxygen demand (estimated by the modified pressure work index) and measured myocardial oxygen uptake are, however, not systematically different from the conscious state to that during anaesthesia.[74 77] Therefore, a specific metabolic effect of anaesthesia in terms of uncoupling myocardial energy conversion is very unlikely.

Under resting conditions myocardial oxygen uptake is approximately 10–11 ml/min per 100 g (figs 10.10, 10.11, and 10.12). As most anaesthetic agents are cardiodepressive either through their direct negative inotropic effects or indirectly through decreasing sympathetic drive, induction with virtually any anaesthetic leads to a decrease in arterial blood pressure and stroke volume index (figs 10.10, 10.11, and 10.12). Ketamine (without supplemental benzodiazepines) might be an exception (fig 10.10). Ketamine is known to cause sympathetic hyperactivity, and an increase in arterial blood pressure and heart rate is observed, whereas stroke volume is decreased (fig 10.10). In general a reflex increase in heart rate is seen with barbiturates, but only a slight increase with etomidate (fig 10.10). Heart rate, on the one hand, and arterial pressure and stroke volume, on the other, have opposing effects

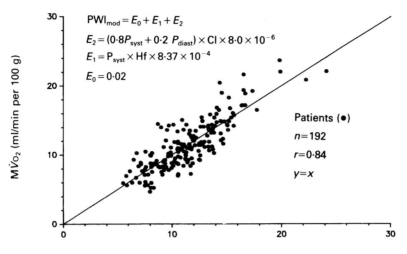

Fig 10.9 Correlation of myocardial oxygen uptake ($M\dot{V}O_2$) and modified pressure work index (PWI_{mod}) as an estimate of myocardial oxygen consumption. PWI_{mod} and $M\dot{V}O_2$ showed a correlation coefficient of 0·84 in patients undergoing coronary artery bypass surgery. Haemodynamic variables required for calculation of myocardial oxygen demand by PWI_{mod} are heart rate (Hf), arterial blood pressure (P_{syst}, P_{diast}), and cardiac index (CI: ml/m^2). The modified pressure work index is currently the most reliable index for estimation of myocardial oxygen demand from haemodynamic variables in patients. (Data from Hoeft et al.[74])

on myocardial oxygen demand. The net effect is, however, an increase in myocardial oxygen consumption with methohexitone and thiopentone, and more so with ketamine, whereas the haemodynamics and myocardial metabolic rate remain more or less unchanged with etomidate[79] (fig 10.10).

Induction of anaesthesia with volatile anaesthetic agents as well as with propofol leads to a decrease in blood pressure and stroke volume. As a result of inhibition of the baroreceptor reflex, however, less increase in heart rate is observed. Accordingly, myocardial oxygen consumption is decreased by almost one third, which is in contrast to classic induction agents (fig 10.11). Induction of anaesthesia with high doses of opiates is associated with a decrease in blood pressure, stroke volume, and a considerable reduction in myocardial oxygen consumption[80] (fig 10.12).

Intense surgical stimulation, such as a sternotomy, results in sympathetic activation that is difficult to block by anaesthesia. Blood pressure control is usually easier to achieve with volatile anaesthetic agents whereas it is difficult to maintain blood pressures in normal ranges even with high dose opiate anaesthesia (figs 10.11 and 10.12).[80] The poor control of blood pressure during opiate based anaesthesia can lead to a significant increase in myocardial oxygen consumption, up to twofold above baseline. Adjuvant measures

289

(such as vasodilators, β blockade, and other anithypertensive drugs) are therefore often employed during opiate based anaesthesia to maintain arterial pressure within its normal limits. In clinical practice it is also very common to supplement opiate based anaesthesia with volatile anaesthetic agents for blood pressure control.

High rates of myocardial oxygen consumption are also likely to occur during the recovery period. A dramatic sympathetic activation occurs during this phase, and observed noradrenaline levels by far exceed levels during

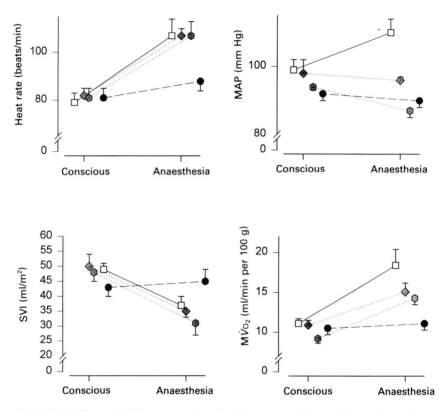

Fig 10.10 Influence of thiopentone, hexobarbitone, etomidate, and ketamine on heart rate, mean arterial blood pressure, stroke volume index, and myocardial oxygen consumption. Induction of anaesthesia with thiopentone (●) and methohexitone (◆) is associated with a decrease in blood pressure (MAP) and stroke volume index (SVI) whereas heart rate and myocardial oxygen consumption ($M\dot{V}O_2$) are increased. Ketamine (□) exerts the most pronounced effect on myocardial oxygen consumption because sympathetic activation leads to an increase in heart rate and blood pressure. However, stroke volume index is decreased by ketamine, too. The haemodynamic effects of etomidate (●) are almost neglible and myocardial oxygen consumption remains unchanged.

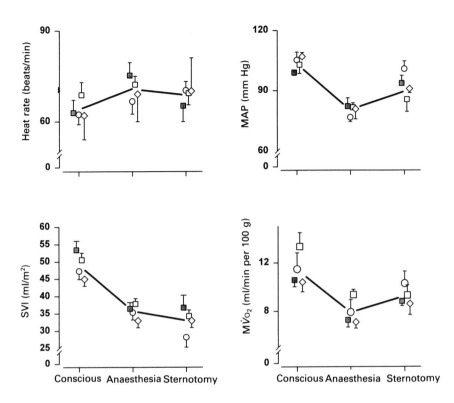

Fig 10.11 Effects of volatile anaesthetic agents and propofol on heart rate, mean arterial pressure, stroke volume index and myocardial oxygen consumption in patients undergoing coronary artery bypass surgery. Induction of anaesthesia with volatile anaesthetic agents or propofol is associated with a decrease of blood pressure, stroke volume index, and only minor changes of heart rate. As a result, myocardial oxygen consumption is decreased, as well. ○, Enflurane; ■, propofol; □, halothane; ◇, isoflurane; —, pooled data. (Data from Hoeft et al.[80])

anaesthesia and surgery (fig 10.13).[81] Although no measurements of myocardial blood flow and myocardial oxygen consumption are available for this critical period, an estimation of myocardial oxygen demand can be made based on the modified pressure work index and data from the literature. Patients who shiver might, in particular, have an extremely high myocardial oxygen demand.[81] This is mainly because of high systemic metabolic rates (fig 10.14), which in turn cause a high cardiac work load. During anaesthesia total body oxygen consumption is in the range of 80–120 ml/min per m² (fig 10.14). Thus, with a haemoglobin of 12 g% and an arteriovenous oxygen extraction of 25% the required cardiac index is 1·5–2·3 l/min per m². For a normal blood pressure (120/80 mm Hg) and a normal heart rate (80 beats/

min) myocardial oxygen demand calculated by the modified pressure work index is in the range 10·4–10·9 ml/min per 100 g, which is the range determined during anaesthesia (figs 10.11 and 10.12). Myocardial oxygen demand also depends on the haemoglobin content of the blood. The lower the haemoglobin content, the higher the required cardiac output and the myocardial oxygen demand (fig 10.14). During the recovery phase from anaesthesia systemic metabolic rates can be extremely high, particularly in shivering patients.[81] On average, a systemic metabolic rate of 260 ml/min per

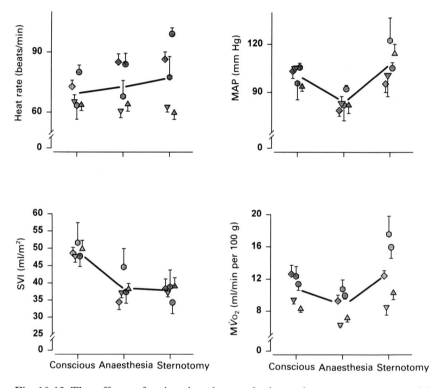

Fig 10.12 The effects of opiate based anaesthesia on heart rate, mean arterial pressure, stroke volume index, and myocardial oxygen consumption in patients undergoing coronary artery bypass surgery. As with volatile anaesthetic agents (fig 10.11) induction of anaesthesia is associated with a decrease in blood pressure and stroke volume index whereas heart rate remains unchanged. Myocardial oxygen consumption is therefore also decreased. Blood pressure control is more difficult to achieve during sternotomy. On average an increase in myocardial oxygen consumption is observed. ◇ , Fentanyl–midazolam; ◉ , high dose fentanyl; ○ , high dose morphine; ▽ , high dose sufentanil; △ , sufentanil–nitrous oxide; —, pooled data. (Data from Hoeft et al.[80])

m^2 is observed during this period in patients after major abdominal surgery (fig 10.14). Myocardial oxygen demand is 13·5 ml/min per m^2 with a haemoglobin of 12 g%, which increases to more than 19·2 ml/min per 100 g at a haemoglobin of 8 g%. Maximal values of up to 480 ml/min per m^2 (fig 10.14) have been observed in shivering patients.[81] In this case a cardiac index of 8·7 l/min per m^2 would be required (if haemoglobin is 12 g% and oxygen extraction ratio is 25%), and the resulting myocardial oxygen demand is 16·9 ml/min per 100 g. A decrease in haemoglobin, as often observed after surgery in the recovery room, would further increase myocardial oxygen demand into a range (>25 ml/min per 100 g) that can hardly be met by healthy patients and which certainly will cause problems in patients with limited coronary blood supply.

Effect of anaesthesia on myocardial efficiency

In technical terms efficiency is the ratio of work performed divided by energy required. In a similar way the efficiency of myocardial oxygen utilisation can be defined as the ratio of external pressure–volume work to myocardial oxygen consumption. Pressure–volume work is by definition the area under the left ventricular pressure–volume loop, which is unfortunately

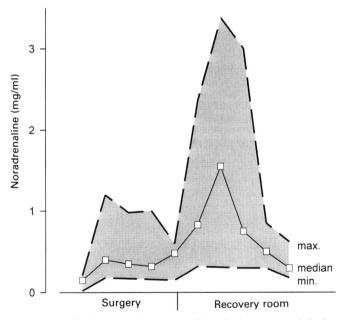

Fig 10.13 Noradrenaline levels during major abdominal surgery and during recovery from surgery. Median and range (min., max.) of noradrenaline plasma levels during and after major abdominal surgery are shown. The most pronounced sympathetic activation occurs during recovery from surgery. (Data from Turner.[81])

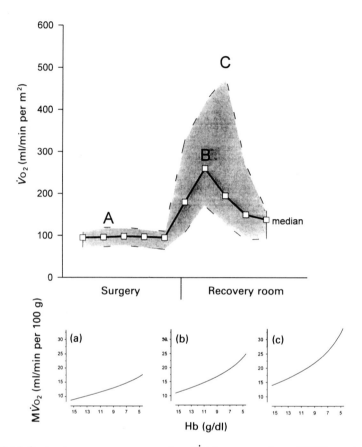

Fig 10.14 Systemic oxygen consumption ($\dot{V}_{O_2}$) measured at STPD, and myocardial energy demand ($M\dot{V}_{O_2}$) during major abdominal surgery and during recovery from surgery. Median and range (shaded area) of systemic oxygen uptake ($\dot{V}_{O_2}$) are shown. $\dot{V}_{O_2}$ measurements were performed in 24 patients by the Fick principle. Note the tremendous increase in $\dot{V}_{O_2}$ in some patients during the recovery period. The insets (a, b, and c) demonstrate myocardial oxygen demand for a typical situation during surgery (a), for median systemic metabolic rate during recovery from anaesthesia and surgery (b), and for a maximal metabolic rate (c) in the same period. In principle, myocardial oxygen demand depends on cardiac output, which in turn depends on haemoglobin concentration. Thus, for each situation (a, b, and c) myocardial energy demand ($M\dot{V}_{O_2}$) is depicted in relation to haemoglobin concentration. During anaesthesia systemic metabolic rate and systemic oxygen consumption are low (about 100 ml/min per m², upper panel, point A). In this situation and for a haemoglobin concentration of 12 g% a myocardial oxygen demand ($M\dot{V}_{O_2}$) of 10 ml/min per 100 g is necessary (inset a), which will increase up to 17 ml/min per 100 g with haemodilution down to 5 g% (see curve in inset a). During recovery from

294

difficult to assess in patients. For clinical purposes, however, a good estimate of external pressure volume work can be obtained from the product of stroke volume and mean systolic pressure during the ejection phase.

It has been known for a long time that myocardial efficiency is not constant but varies with preload, afterload, and contractility. Evans and Matsuoka[82] demonstrated as early as 1915 that an increase of cardiac work caused by an increase in blood pressure requires a higher increase in oxygen consumption than the same increase in cardiac work caused by an increase in stroke volume. Recently, theoretical models have been developed which try to relate the efficiency of myocardial oxygen use to haemodynamics, that is, to indices of preload, afterload, and contractility.[83-85] Although the approaches for estimation of myocardial efficiency differ in the way myocardial oxygen demand is estimated from haemodynamic indices, similar results have been obtained. In principle, myocardial efficiency is improved by an increase in preload and/or by a decrease in afterload. The most notable implication of the theoretical models is the hypothesis that myocardial performance can be optimised with respect to myocardial efficiency: for a given preload and afterload a maximal efficiency is achieved when contractility is neither too low nor too high, that is, when contractility is ideally tuned to an optimal value. In fact, there is a growing body of evidence that preload, afterload, and contractility are optimised under resting conditions at the point of maximal efficiency.[83 85] The question of whether afterload is tuned to a given preload and contractility, or whether all three parameters are adjusted simultaneously is only interesting from an academic point of view. Normally, myocardial performance (contractility) and vascular properties (preload and afterload) are well matched with respect to optimisation of myocardial efficiency. Burkhoff and Sagawa[83] coined the terms "ventriculoarterial coupling" and "ventricular–vascular matching" to describe this physiologically important relationship.

From this point of view it is very interesting that induction of anaesthesia is associated with a decrease in efficiency of myocardial oxygen use (fig 10.15). As outlined above, induction of anaesthesia with volatile anaesthetic agents as well as with intravenous anaesthetic agents leads to decreased sympathetic drive, associated with a decrease in cardiac performance and myocardial oxygen consumption. In fact, myocardial oxygen consumption is not de-

---

Fig. 10.14 (contd) surgery and anaesthesia median systemic oxygen consumption was 260 ml/min per m^2 (upper panel, point B). As a result, required M$\dot{V}$O$_2$ is increased to about 13–23 ml/min per 100 g, depending on haemoglobin concentration (inset b). In some patients, very high values of myocardial oxygen have been observed, up to 480 ml/min per m^2 (upper panel, point C). During these conditions M$\dot{V}$O$_2$ is already 17·5 ml/min per 100 g for a haemoglobin concentration of 12 g% and will be tremendously increased by additional haemodilution up to 32 ml/min per 100 g at a haemoglobin of 5 g% (inset c). (Data from Turner.[81])

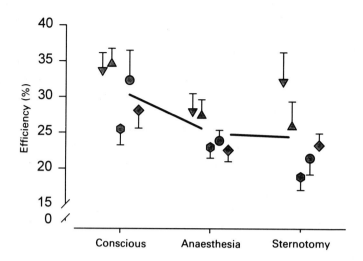

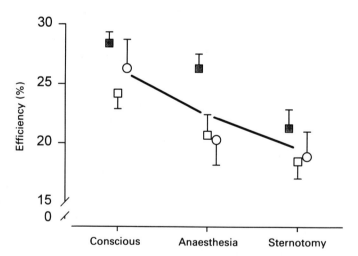

Fig 10.15 Effects of anaesthesia on myocardial efficiency. Efficiency of myocardial oxygen use is calculated from the ratio of external myocardial work (mean systolic pressure × cardiac index) to myocardial oxygen consumption. Induction and maintenance of anaesthesia with any anaesthetic agent is associated with decreased myocardial efficiency. Upper: ◆, fentanyl–midazolam; ●, high dose fentanyl; ●, high dose morphine; ▼, high dose sufentanil; ▲, sufentanil–nitrous oxide; —, pooled data. Lower: ○, enflurane; □, halothane; ■, propofol; —, pooled data.

creased in proportion to the decrease of external myocardial work (fig 10.15). As a result, efficiency is decreased, regardless of the type of anaesthesia[80] (fig 10.15). Theoretically, an increase in efficiency could also occur because of afterload (blood pressure) decrease. However, the decrease in contractility and stroke volume outweigh the former effect, that is, contractility and afterload do not match preload conditions after induction of anaesthesia. In terms of "ventricular–vascular matching," stroke volumes and contractility are too low. It is somewhat surprising that this effect is seen not only with anaesthetic agents that are well known to have direct negative inotropic properties (that is, halothane and enflurane) but also to the same extent with anaesthetic agents that supposedly have no direct negative inotropic effects (that is, opiates).[80] This finding indicates that, under in vivo conditions, even opiate anaesthesia is associated with a decrease in contractility, presumably because of decreased or inadequate sympathetic drive.

As pointed out, surgical stimulation such as a sternotomy is associated with sympathetic activation and an increase in blood pressure. There is evidence that during anaesthesia this sympathetic activation has a different pattern than under conscious conditions. In general, increases in heart rate are not very pronounced, and sometimes heart rate even decreases (because of the attempt to block the cardiovascular response by deepening anaesthesia). In contrast significant increases in blood pressure can be observed, in particular during opiate based anaesthesia. Although sympathetic activation should enhance myocardial contractility, stroke volume indices and myocardial efficiency of oxygen use remain decreased. These findings also suggest that anaesthesia significantly interferes with cardiovascular control mechanisms because optimal tuning of the system is obviously not achieved during volatile as well as during opiate anaesthesia. Thus there is substantial evidence that, under in vivo conditions, the direct negative inotropic effects of anaesthetic agents might be of minor importance compared with the central effects of anaesthesia on cardiovascular control mechanisms.

Effects of anaesthetic agents on coronary blood flow

With the exception of isoflurane, autoregulation of coronary blood flow is not affected by anaesthetic agents, that is, myocardial blood flow is adjusted to match myocardial oxygen demand. As a result myocardial blood flow decreased with induction of anaesthesia in conjunction with the decrease in myocardial oxygen demand, and coronary sinus oxygen saturation remains practically unchanged[86] (fig 10.16). In contrast isoflurane causes coronary vasodilatation with an increase in coronary sinus oxygen saturation.[86] Halothane and enflurane are also coronary vasodilators, but to a lesser degree.[86] Many studies have been performed to investigate whether the coronary vasodilator properties of isoflurane can cause a coronary steal phenomenon. In most studies that demonstrated myocardial ischaemia during isoflurane, however, high doses were used with considerable concomi-

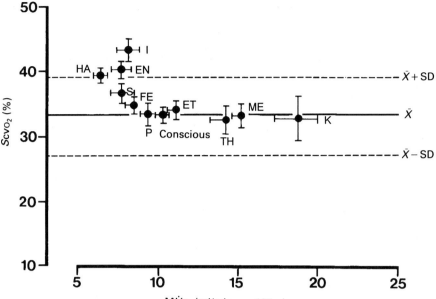

Fig 10.16 Coronary venous oxygen saturation ($Scvo_2$) in conscious patients (A) and after induction of anaesthesia with ketamine (K), methohexitone (ME), thiopentone (TH), etomidate (ET), isoflurane (I), halothane (H), enflurane (EN), propofol (P), sufentanil (S), and fentanyl (FE). With the exception of isoflurane coronary venous oxygen saturation remains more or less unchanged compared with the conscious state, that is, autoregulatory control of coronary blood flow is not affected by most anaesthetic agents. Halothane, enflurane, and more so isoflurane are coronary vasodilators. (Modified from Hoeft et al.[86])

tant arterial hypotension. It is now commonly accepted that isoflurane can be used safely in patients with coronary artery disease as long as high doses and arterial hypotension are avoided.[87] Thus, in case there is a hypertensive response to surgical stimuli during opiate based anaesthesia, supplemental isoflurane can be used safely for blood pressure control.

Central and peripheral circulation

Anaesthesia exerts direct and indirect effects on the peripheral circulation. As with the heart it is difficult to discriminate direct and indirect effects under in vivo conditions. Decreased sympathetic drive, which is associated with virtually any anaesthetic technique, will also affect peripheral vascular tone. This can be expected to alter distribution of vascular resistances and blood flows, and that of intravascular blood volume. In addition, many anaesthetic agents exert direct effects on vascular smooth muscle, either by direct vasodilatation or by altering the response to other factors that modulate vascular tone.

Direct effects of anaesthetic agents on vascular smooth muscle

Volatile anaesthetic agents are known to cause mild vasodilatation under in vivo conditions. This is the result of both diminished vascular smooth muscle sensitivity to circulating catecholamines and diminished neurovascular tone. Larach et al[88] found that halothane selectively attenuates α_2-adrenoreceptor mediated vasoconstriction. It was suggested that this is the result of interference with calcium entry through smooth muscle membranes. More recent investigations have demonstrated that volatile anaesthetic agents might additionally attenuate the pressure response to α_1-adrenoceptor mediated vasoconstriction, and that this effect is not mediated by blockade of calcium influx through voltage dependent channels.[89] The attenuation of α_1 and α_2 responsiveness most probably contributes to in vivo effects of volatile anaesthetic agents because stimulation of α_1 and α_2-adrenoceptors contributes to basal vascular tone.

As outlined above, the vasodilator effects of volatile anaesthetic agents can differ within the circulation. For instance, halothane, like glyceryl trinitrate, is a more potent dilator of large coronary arteries, whereas isoflurane is a more potent dilator of small coronary arteries.[90] Only isoflurane will cause a significant increase in coronary blood flow, because under in vivo conditions dilatation of large coronary arteries is counteracted by the metabolic control of coronary blood flow at the level of the arterioles and the microcirculation.

Many in vivo studies indicate that propofol has a vasodilating effect. It is still, however, controversial whether this effect results from a direct vasodilating action of propofol or from a reduction in sympathetic outflow. Park et al[91] as well as Nakamura et al[92] found that propofol in concentrations of 0·1 mmol/l causes vasodilatation of isolated vascular rings. These are concentrations found in clinical practice. However, 97–99% of this is bound to plasma proteins. Nakamura therefore concluded that clinically relevant concentrations of propofol do not have direct vasodilator effects.[92]

Effects of anaesthesia on blood volume distribution

From the physiological point of view, the vascular system can be divided into two parts:

1 The low pressure system which comprises all postarteriolar vessels, the right heart, the pulmonary vascular system, and the left heart during diastole.
2 The high pressure system which includes the left ventricle during systole, systemic arteries, and arterioles.

The low pressure system holds about 85% of the total intravascular blood volume, one third of which is in the intrathoracic compartment and two thirds are in the extrathoracic low pressure system. According to the definition by Gauer and Henry,[93] the central blood volume that represents the intravascular blood content between the pulmonary and the aortic valve, is part of the intrathoracic blood volume. Intrathoracic and central blood volumes hold a key position within the circulation because they serve as a reservoir for the left ventricle.[94] It is common clinical practice to evaluate changes in intrathoracic and central blood volumes by corresponding changes in central venous and pulmonary capillary wedge pressure.[94] This practice is based on the early work of Gauer and Henry, who demonstrated changes of central venous pressure during blood withdrawal and retransfusion in spontaneously breathing healthy volunteers.[95 96] According to their data the compliance of the low pressure system is about 2·3 ml/mm Hg per kg, that is, a 1 mm Hg change in central venous pressure corresponds to a 200 ml change in intravascular blood volume. There are, however, several problems that complicate the applicability of blood pressure measurements in the low pressure system for evaluation of intravascular volume status during anaesthesia:

1 Already Gauer and Henry demonstrated a considerable interindividual variability of low pressure compliance.
2 The compliance of the low pressure system is naturally affected by vascular smooth muscle tone. When adrenergic drive is enhanced by infusion of noradrenaline the compliance decreases to 1·7 ml/mm Hg per kg and lower.[97] Consequently, it has been shown that sympathetic tone influences central venous pressure as a result of changes in effective compliance.[98]
3 Mechanical ventilation with positive airway pressure, and in particular with positive end expiratory pressure (PEEP), will alter the relationship of central venous pressure, pulmonary capillary wedge pressure, and intrathoracic volume status.[94] It has repeatedly been demonstrated that changes in central venous pressure do not correlate with changes in pulmonary capillary wedge pressure in patients with impaired left ventricular function.[99]

Direct measurements of intrathoracic or central blood volume by indicator dilution techniques seem therefore to be more adequate for evaluation of intravascular volume status, in particular in patients undergoing cardiac surgery, in which myocardial dysfunction and a critical dependence on adequate intravascular filling can be anticipated.[100]

Surprisingly, only very few studies have been performed on the impact of anaesthesia on intrathoracic blood volume and left ventricular preload. It is common practice to give additional fluids with induction of anaesthesia to compensate for decreases in blood pressure. It has, however, not been systematically investigated to what extent the commonly observed decrease in blood pressure is the result of a volume shift between the intrathoracic and extrathoracic compartments or a decrease in contractility. In general, both can be expected with decreased sympathetic drive. Hedenstierna et al[101] as well as Krayer et al[102] found that, compared with the conscious state, anaesthesia with muscle paralysis and mechanical ventilation leads to a decrease in thoracic volume associated with a decrease in functional residual capacity. Both groups presented different results, however, with respect to the intrathoracic blood volume. Krayer et al measured total thoracic cavity volume by three dimensional X-ray computed tomography, and functional residual capacity by inert gas clearance techniques. From the difference in both they calculated an increase in intrathoracic blood volume after induction of anaesthesia. In contrast Hedenstierna et al measured a decrease in intrathoracic blood volume using a double indicator dilution technique. The results of Hedenstierna et al seem to be more plausible, taking into account the known effects of anaesthesia on the sympathetic system and the impact of mechanical ventilation on intrathoracic pressures. A volume redistribution from the intrathoracic to the extrathoracic compartment with induction of anaesthesia would support the clinical practice, where hypotension after intubation is treated by intravenous fluids. Different anaesthetic techniques could, however, possibly explain the different results of Krayer et al and Hedenstierna et al. Krayer et al used fentanyl/thiopentone anaesthesia, whereas Hedenstierna and co-workers used halothane anaesthesia.[101][102] Currently, there are no systematic data available on how different types of anaesthesia affect the expected redistribution of intravascular blood volume from the intrathoracic to the extrathoracic compartment.

It is well known that both spinal and epidural anaesthesia cause a loss of sympathetic innervation in the corresponding areas. The impact of regional sympathectomy by spinal and epidural anaesthesia has been investigated by Arndt and co-workers[103] in a very elegant way using labelled erythrocytes and whole body scintigraphy. Regional anaesthesia elicits a redistribution of blood to the denervated musculature and skin at the expense of cardiac filling. The capacitance vessels of the remaining innervated muscles and skin areas, usually of the upper extremities, might constrict in a compensatory manner. The data of Arndt and co-workers[103] also suggest that compensatory vasoconstriction might occur in the splanchnic area, the mechanism of which is, however, unknown. In patients with compromised compensatory mechanisms central blood volume might decrease dramatically. On the basis of these findings Lipfert and Arndt[104] concluded that the poor outcome of resuscitation attempts in case of cardiac arrests during spinal anaesthesia[105] is largely the result of insufficient filling of the central vascular system.

Conclusion

In summary, there is evidence that regional as well as general anaesthesia is associated with a redistribution of blood volume from the intrathoracic to the

301

extrathoracic compartment. Little is known about the time course of volume distribution during surgery and especially during recovery from anaesthesia. This, as well as the influence of various anaesthetic techniques on intravascular volume distribution, is certainly a subject that merits further investigations.

1 Sebel PS, Bovill JG. Cardiovascular effects of sufentanil anesthesia. *Anesth Analg* 1982; **61**: 115–19.
2 Bovill JG, Sebel PS, Stanley TH. Opioid analgesics in anesthesia: With special reference to their use in cardiothoracic anesthesia. *Anesthesiology* 1984; **61**: 731–55.
3 Skarvan K, Schwinn W. Haemodynamic interactions between midazolam and alfentanil in patients with coronary disease *Anaesthetist* 1986; **35**: 17–23.
4 Tomicheck RC, Rosow CE, Philbin DM, Moss J, Teplick RS, Schneider RC. Diazepam–fentanyl interaction—hemodynamic and hormonal effects in coronary artery surgery. *Anesth Analg* 1985; **62**: 881–4.
5 Strauer BE. Contractile response to morphine, piritramide, meperidine and fentanyl: A comparative study of effects on the isolated ventricular myocardium. *Anesthesiology* 1972; **37**: 304–10.
6 Hug CC Jr. Does opioid "anesthesia" exist. *Anesthesiology* 1990; **73**: 1–4.
7 Ebert TJ, Muzi M, Berens R, Goff D, Kampine J. Sympathetic responses to induction of anaesthesia in humans with propofol or etomidate. *Anesthesiology* 1992; **76**: 725–33.
8 Wallin BG, Fagius J. Peripheral sympathetic neural activity in conscious humans. *Annu Rev Physiol* 1988; **50**: 565–76.
9 Ebert TJ, Kampine JP. Nitrous oxide augments sympathetic outflow: Direct evidence from human peroneal nerve recordings. *Anesth Analg* 1989; **69**: 444–9.
10 Sellgren J, Ponten J, Wallin BG. Characteristics of muscle sympathetic nerve activity during general anaesthesia in humans. *Acta Anaesthesiol Scand* 1992; **36**: 336–45.
11 Sellgren J, Ponten J, Wallin G. Percutaneous recordings of muscle nerve sympathetic nerve activity during propofol, nitrous oxide, and isoflurane anesthesia in humans. *Anesthesiology* 1990; **73**: 20–7.
12 Ebert TJ, Kanitz DD, Kampine JP. Inhibition of sympathetic neural outflow during thiopental anesthesia in humans. *Anesth Analg* 1990; **71**: 319–26.
13 Griffiths R and Norman RI. Effects of anesthetics on uptake, synthesis and release of transmitters. *Br J Anaesth* 1993; **71**: 96–107.
14 Goldstein DS, McCarty R, Polinsky RJ, Kopin IJ. Relationship between plasma norepinephrine and sympathetic nerve activity. *Hypertension* 1983; **5**: 552–9.
15 Honda T, Ninomiya I, Azumi T. Changes in AdSNA and arterial catecholamines to coronary occlusion in cats. *Am J Physiol* 1988; **255** (*Heart Circ Physiol* 24): H704–10.
16 Esler M, Jennings G, Korner P. Assessment of human sympathetic nervous system activity from measurements of norepinephrine turnover. *Hypertension* 1988; **11**: 3–20.
17 Wallin B, Sundlöf G, Eriksson B. Plasma noradrenaline correlates to sympathetic muscle nerve activity in normotensive man. *Acta Physiol Scand* 1981; **111**: 69–73.
18 Pocock G, Richards CD. Cellular mechanisms in general anaesthesia. *Br J Anaesth* 1991; **66**: 116–28.
19 Philbin DM, Rosow CE, Schneider RC, Koski G, D'Ambra MN. Fentanyl and sufentanil anesthesia revisited: How much is enough. *Anesthesiology* 1990; **73**: 5–11.
20 Sonntag H, Stephan H, Lange H, Rieke H, Kettler D, Martschausky N. Sufentanil does not block sympathetic responses to surgical stimuli in patients having CABG. *Anesth Analg* 1989; **68**: 584–92.
21 Liem TH, Booij LHDJ, Gielen MJM, Hasenbos MAWM, van Egmond J. Coronary artery bypass grafting using two different anesthetic techniques: Part 3: Adrenergic responses. *J Cardiothorac Vasc Anesth* 1992; **6**: 162–7.
22 Ebert TJ, Muzi M. Sympathetic hyperactivity during desflurane anesthesia in healthy volunteers. *Anesthesiology* 1993; **79**: 444–53.
23 Yli-Hankala A, Randell T, Seppälä T, Lindgren L. Increases in hemodynamic variables and catecholamine levels after rapid increase in isoflurane concentration. *Anesthesiology* 1993; **78**: 266–71.

24 Kotrly KJ, Ebert TJ, Vucins E, Igler FO, Barney JA, Kampine JP. Baroreceptor reflex control of the heart rate during isoflurane anesthesia in humans. *Anesthesiology* 1984; **60**: 173–9.

25 Skovstedt P, Price ML, Price HL. The effect of short acting barbiturates on arterial pressure, preganglionic sympathetic activity and barostatic reflexes. *Anesthesiology* 1970; **33**: 10–18.

26 Kotrly KJ, Ebert TJ, Vucins EJ, Roerig DL, Stadnicka A, Kampine JP. Effects of fentanyl–diazepam–nitrous oxide anesthesia on arterial baroreflex control of heart rate in man. *Br J Anaesth* 1986; **58**: 406–14.

27 Komai H, Rusy BF. Differences in the myocardial depressant action of thiopental and halothane. *Anesth Analg* 1984; **63**: 313–18.

28 Kissin I, Motomura S, Aultmann DF, Reves JF. Inotropic and anesthetic potencies of etomidate and thiopental in dogs. *Anesth Analg* 1983; **62**: 961–5.

29 Roewer N, Proske O, Schulte am Esch J. The effects of midazolam on the mechanical and electrical properties of the isolated ventricular myocardium. *Anaesth-Intensivther-Notfallmed* 1990; **25**: 354–61.

30 Azuma M, Matsumura C, Kemmotsu O. Inotropic and electrophysiology effects of propofol and thiamylal in isolated papillary muscles of the guinea pig and the rat. *Anesth Analg* 1993; **77**: 557–63.

31 Mattheusen M, Housmans PR. Mechanisms of the direct, negative inotropic effect of etomidate in isolated ferret ventricular myocardium. *Anesthesiology* 1993; **79**: 1284–95.

32 Stowe DF, Bosjnak ZJ, Kampine JP. Comparison of etomidate, ketamine, midazolam, propofol and thiopental on function and metabolism of isolated hearts. *Anesth Analg* 1992; **74**: 547–58.

33 Park WK, Lynch C III. Propofol and thiopentone depression of myocardial contactility. A comparative study of mechanical and electrophysiological effects in isolated guinea pig ventricular muscle. *Anesth Analg* 1992; **74**: 395–405.

34 Rusy BF, Komai H. Anesthetic depression of myocardial contractility. A review of possible mechanisms. *Anesthesiology* 1987; **67**: 745–66.

35 Riou B, Viars P, Lecarpentier Y. Effects of ketamine on the cardiac papillary muscle of normal hamsters and those with cardiomyopathy. *Anesthesiology* 1990; **73**: 910–18.

36 Cook DJ, Carton EG, Housmans PR. Mechanisms of the positive inotropic effect of ketamine in isolated ferret ventricular papillary muscle. *Anesthesiology* 1991; **74**: 880–8.

37 Kongsayreepong S, Cook DJ, Housmans PR. Mechanisms of the direct, negative inotropic effect of ketamine in isolated ferret and frog ventricular myocardium. *Anesthesiology* 1993; **79**: 313–22.

38 Dowdy EG, Kaya K. Studies of the mechanisms of cardiovascular responses to CI–581. *Anesthesiology* 1968; **29**: 931.

39 Urthaler F, Walker AA, James TN. Comparison of the inotropic action of morphine and ketamine studies in canine artery muscle. *J Thorac Cardiovasc Surg* 1976; **72**: 142.

40 Lynch C III, Frazer MJ. Depressant effects of volatile anesthetics upon rat and amphibian myocardium: Insights into anesthetic mechanisms of action. *Anesthesiology* 1989; **70**: 511–22.

41 Wolf WJ, Neal MB, Mathew BP, Bee DE. Comparison of the in vitro myocardial depressant effects of isoflurane and halothane anesthesia. *Anesthesiology* 1988; **69**: 660–6.

42 Kemmotsu O, Hashimoto Y, Shimosato S. Inotropic effects of isoflurane on mechanics of contraction in isolated cat paillary muscles from normal and failing hearts. *Anesthesiology* 1973; **39**: 402–15.

43 Kemmotsu O, Hashimoto Y, Shimosato S. The effects of fluroxene and enflurane on contractile performance of isolated papillary muscles from failing hearts. *Anesthesiology* 1974; **40**: 253–60.

44 Lynch C III. Differential depression of myocardial contractility by volatile anesthetics in vitro: Comparison with uncouplers of excitation–contraction coupling. *J Cardiovasc Pharmacol* 1990; **15**: 655–65.

45 Stowe DF, Monroe SM, Marijic J, Bosnjak ZJ, Kampine JP. Comparison of halothane, enflurane, and isoflurane with nitrous oxide on contractility and oxygen supply and demand in isolated hearts. *Anesthesiology* 1991; **75**: 1062–74.

46 Lawson D, Frazer MJ, Lynch C III. Nitrous oxide effects on isolated myocardium: a reexamination in vitro. *Anesthesiology* 1990; **73**: 930–43.
47 Bovill JG, Boer F. Opiods in cardiac anesthesia. In: Kaplan J, ed, *Cardiac anesthesia*, 3rd edn. Philadelphia: WB Saunders, 1993; 467–511.
48 Sagawa K. The ventricular pressure–volume diagramm revisited. *Circ Res* 1978; **46**: 677–87.
49 Frank O. Die Grundform des arteriellen Pulses. *Z Biol* 1895; **36**: 483–526.
50 Pagel PS, Kampine JP, Schmeling WT, Warltier DC. Reversal of volatile anesthetic induced depression of myocardial contractility by extracellular calcium also enhances left ventricular diastolic function. *Anesthesiology* 1993; **78**: 1241–54.
51 Heinrich H, Fontaine L, Fösel TH, Spilker D, Winter H, Ahnefeld FW. Echocardiographic assessment of the negative inotropic effects of halothane, enflurane and isoflurane. *Anaesthetist* 1986; **35**: 465–72.
52 Mulier JP, Wouters P, Van Aken H, Vermaut G, Vandermersch M. Cardiodyamic effects of propofol in comparison with thiopental: Assessment with transesophageal echocardiographic approach. *Anesth Analg* 1991; **72**: 28–35.
53 Asanoi A, Sasayaema S, Kameyama T. Ventriculo arterial coupling in normal and failing heart in humans. *Circ Res* 1989; **65**: 483–93.
54 Grossman W, Braunwald E, Mann T, McLaurin LP, Green LH. Contractile state of the left ventricle in man as evaluated from end-systolic pressure–volume relations. *Circulation* 1977; **56**: 845–52.
55 Pagel PS, Kampine JP, Schmeling WT, Warltier DC. Comparison of end systolic pressure–length relations and preload recruitable stroke work as indices of myocardial contractility in the conscious and anesthetized chronically instrumented dog. *Anesthesiology* 1990; **73**: 278–90.
56 Pagel PS, Kampine JP, Schmeling WT, Warltier DC. Effects of nitrous oxide on myocardial contractility as evaluated by the preload recruitable stroke work relationship in chronically instrumented dogs. *Anesthesiology* 1990; **73**: 1148–57.
57 Pagel PS, Kampine JP, Schmeling WT, Warltier DC. Influence of volatile anesthetics on myocardial contractility in vivo: desflurane versus isoflurane. *Anesthesiology* 1991; **74**: 900–7.
58 Lowenstein E, Park KW, Reiz S. Effects of inhalation anesthetics on systemic hemodynamics and the coronary circulation. In: Kaplan J, ed, *Cardiac anesthesia*, 3rd edn. Philadelphia: WB Saunders, 1993: 441–66.
59 Opie LH. Effects of regional ischemia on metabolism of glucose and fatty acids. Relative rates of aerobic and anaerobic energy production during myocardial infarction and comparison with effects of anoxia. *Circ Res* 1976 **38**: I52–68;
60 Marcus ML, Wilson RF, White CW. Methods of measurement of myocardial blood flow in patients: a critical review. *Circulation* 1987; **76**: 245–53.
61 Kety SS, Schmidt CF. Measurement of cerebral blood flow by inert gas inhalation and inlet-outlet detection of the tracer. *Am J Physiol* 1945; **143**: 53–63.
62 Bing RJ, Hammond MM, Handelsann JC, *et al*. The measurement of coronary blood flow, oxygen consumption and efficiency of the left ventricle in man. *Am Heart J* 1949; **38**: 1–24.
63 Tauchert M, Kochsiek K, Heiss HW. Measurement of coronary blood flow in man by the argon method. In Maseri A, ed, *Myocardial blood flow in man*. Turin: Minerva Medica. 1970: 859.
64 Wolpers HG, Hoeft A, Korb H, Lichtlen PR, Hellige G. Heterogeneity of myocardial blood flow under normal conditions and its dependence on arterial P_{O_2}. *Am J Physiol* 1990; **258**: H549–55.
65 Wolpers HG, Hoeft A, Korb H, Lichtlen PR, Hellige G. Transport of inert gases in mammalian myocardium: comparison with a convection diffusion model. *Am J Physiol* 1990; **259**: H167–73.
66 Wolpers HG, Böck J, Hoeft A, Korb H, Hellige G. Measurement of coronary blood flow by the inert gas method-comparison of indicator gases. *Z Kardiol* 1987; **76**: 95–101.
67 Sonntag H, Merin RG, Donath U, Radke J, Schenk HJD. Myocardial metabolism and oxygenation in man awake and during halothane anesthesia. *Anesthesiology* 1979; **51**: 204–10.
68 Sonntag H, Larsen R, Hilfiker O, Kettler D, Brockschnieder B. Myocardial blood flow and

oxygen consumption during high-dose fentanyl anesthesia in patients with coronary artery disease. *Anesthesiology 1982;* **56**: 417–22.

69 Stephan H, Sonntag H, Schenk JD, Kettler D, Khambatta H. Effects of propofol on cardiovascular dynamics, myocardial blood flow and myocardial metabolism in patients with coronary artery disease. *Br J Anaesth* 1986; **58**: 969–75.

70 Hilfiker O, Larsen R, Sonntag H. Myocardial blood flow and oxygen consumption during halothane nitrous oxide anaesthesia for coronary revascularization. *Br J Anaesth* 1983; **55**: 927–32.

71 Hilfiker O, Larsen R, Brockschnieder B, Sonntag H. Morphine anaesthesia-coronary blood flow and oxygen consumption in patients with coronary artery disease. *Anaesthesist* 1982; **31**: 371–6.

72 Larsen R, Hilfiker O, Philbin DM, Sonntag H. Myocardial metabolism during enflurane-nitrous oxide anaesthesia in patients with coronary artery disease. *Anaesthesist* 1986; **35**: 10–16.

73 Larsen R, Hilfiker O, Philbin DM, Sonntag H. Isoflurane: Coronary blood flow and myocardial metabolism patients with coronary artery disease. *Anaesthesist* 1986; **35**: 284–90.

74 Hoeft A, Sonntag H, Stephan H, Kettler D. Validation of myocardial oxygen demand indices in patients awake and during anesthesia. *Anesthesiology* 1991; **75**: 49–56.

75 Rhode E. Über den Einfluß der mechanischen Bedingungen auf die Tätigkeit und den Sauerstoffverbrauch des Warmblüterherzens. *Archiv für experimentelle Pathologie und Pharmakologie* 1915; **68**: 401–34.

76 Baller D, Bretschneider HJ, Hellige G. Validity of myocardial oxygen consumption parameters. *Clin Cardiol* 1979; **2**: 317–27.

77 Rooke GA, Feigl EO. Work as a correlate of canine left ventricular oxygen consumption, and the problem of catecholamine wasting. *Circ Res* 1982; **50**: 273–86.

78 Rooke GA. Low dose halothane anesthesia does not affect the hemodynamic estimation of myocardial oxygen consumption in dogs. *Anesthesiology* 1990; **72**: 682–93.

79 Kettler D, Sonntag H. Intravenous anaesthetics: Coronary blood flow and myocardial oxygen consumption. *Acta Anaesthesiol Belg* 1974; **25**: 384–401.

80 Hoeft A, Sonntag H, Stephan H, Kettler D. Influence of anesthesia on efficiency of cardiac work in patients undergoing coronary artery bypass surgery. *Anesth Analg* 1994 (in press).

81 Turner E. Pathophysiologie der Aufwachphase. *Anästhesiologie und Intensivmedizin* (Bd 179), Berlin: Springer Verlag) 1986.

82 Evans CL, Matsuoka Y. The effect of various mechanical conditions on the gaseous metabolism abnd efficiency of the mammalian heart. *J Physiol (Lond)* 1915; **49**: 378–405.

83 Burkhoff D, Sagawa K. Ventricular effiency predicted by an analytical model. *Am J Physiol* 1986; **250**: R1021–7.

84 Suga H, Igarashi Y, Yamada O, Goto Y. Mechanical efficiency of the left ventricle as a function of preload, afterload, and contractility. *Heart and Vessels* 1985; **1**: 3–8.

85 Hoeft A, Koeb H, Hellige G, Sonntag H. Energetics and efficiency of cardiac pump work. *Anaesthesist* 1991; **40**: 465–78.

86 Hoeft A, Sonntag H, Stephan H. Coronary flow and myocardial oxygen balance in anesthesia. *Anaesth-Intensivther-Notfallmed* 1993; **26**: 398–407.

87 Priebe HJ. Coronary circulation and factors affecting coronary "steal". *Eur J Anaesth* 1991; **8**: 177–95.

88 Larach DR, Schuler HG, Derr JA, Larach MG, Hensley FA, Zelis R. Halothane selectively attenuates α_2-adrenoreceptor mediated vasoconstriction, in vivo and in vitro. *Anesthesiology* 1987; **66**: 781–91.

89 Kenny D, Pelch LR, Brooks HL, Kampine JP, Schmeling WT, Warltier DC. Calcium channel modulation of α_1 and α_2 adrenergic pressor responses in conscious and anesthetized dogs. *Anesthesiology* 1990; **72**: 874–881.

90 Nakamura K, Toda H, Hatano Y, Mori K. Comparison of the direct effects of sevoflurane, isoflurane and halothane on isolated canine coronary arteries. *Can J Anaesth* 1993; **40**: 257–61.

91 Park WK, Lynch C III, Johns RA. Effects of propofol and thiopental in isolated rat aorta and pulmonary artery. *Anesthesiology* 1992; **77**: 956–63.

92 Nakamura K, Hatano Y, Hirakata H, Nishiwada M, Toda H, Mori K. Direct vasoconstrictor and vasodilator effects of propofol in isolated dog arteries. *Br J Anaesth* 1992; **68**: 193–7.

305

93 Gauer OH, Henry JP. Circulatory basis of fluid volume control. *Physiol Rev* 1963; **43**: 423–81.

94 Arndt JO. The low pressure system: the integrated function of veins. *Eur J Anaesth* 1986; **3**: 343–70.

95 Henry JP, Gauer OH, Sieker HO. The effects of moderate changes of blood volume on left and right atrial pressure. *Circ Res* 1956; **4**: 91–4.

96 Gauer OH, Henry JP, Behn C. Changes in central venous pressure after moderate hemorrhage and tranfusion in man. *Circ Res* 1956; **4**: 79–90.

97 Echt M, Düweling J, Gauer OH Lange L. Effective compliance of the total vascular bed and the intrathoracic compartment derived from changes in central venous pressure induced by volume changes in man. *Circ Res* 1974; **34**: 61–8.

98 Bonica JJ Kennedy WF, Nakamatsu TJ, Gerbershagen HU. Circulatory effects of peridural block: III effects of acute blood loss. *Anesthesiology* 1972; **36**: 219–27.

99 Mangano DT. Monitoring pulmonary artery pressure in coronary artery disease. *Anesthesiology* 1980; **53**: 364–70.

100 Hoeft A, Schorn B, Weyland A, *et al*. Bedside assessment of intravascular volume status in patients undergoing cardiac surgery. *Anesthesiology* 1994 (in press).

101 Hedenstierna G, Strandberg A, Brismar B, Lundquist H, Svensson L, Tokics L. Functional residual capacity, thoracoabdominal dimensions and central blood volume during general anesthesia with muscle paralysis and mechanical ventilation. *Anesthesiology* 1985; **62**: 247–54.

102 Krayer S, Rehder K, Beck KC, Cameron PD, DIdsier EP, Hofman EA. Quantification of thoracic volumers by three dimensional imaging. *J Appl Physiol* 1987; **62**: 591–8.

103 Arndt JO, Höck A, Stanton-Hicks M, Stühmeier KD. Peridural anesthesia and the distribution of blood in supine humans. *Anesthesiology* 1985; **63**: 616–23.

104 Lipfert P, Arndt JO. Major conduction anaesthesia, Pathogenesis, prophylaxis, and therapy of circulatory complications. *Anaesthesist* 1993; **42**: 773–87.

105 Caplan RA, Ward RJ, Posner K, Cheney FW. Unexpected cardiac arrest during spinal anesthesia: A closed claims analysis of predisposing factors. *Anesthesiology* 1988; **68**: 5–11.

Index